HERBAL SIMPLES

HERBAL SIMPLES
APPROVED
FOR MODERN USES OF CURE.

by

W. T. FERNIE, M.D.

SECOND EDITON

"Medicine is mine; what herbs annd Simples grow In
fields and forests, all their powers I know."
DRYDEN.

GYAN

Published by

GYAN

Gyan Publishing House
5, Ansari Road
Daryaganj, New Delhi-110002
Phone: 011-47034999, 9811692060
E-mail: books@gyanbooks.com

Distribution Network
gyanbooks.com
India, USA, Canada, UK, Australia, France

ISBN : 978-81-212-6077-0 (PB)
First Published, 1897

2nd Impression 2021

Printed at: Gyan Press, Delhi.

The Music of India
Author: W. T. Fernie

HERBAL SIMPLES

APPROVED

FOR MODERN USES OF CURE.

BY

W. T. FERNIE, M.D.

SECOND EDITION.

"Medicine is mine; what herbs and *Simples* grow
In fields and forests, all their powers I know."

DRYDEN.

"And now Iapis had appeared,
Blest leech! to Phœbus'-self endeared
Beyond all men below;
On whom the fond, indulgent God
His augury had fain bestowed,
His lyre—his sounding bow!
But he, the further to prolong
A fellow creature's span,
The humbler art of Medicine chose,
The knowledge of each plant that grows,
Plying a craft not known to song,
An unambitious man!"

PREFACE TO THE FIRST EDITION.

It may happen that one or another enquirer taking up this book will ask, to begin with, "What is a Herbal Simple?" The English word "Simple," composed of two Latin words, *Singula plica* (a single fold), means "Singleness," whether of material or purpose.

From primitive times the term "Herbal Simple" has been applied to any homely curative remedy consisting of one ingredient only, and that of a vegetable nature. Many such a native medicine found favour and success with our single-minded forefathers, this being the "reverent simplicity of ancienter times."

In our own nursery days, as we now fondly remember, it was: "Simple Simon met a pieman going to the fair; said Simple Simon to the pieman, 'Let me taste your ware.'" That ingenuous youth had but one idea, connected simply with his stomach; and his sole thought was how to devour the contents of the pieman's tin. We venture to hope our readers may be equally eager to stock their minds with the sound knowledge of Herbal Simples which this modest Manual seeks to provide for their use.

Healing by herbs has always been popular both

with the classic nations of old, and with the British islanders of more recent times. Two hundred and sixty years before the date of Hippocrates (460 B.C.) the prophet Isaiah bade King Hezekiah, when sick unto death, "take a lump of Figs, and lay it on the boil; and straightway the King recovered."

Iapis, the favourite pupil of Apollo, was offered endowments of skill in augury, music, or archery. But he preferred to acquire a knowledge of herbs for service of cure in sickness; and, armed with this knowledge, he saved the life of Æneas when grievously wounded by an arrow. He averted the hero's death by applying the plant "Dittany," smooth of leaf, and purple of blossom, as plucked on the mountain Ida.

It is told in *Malvern Chase* that Mary of Eldersfield (1454), "whom some called a witch," famous for her knowledge of herbs and medicaments, "descending the hill from her hut, with a small phial of oil, and a bunch of the 'Danewort,' speedily enabled Lord Edward of March, who had just then heavily sprained his knee, to avoid danger by mounting 'Roan Roland' freed from pain, as it were by magic, through the plant-rubbing which Mary administered."

In Shakespeare's time there was a London street, named Bucklersbury (near the present Mansion House), noted for its number of druggists who sold Simples and sweet-smelling herbs. We read, in

The Merry Wives of Windsor, that Sir John Falstaff flouted the effeminate fops of his day as "Lisping hawthorn buds that smell like Bucklersbury in simple time."

Various British herbalists have produced works, more or less learned and voluminous, about our native medicinal plants; but no author has hitherto radically explained the why and wherefore of their ultimate curative action. In common with their early predecessors, these several writers have recognised the healing virtues of the herbs, but have failed to explore the chemical principles on which such virtues depend. Some have attributed the herbal properties to the planets which rule their growth. Others have associated the remedial herbs with certain cognate colours, ordaining red flowers for disorders of the blood, and yellow for those of the liver. "The exorcised demon of jaundice," says Conway, "was consigned to yellow parrots; that of inflammatory disease to scarlet, or red weeds." Again, other herbalists have selected their healing plants on the doctrine of allied signatures, choosing, for instance, the Viper's Bugloss as effectual against venomous bites, because of its resembling a snake; and the sweet little English Eyebright, which shows a dark pupil in the centre of its white ocular corolla, as of signal benefit for sore and inflamed eyes.

Thus it has continued to happen that until the

last half-century Herbal Physic has remained only speculative and experimental, instead of gaining a solid foothold in the field of medical science. Its claims have been merely empirical, and its curative methods those of a blind art :—

> "Si vis curari, de morbo nescio quali,
> Accipias herbam ; sed quale nescio ; nec quâ
> Ponas ; nescio quo ; curabere, nescio quando."

> "Your sore, I know not what, be not foreslow
> To cure with herbs, which, where, I do not know ;
> Place them, well pounc't, I know not how, and then
> You shall be perfect whole, I know not when."

Happily now-a-days, as our French neighbours would say, *Nous avons changé tout cela*, "Old things are passed away ; behold all things are become new !" Herbal Simples stand to-day safely determined on sure ground by the help of the accurate chemist. They hold their own with the best, and rank high for homely cures, because of their proved constituents. Their manifest healing virtues are shown to depend on medicinal elements plainly disclosed by analysis. Henceforward the curtain of oblivion must fall on cordial waters distilled mechanically from sweet herbs, and on electuaries artlessly compounded of seeds and roots by a Lady Monmouth, or a Countess of Arundel, as in the Stuart and Tudor times. Our Herbal Simples are fairly entitled at last to independent promotion from the shelves of the amateur still-room, from the rustic ventures of the village grandam, and from the shallow practices of self styled botanical doctors in the back streets of our cities.

"I do remember an apothecary,—
And hereabouts he dwells,---whom late I noted
In tatter'd weeds, with overwhelming brows,
Culling of Simples; meagre were his looks;
And in his needy shop a tortoise hung,
An alligator stuff'd, and other skins
Of ill-shap'd fishes; and about his shelves
A beggarly account of empty boxes,
Green earthen pots, bladders, and musty seeds,
Remnants of packthread, and old cakes of roses
Were thinly scattered to make up a show."
Romeo and Juliet, Act V. Sc. 1.

Chemically assured, therefore, of the sterling curative powers which our Herbal Simples possess, and anxious to expound them with a competent pen, the present author approaches his task with a zealous purpose, taking as his pattern, from the *Comus* of Milton:—

"A certain shepherd lad
Of small regard to see to, yet well skilled
In every virtuous plant, and healing herb;
He would beg me sing;
Which, when I did, he on the tender grass
Would sit, and hearken even to constancy;
And in requital ope his leathern scrip,
And show me *Simples*, of a thousand names,
Telling their strange, and vigorous faculties."

Shakespeare said, three centuries ago, "throw physic to the dogs." But prior to him, one Doctor Key, self styled Caius, had written in the Latin tongue (*tempore* Henry VIII.), a Medical History of the British Canine Race. His book became popular, though abounding in false concords; insomuch that from then until now medical classics have been held by scholars in poor repute for grammar, and sound construction. Notwithstanding which risk, many a passage is quoted here of ancient Herbal lore in the past tongues of Greece, Rome, and the Gauls. It is fondly hoped that the apt lines thus borrowed from old faultless sources will escape reproach for a defective modern rendering in Dog Latin, Mongrel Greek, or the "French of Stratford atte bowe."

Lastly, quaint old Fuller shall lend an appropriate Epilogue. "I stand ready," said he (1672), "with a pencil in one hand, and a spunge in the other, to add, alter, insert, efface, enlarge, and delete, according to better information. And if these my pains shall be found worthy to passe a second Impression, my faults I will confess with shame, and amend with thankfulnesse, to such as will contribute clearer intelligence unto me."

1895.

PREFACE TO THE SECOND EDITION.

On its First Reading, a Bill drafted in Parliament meets with acquiescence from the House on both sides mainly because its merits and demerits are to be more deliberately questioned when it comes up again in the future for a second closer Reading. Meanwhile its faults can be amended, and its omissions supplied: fresh clauses can be introduced: and the whole scheme of the Bill can be better adapted to the spirit of the House inferred from its first reception.

In somewhat similar fashion the Second Edition of "Herbal Simples" is now submitted to a Parliament of readers with the belief that its ultimate success, or failure of purpose, is to depend on its present revised contents, and the amplified scope of its chapters.

The criticisms which public journalists, not a few, thought proper to pass on its First Edition have been attentively considered herein. It is true their comments were in some cases so conflicting as to be difficult of practical appliance. The fabled old man and his ass stand always in traditional warning against futile attempts to satisfy inconsistent objectors, or to carry into effect suggestions made by irreconcilable censors. "*Quot homines, tot sententiæ*," is an adage signally verified when a fresh venture is made on the waters of chartered opinion. How shall the perplexed navigator steer his course when monitors in office accuse him on the one hand of lax precision throughout, and belaud him on the other for careful observance of detail? Or how shall he trim his sails when a contemptuous Standard-bearer, strangely uninformed on the point, ignores, as a leader of any repute, "one Gerard," a former famous Captain of the Herbal fleet? With the would-be Spectator's lament that Gerard's graphic drawings are regrettedly wanting here, the author is fain to concur. He feels that the absence of appropriate cuts to depict the various herbs is quite a deficiency: but the hope is inspired that a still future Edition may serve to supply this need. Certain botanical mistakes pointed out with authority by the *Pharmaceutical Journal* have here been duly corrected: and as many as fifty additional Simples will be found described in the present Enlarged Edition. At the same time a higher claim than hitherto made for the paramount importance of the whole subject is now courageously advanced.

To all who accept as literal truth the Scriptural account of the Garden of Eden it must be evident how intimately man's welfare from the first was made to depend on his uses of trees and herbs. The labour of earning his bread in the sweat of his brow by tilling the ground: and the penalty of thorns and thistles produced thereupon, were alike incurred by Eve's disobedience in plucking the forbidden fruit: and a signified possibility of man's eventful share in the tree of life, to "put forth his hand, and eat, and live for ever," has been more than vaguely revealed. So that with almost a sacred mission, and with an exalted motive of supreme usefulness, this Manual of healing Herbs is published anew, to reach, it is hoped, and to rescue many an ailing mortal.

Against its main principle an objection has been speciously raised, which at first sight appears of subversive weight; though, when further examined, it is found to be clearly fallacious. By an able but carping critic it was alleged that the mere chemical analysis of old-fashioned Herbal Simples makes their medicinal actions no less empirical than before: and that a pedantic knowledge of their constituent parts, invested with fine technical names, gives them no more scientific a position than that which our fathers understood.

But, taking, for instance, the herb Rue, which was formerly brought into Court to protect a Judge and the Bench from gaol fever, and other infectious disease; no one knew at the time by what particular virtue the Rue could exercise this salutary power. But more recent research has taught, that the essential oil contained in this, and other allied aromatic herbs, such as Elecampane,

Rosemary, and Cinnamon, serves by its germicidal principles (stearoptens, methyl-ethers, and camphors), to extinguish bacterial life which underlies all contagion. In a parallel way the antiseptic diffusible oils of Pine, Peppermint, and Thyme, are likewise employed with marked success for inhalation into the lungs by consumptive patients. Their volatile vapours reach remote parts of the diseased air-passages, and heal by destroying the morbid germs which perpetuate mischief therein. It need scarcely be said the very existence of these causative microbes, much less any mode of cure by their abolishment, was quite unknown to former Herbal Simplers.

Again, in past times a large number of our native plants acquired a well-deserved, but purely empirical celebrity, for curing scrofula and scurvy. But later discovery has shown that each of these several herbs contains lime, and earthy salts, in a subtle form of high natural sub-division: whilst, at the same time, the law of cure by medicinal similars has established the cognate fact that to those who inherit a strumous taint, infinitesimal doses of these earth salts are incontestably curative. The parents had first undergone a gradual impairment of health because of calcareous matters to excess in their general conditions of sustenance; and the lime proves potent to cure in the offspring what, through the parental surfeit, was entailed as a heritage of disease. Just in the same way the mineral waters of Missisquoi, and Bethesda, in America, through containing siliceous qualities so sublimated as almost to defy the analyst, are effective to cure cancer, albuminuria, and other organic complaints.

Nor is this by any means a new policy of cure. Its barbaric practice has long since obtained, even in African wilds, where the native snake doctor inoculates with his prepared snake poison to save the life of a victim otherwise fatally bitten by another snake of the same deadly virus. To Ovid, of Roman fame (20 B.C.), the same sanative axiom was also indisputably known as we learn from his lines:—

> "Tunc observatas augur descendit in herbas;
> Usus et auxilio est anguis ab angue dato."

> "Then searched the Augur low mid grass close scanned
> For snake to heal a snake-envenomed hand."

And with equal cogency other arguments, which are manifold, might be readily adduced, as of congruous force, to vindicate our claim in favour of analytical knowledge over blind experience in the methods of Herbal cure, especially if this be pursued on the broad lines of enlightened practice by similars.

So now, to be brief, and to change our allegory, "on the banks of the Nile," as Mrs. Malaprop would have pervertingly put it, with "a nice derangement of epitaphs," we invite our many guests to a simple "dinner of herbs." Such was man's primitive food in Paradise: "every green herb bearing seed, and every tree in the which is the fruit of a tree yielding seed:" "the green herb for meat for every beast of the earth, and every fowl of the air." What better Preface can we indite than a grace to be said before sitting down to the meal? "Sallets," it is hoped, will be found "in the lines to make the matter savoury." Far be it from our object to preach a prelude of texts, or to weary those at our board with a meaningless long benediction. "'Tis not so plain as the old Hill of Howth," said tender-hearted witty Tom Hood, with serio-comic truth, "a man has got his belly full of meat, because he talks with victuals in his mouth." Rather would we choose the "russet Yeas and honest kersey Noes" of sturdy yeoman speech; and cheerfully taking the head of our well-stocked table, ask in homely terms that "God will bless these the good creatures of His Herbal Simples to our saving uses, and us to His grateful service."

1897.

CONTENTS.

HERBAL SIMPLES

APPROVED

FOR MODERN USES OF CURE.

INTRODUCTION.

THE art of *Simpling* is as old with us as our British hills. It aims at curing common ailments with simple remedies culled from the soil, or got from home resources near at hand.

Since the days of the Anglo-Saxons such remedies have been chiefly herbal; insomuch that the word "drug" came originally from their verb *drigan*, to dry, as applied to medicinal plants.

These primitive Simplers were guided in their choice of herbs partly by watching animals who sought them out for self-cure, and partly by discovering for themselves the sensible properties of the plants as revealed by their odour and taste; also by their supposed resemblance to those diseases which nature meant them to heal.

John Evelyn relates in his *Acetaria* (1725) that "one Signor Faquinto, physician to Queen Anne (mother to the beloved martyr, Charles the First), and formerly physician to one of the Popes, observing scurvy and dropsy to be the epidemical and dominant diseases of this nation, went himself into the hundreds of Essex, reputed the most unhealthy county of this island, and used to follow the sheep and cattle on purpose to observe what plants they chiefly fed upon; and of these Simples he composed an excellent electuary of marvellous effects against these same obnoxious infirmities." Also, in like manner, it was noticed by others that "the dog, if out of condition, would seek for certain grasses of an emetic or purgative sort; sheep and cows, when ill, would devour curative plants; an anima. suffering from rheumatism would remain as much as it could in the sunshine; and creatures infested by parasites would roll themselves frequently in the dust." Again, William Coles in his *Nature's Paradise*, or, *Art of Simpling* (1657), wrote thus: "Though sin and Sathan have plunged mankinde into an ocean of infirmities, yet the mercy of God, which is over all His works, maketh grass to grow upon the mountaines, and Herbes for the use of men; and hath not only stamped upon them a distinct forme, but also given them particular signatures, whereby a man may read even in legible characters the use of them."

The present manual of our native Herbal Simples seeks rather to justify their uses on the sound basis of accurate chemical analysis, and precise elementary research. Hitherto medicinal herbs have come down to us from early times as possessing only a traditional value, and as exercising merely empirical effects. Their selection has been commended solely by a shrewd discernment, and by the practice of successive centuries. But to-day a closer analysis in the laboratory, and skilled provings by experts have resolved the several plants into their component parts, and have chemically determined the medicinal nature of these parts, both singly and collectively. So that the study and practice of curative British herbs may now fairly take rank as an exact science, and may command the full confidence of the sick for supplying trustworthy aid and succour in their times of bodily need.

Scientific reasons which are self-convincing may be readily adduced for prescribing all our best known native herbal medicines. Among them the Elder, Parsley, Peppermint, and Watercress may be taken as familiar examples of this leading fact. Almost from time immemorial in England a "rob" made from the juice of Elderberries simmered and thickened with sugar, or mulled Elder wine concocted from the fruit, with raisins, sugar, and spices, has been a popular remedy in this country, if taken hot at bedtime, for a recent cold, or for a sore throat. But only of late has chemistry explained that Elderberries furnish "viburnic acid," which induces sweating, and is specially curative of inflammatory bronchial soreness. So likewise Parsley, besides being a favourite pot herb, and a garnish for cold meats, has been long popular in rural districts as a tea for catarrh of the bladder or kidneys; whilst the bruised leaves have been extolled as a poultice for swellings and open sores. At the same time, a saying about the herb has commonly prevailed that it "brings death to men, and salvation to women." Not, however, until recently has it been learnt that the sweet-smelling plant yields what chemists call "apiol," or Parsley-Camphor, which, when given in moderation, exercises a quieting influence on the main sensific centres of life—the head and the spine. Thereby any feverish irritability of the urinary organs inflicted by cold, or other nervous shock, would be subordinately allayed. Thus likewise the Parsley-Camphor (whilst serving, when applied externally, to usefully stimulate indolent wounds) proves especially beneficial for female irregularities of the womb, as was first shown by certain French doctors in 1849.

Again, with respect to Peppermint, its cordial water, or its lozenges taken as a confection, have been popular from the days of our grandmothers for the relief of colic in the bowels, or for the stomach-ache of flatulent indigestion. But this practice has obtained simply because the pungent herb was found to diffuse grateful aromatic warmth within the stomach and bowels, whilst promoting the expulsion of wind; whereas we now know that an active principle "menthol" contained in the plant, and which may be extracted from it as a camphoraceous oil, possesses in a marked degree antiseptic and sedative properties which are chemically hostile to putrescence, and preventive of dyspeptic fermentation.

Lastly, the Watercress has for many years held credit with the common people for curing scurvy and its allied ailments; while its juices have been further esteemed as of especial use in arresting tubercular consumption of the lungs; and yet it has remained for recent analysis to show that the Watercress is chemically rich in "antiscorbutic salts," which tend to destroy the germs of tubercular disease, and which strike at the root of scurvy generally. These salts and remedial principles are "sulphur," "iodine," "potash," "phosphatic earths," and a particular volatile essential oil known as "sulphocyanide of allyl," which is almost identical with the essential oil of White Mustard.

Moreover, many of the chief Herbal Simples indigenous to Great Britain are further entitled for a still stronger reason to the fullest confidence of both doctor and patient. It has been found that when taken experimentally in varying quantities by healthy provers, many single medicines will produce symptoms precisely according with those of definite recognized maladies; and the same herbs, if administered curatively, in doses sufficiently small to avoid producing their toxical effects, will speedily and surely restore the patient to health by dispelling the said maladies. Good instances of such homologous cures are afforded by the common Buttercup, the wild Pansy, and the Sundew of our boggy marshes. It is widely known that the field Buttercup (*Ranunculus bulbosus*), when pulled from the ground, and carried in the palm of the hand, will redden and inflame the skin by the acrimony of its juices; or, if the bruised leaves are applied to any part they will excite a blistering of the outer cuticle, with a discharge of watery fluid from numerous small vesicles, whilst the tissues beneath become red, hot, and swollen; and these combined symptoms precisely represent "shingles,"—a painful skin disease given to arise from a depraved state of the bodily system, and from a faulty supply of nervous force. These shingles appear as a crop of sore angry blisters, which commonly surround the walls of the chest either in part or entirely; and modern medicine teaches that a medicinal tincture of the Buttercup, if taken in small doses, and applied, will promptly and effectively cure the same troublesome ailment; whilst it will further serve to banish a neuralgic or rheumatic stitch occurring in the side from any other cause.

And so with respect to the Wild Pansy (*Viola tricolor*), we read in Hahnemann's commentary on the proved plant: "The Pansy Violet excites certain cutaneous eruptions about the head and face, a hard thick scab being formed, which is cracked here and there, and from which a tenacious yellow matter exudes, and hardens into a substance like gum." This is an accurate picture of the diseased state seen often affecting the scalp of unhealthy children, as milk-crust, or, when aggravated, as a disfiguring eczema, and concerning the same Dr. Hughes of Brighton, in his authoritative modern treatise, says, "I have rarely needed any other medicine than the *Viola tricolor* for curing milk-crust, which is the plague of children," and "I have given it in the adult for recent impetigo (a similar disease of the skin), with very satisfactory results."

Finally, the Sundew (*Drosera rotundifolia*), which is a common little plant growing on our bogs, and marshy places, is found to act in the same double fashion of cause or cure according to the quantity taken, or administered. Farmers well know that this small herb when devoured by sheep in their pasturage will bring about a violent chronic cough, with waste of substance: whilst the Sundew when given experimentally to cats has been found to stud the surface of their lungs with morbid tubercular matter, though this is a form of disease to which cats are not otherwise liable. In like manner healthy human provers have become hoarse of voice through taking the plant, and troubled with a severe cough, accompanied with the expectoration of abundant yellow mucus, just as in tubercular mischief beginning at the windpipe. Meantime it has been well demonstrated (by Dr. Curie, and others) that at the onset of pulmonary consumption in the human subject a cure may nearly always be brought about, or the symptoms materially improved, by giving the tincture of *Sundew* throughout several weeks—from four to twenty drops in the twenty-four hours. And it has further become an established fact that the same tincture will serve with remarkable success to allay the troublesome spasms of Whooping Cough in its second stage, if given in small doses, repeated several times a day.

From these several examples, therefore, which are easy to be understood, we may fairly conclude that positive remedial actions are equally exercised by other Herbal Simples, both because of their chemical constituents and by reason of their curing in many cases according to the known law of medicinal correspondence.

Until of late no such an assured position could be rightly claimed by our native herbs, though pretentions in their favour have been widely popular since early English times. Indeed, Herbal physic has engaged the attention of many authors from the primitive days of Dioscorides (A.D. 60) to those of Elizabethan Gerard, whose exhaustive and delightful volume published in 1587 has remained ever since in paramount favour with the English people. Its quaint fascinating style, and its queer astrological notions, together with its admirable woodcuts of the plants described, have combined to make this comprehensive Herbal a standing favourite even to the present day.

Gerard had a large physic-garden near his house in Old Bourne (Holborn), and there is in the British Museum a letter drawn up by his hand asking Lord Burghley, his patron, to advise the establishment by the University of Cambridge in their grounds of a Simpling Herbarium. Nevertheless, we are now told (H. Lee, 1883) that Gerard's "ponderous book is little more than a translation of Dodonœus, from which comparatively un-read author whole chapters have been taken verbatim without acknowledgment."

No English work on herbs and plants is met with prior to the sixteenth century. In 1552 all books on astronomy and geography were ordered to be destroyed, because supposed to be infected with magic. And it is more than probable that any publications extant at that time on the virtues of herbs (then associated by many persons with witchcraft), underwent the same fate. In like manner King Hezekiah long ago "fearing lest the Herbals of Solomon should come into profane hands, caused them to be burned," as we learn from that "loyal and godly herbalist," Robert Turner.

During the reigns of Edward the Sixth and Mary, Dr. William Bulleyn ranked high as a physician and botanist. He wrote the first *Boke of Simples*, which remains among the most interesting literary productions of that era as a record of his acuteness and learning. It advocates the exclusive employment of our native herbal medicines. Again, Nicholas Culpeper, "student in physick," whose name is still a household word with many a plain thinking English person, published in 1652, for the benefit of the Commonwealth, his "*Compleat Method* whereby a man may cure himself being sick, for threepence charge, with such things only as grow in England, they being most fit for English bodies." Likewise in 1696 the Honourable Richard Boyle, F.R.S., published "*A Collection of Choice, Safe, and Simple English Remedies*, easily prepared, very useful in families, and fitted for the service of country people."

Once more, the noted John Wesley gave to the world in 1769 an admirable little treatise on *Primitive Physic, or an Easy and Natural Method for Curing most Diseases;* the medicines on which he chiefly relied being our native plants. For asthma, he advised the sufferer to "live a fortnight on boiled Carrots only"; for "baldness, to wash the head with a decoction of Boxwood";

for "blood-spitting to drink the juice of Nettles"; for "an open cancer, to take freely of Clivers, or Goosegrass, whilst covering the sore with the bruised leaves of this herb"; and for an ague, to swallow at stated times "six middling pills of Cobweb."

In Wesley's day tradition only, with shrewd guesses and close observation, led him to prescribe these remedies. But now we have learnt by patient chemical research that the Wild Carrot possesses a particular volatile oil, which promotes copious expectoration for the relief of asthmatic cough; that the Nettle is endowed in its stinging hairs with "formic acid," which avails to arrest bleeding; that Boxwood yields "buxine," a specific stimulant to those nerves of supply which command the hair bulbs; that Goosegrass or Clivers is of astringent benefit in cancer, because of its "tannic," "citric," and "rubichloric acids"; and that the Spider's Web is of real curative value in ague, because it affords an albuminous principle "allied to and isomeric with quinine."

Long before this middle era in medicine, during quite primitive British times, the name and office of "Leeches" were familiar to the people as the first doctors of physic; and their *parabilia* or "accessibles" were worts from the field and the garden; so that when the Saxons obtained possession of Britain, they found it already cultivated and improved by what the Romans knew of agriculture and of vegetable productions. Hence it had happened that Rue, Hyssop, Fennel, Mustard, Elecampane, Southernwood, Celandine, Radish, Cummin, Onion, Lupin, Chervil, Fleur de Luce, Flax (probably), Rosemary, Savory, Lovage, Parsley, Coriander, Alexanders, or Olusatrum, the black pot herb, Savin, and other useful herbs, were already of common growth for kitchen uses, or for medicinal purposes.

And as a remarkable incidental fact antiquity has bequeathed to us the legend, that goats were always exceptionally wise in the choice of these wholesome herbs; that they are, indeed, the herbalists among quadrupeds, and known to be "cunning in simples." From which notion has grown the idea that they are physicians among their kind, and that their odour is wholesome to the animals of the farmyard generally. So that in deference, unknowingly, to this superstition, it still happens that a single Nanny or a Betty is freakishly maintained in many a modern farmyard, living at ease, rather than put to any real use, or kept for any particular purpose of service. But in case of stables on fire, he or she will face the flames to make good an escape, and then the horses will follow.

It was through chewing the beans of Mocha, and becoming stupefied thereby, that unsuspicious goats first drew the attention of Mahomedan monks to the wonderful properties of the Coffee berry.

Next, coming down to the first part of the present century, we find that purveyors of medicinal and savoury herbs then wandered over the whole of England in quest of such useful simples as were in constant demand at most houses for the medicine-chest, the store-closet, or the toilet-table. These rustic practitioners of the healing art were known as "green men," who carried with them their portable apparatus for distilling essences, and for preparing their herbal extracts. In token of their having formerly officiated in this capacity, there may yet be seen in London and elsewhere about the country, taverns bearing the curious sign of "The Green Man and (his) Still."

It is told of a certain French writer not long since, that whilst complacently describing our British manners and customs, he gravely translated this legend of the signboard into "*L'homme vert, et tranquil.*"

Passing on finally to our own times at the close of the nineteenth century, we are able now-a-days, as has been already said, to avail ourselves of precise chemical research by apparatus far in advance of the untutored herbalist's still. He prepared his medicaments and his fragrant essences, merely as a mechanical art, and without pretending to fathom their method of physical action. But the skilled expert of to-day resolves his herbal simples into their ultimate elements by exact analysis in the laboratory, and has learnt to attach its proper medicinal virtue to each of these curative principles. It has thus come about that Herbal Physic under competent guidance, if pursued with intelligent care, is at length a reliable science of fixed methods, and crowned with sure results.

Moreover, in this happy way is at last vindicated the infinite superiority felt instinctively by our forefathers of home-grown herbs over foreign and far-fetched drugs; a superiority long since expressed by Ovid with classic felicity in the passage:—

> "Ætas cui facimus *aurea* nomen,
> Fructibus arbuteis, et humus quas educat herbis
> Fortunata fuit."—*Metamorphos., Lib. XV.*

> "Happy the age, to which we moderns give
> The name of 'golden,' when men chose to live
> On woodland fruits; and for their medicines took
> Herbs from the field, and simples from the brook."

or, as epitomised in the time-worn Latin adage:—

> "Qui potest mederi *simplicibus* frustra quærit composita."

> "If *simple* herbs suffice to cure,
> 'Tis vain to compound drugs endure."

In the following pages our leading Herbal Simples

are reviewed alphabetically; whilst, to ensure accuracy, the genus and species of each plant are particularised.

Most of these herbs may be gathered fresh in their proper season by persons who have acquired a knowledge of their parts, and who live in districts where such plants are to be found growing; and to other persons who inhabit towns, or who have no practical acquaintance with Botany, great facilities are now given by our principal druggists for obtaining from their stores concentrated fresh juices of the chief herbal simples.

Again, certain preparations of plants used only for their specific curative methods are to be got exclusively from the Homœopathic chemist, unless gathered at first hand. These, not being officinal, fail to find a place on the shelves of the ordinary Pharmaceutical druggist. Nevertheless, when suitably employed, they are of singular efficacy in curing the maladies to which they stand akin by the law of similars. For convenience of distinction here, the symbol H. will follow such particular preparations, which number in all some seventy-five of the simples described. At the same time any of the more common extracts, juices, and tinctures (or the proper parts of the plants for making these several medicaments), may be readily purchased at the shop of every leading druggist.

It has not been thought expedient to include among the Simples for homely uses of cure such powerfully poisonous plants as Monkshood (*Aconite*), Deadly Nightshade (*Belladonna*), Foxglove (*Digitalis*), Hemlock or Henbane (except for some outward uses), and the like dangerous herbs, these being beyond the province of domestic medicine, whilst only to be administered under the advice and guidance of a qualified prescriber.

The chief purpose held in view has been to reconsider those safe and sound herbal curative remedies and medicines which were formerly most in vogue as homely simples, whether to be taken or to be outwardly applied. And the main object has been to show with what confidence their uses may be now resumed, or retained under the guidance of modern chemical teachings, and of precise scientific provings. This question equally applies, whether the Simples be employed as auxiliaries by the physician in attendance, or are welcomed for prompt service in a household emergency as ready at hand when the doctor cannot be immediately had.

Moreover, such a Manual as the present of approved Herbal Remedies need not by any means be disparaged by the busy practitioner, when his customary medicines seem to be out of place, or are beyond speedy reach; it being well known that a sick person is always ready to accept with eagerness plain assistant remedies sensibly advised from the garden, the store-closet, the spice-box, or the field.

> "Of simple medicines, and their powers to cure,
> A wise physician makes his knowledge sure;
> Else for the household in his healing art
> He stands ill-fitted to take useful part."

So said Oribasus (freely translated) as long ago as the fourth century, in classic terms prophetic of later times, *Simplicium medicamentorum et facultatum quæ in eis insunt cognitio ita necessaria est ut sine eâ nemo rite medicari queat*

But after all has been said and done, none the less must it be finally acknowledged in the pathetic utterance of King Alfred's Anglo-Saxon proverb, *Nis no wurt woxen on woode ne on felde, per enure mage be lif uphelden.*

"No wort is waxen in wood or wold,
Which may for ever man's life uphold."

Neither to be discovered in the quaint Herbals of primitive times, nor to be learnt by the advanced chemical knowledge of modern plant lore, is there any panacea for all the ills to which our flesh is heir, or an elixir of life, which can secure for us a perpetual immunity from sickness. *Contra vim mortis nullum medicamentum in hortis*, says the rueful Latin distich :—

"No healing herb can conquer death,
And so for always give us breath."

To sum up which humiliating conclusion good George Herbert has put the matter thus with epigrammatic conciseness :—

"St. Luke was a saint and a physician, yet he is dead!"

But none the less bravely we may still take comfort each in his mortal frailty, because of the hopeful promise preached to men long since by the son of Sirach, "A faithful friend is the Medicine of life; they that fear the Lord shall find Him."

HERBAL SIMPLES.

ACORN.

THIS is the well-known fruit of our British Oak, to which tree it gives the name—*Aik*, or *Eik*, Oak.

The Acorn was esteemed by Dioscorides, and other old authors, for its supposed medicinal virtues. As an article of food it is not known to have been habitually used at any time by the inhabitants of Britain, though acorns furnished the chief support of the large herds of swine on which our forefathers subsisted. The right of maintaining these swine in the woods was called "panage," and formed a valuable property.

The earliest inhabitants of Greece and Southern Europe who lived in the primeval forests were supported almost wholly on the fruit of the Oak. They were described by classic authors as fat of person, and were called "balanophagi"—acorn eaters.

During the great dearth of 1709 the French were driven to eat bread of acorns steeped in water to destroy the bitterness, and they suffered therefrom injurious effects, such as obstinate constipation, or destructive cholera.

It is worth serious notice medically that in years remarkable for a large yield of Acorns disastrous losses have occurred among young cattle from outbreaks of acorn poisoning, or the acorn disease. Those up to two years old suffered most severely, but sheep, pigs and deer were not affected by this acorn malady. Its symptoms are progressive wasting, loss of appetite, diarrhœa, sore places inside the mouth, discharge from the eyes and nostrils, excretion of much pale urine, and no fever, but a fall of temperature below the normal standard. Having regard to which train of symptoms it is fair to suppose the acorn will afford in the human subject a useful specific medicine for the marasmus, or wasting atrophy of young children who are scrofulous. The fruit should be given in the form of a tincture, or vegetable extract, or even admixed (when ground) sparingly with wheaten flour in bread. The dose should fall short of producing any of the above symptoms, and the remedy should be steadily pursued for many weeks.

The tincture should be made of saturated strength with spirit of wine on the bruised acorns, to stand for a fortnight before being decanted. Then the dose will be from twenty to thirty drops with water three or four times a day.

The Acorn contains chemically starch, a fixed oil, citric acid, uncrystallizable sugar, and another special sugar called "quercit."

Acorns, when roasted and powdered, have been sometimes employed as a fair substitute for coffee. By distillation they will yield an ardent spirit.

Dr. Burnett strongly commends a "distilled spirit of acorns" as an antidote to the effects of alcohol, where the spleen and kidneys have already suffered, with induced dropsy. It acts on the principle of similars, ten drops being given three times a day in water.

In certain parts of Europe it is customary to place acorns in the hands of the newly dead; whilst in other districts an apple is put into the palm of a child when lying in its little coffin.

The bark of an oak tree, and the galls, or apples, produced on its leaves, or twigs, by an insect named cynips, are very astringent, by reason of the gallo-tannic acid which they furnish abundantly. This acid, given as a drug, or the strong decoction of oak bark which contains it, will serve to restrain bleedings if taken internally; and finely powdered oak bark, when inhaled pretty frequently, has proved very beneficial against consumption of the lungs in its early stages. Working tanners are well known to be particularly exempt from this disease, probably through their constantly inhaling the peculiar aroma given off from the tan pits; and a like effect may be produced by using as snuff the fresh oak bark dried and reduced to an impalpable powder, or by inhaling day after day the steam given off from recent oak bark infused in boiling water.

Marble galls are formed on the back of young twigs, artichoke galls at their extremities, and currant galls by spangles on the under surface of the leaves. From these spangles females presently emerge, and lay their eggs on the catkins, giving rise to the round shining currant galls.

The Oak—*Quercus robur*—is so named from the Celtic "quer," beautiful; and "cuez," a tree. "Drus," another Celtic word for tree, and particularly for the Oak, gave rise to the terms Dryads and Druids. Among the Greeks and Romans a chaplet of oak was one of the highest honours which could be conferred on a citizen. Ancient oaks exist in several parts of England, which are traditionally called Gospel oaks, because it was the practice in times long past when beating the bounds of a parish to read a portion of the Gospel on Ascension Day beneath an oak tree which was growing on the boundary line of the district. Cross oaks were planted at the juncture of cross roads, so that persons suffering from ague might peg a lock of their hair into the trunks, and by wrenching themselves away might leave the hair and the malady in the tree together. A strong decoction of oak bark is most usefully applied for prolapse of the lower bowel.

Oak Apple day (May 29th) is called in Hampshire "Shikshak" day.

AGRIMONY.

THE Agrimony is a Simple well known to all country folk, and abundant throughout England in the fields and woods, as a popular domestic medicinal herb. It belongs to the Rose order of plants, and blossoms from June to September with small yellow flowers, which sit close along slender spikes a foot high, smelling like apricots, and called by the rustics "Church Steeples." Botanically it bears the names *Agrimonia Eupatoria*, of which the first is derived from the Greek, and means "shining," because the herb is thought to cure cataract of the eye; and the second bears reference to the liver, as indicating the use of this plant for curing diseases of that organ. Chemists have determined that the Agrimony possesses a particular volatile oil, and yields nearly five per cent. of tannin, so that its use in the cottage for gargles, and as an astringent application to indolent wounds, is well justified. The herb does not seem really to own any qualities for acting medicinally on the liver. More probably the yellow colour of its flowers, which, with the root, furnish a dye of a bright nankeen hue, has given it a reputation in bilious disorders, according to the doctrine of signatures, because the bile is also yellow. Nevertheless, Gerard says: "A decoction of the leaves is good for them that have naughty livers." By pouring a pint of boiling water on a handful of the plant—stems, flowers and leaves—an excellent gargle may be made for a relaxed throat; and a teacupful of the same infusion may be taken cold three or four times in the day for simple looseness of the bowels; also for passive losses of blood. In France, Agrimony tea is drank as a beverage at table. This herb formed an ingredient of the genuine arquebusade water, as prepared against wounds inflicted by an arquebus, or hand-gun, and it was mentioned by Philip de Comines in his account of the battle of Morat, 1476. When the Yeomen of the Guard were first formed in England—1485—half were armed with bows and arrows, whilst the other half carried arquebuses. In France the *eau de arquebusade* is still applied for sprains and bruises, being carefully made from many aromatic herbs. Agrimony was at one time included in the London *Materia Medica* as a vulnerary herb. It bears the title of Cockleburr, or Sticklewort, because its seed vessels cling by the hooked ends of their stiff hairs to any person or animal coming into contact with the plant. A strong decoction of the root and leaves, sweetened with honey, has been taken successfully to cure scrofulous sores, being administered two or three times a day in doses of a wineglassful persistently for several months. Perhaps the special volatile oil of the plant, in common with that contained in other herbs similarly aromatic, is curatively antiseptic. Pliny called it a herb "of princely authoritie."

The *Hemp Agrimony*, or St. John's Herb, belongs to the Composite order of plants, and grows on the margins of brooks, having hemp-like leaves, which are bitter of taste and pungent of smell, as if it were an umbelliferous herb. Because of these hempen leaves it was formerly called "Holy Rope," being thus named after the rope with which Jesus was bound. They contain a volatile oil, which acts on the kidneys; likewise some tannin, and a bitter chemical principle, which will cut short the chill of intermittent fever, or perhaps prevent it. Provers of the plant have found it produce a "bilious fever," with severe headache, redness of the face, nausea. soreness over the liver, constipation, and high-coloured urine. Acting on which experience, a tincture, prepared (H.) from the whole plant, may be confidently given in frequent small well-diluted doses with water for influenza, or for a similar feverish chill, with break-bone pains, prostration, hot dry skin, and some bilious vomiting. Likewise a tea made with boiling water poured on the dried leaves will give prompt relief if taken hot at the onset of a bilious catarrh, or of influenza. This plant also is named *Eupatorium* because it refers, as Pliny says, to Eupator, a king of Pontus. In Holland it is used for jaundice, with swollen feet; and in America it belongs to the tribe of *bone-sets.* The Hemp Agrimony grows with us in moist, shady places, with a tall reddish stem, and with terminal crowded heads of dull lilac flowers. Its distinctive title is *Cannabinum*, or "Hempen," whilst by some it is known as "Thoroughwort."

ANEMONE (Wood).

THE *Wood Anemone*, or medicinal English *Pulsatilla*, with its lovely pink white petals, and drooping blossoms, is one of our best known and most beautiful spring flowers. Herbalists do not distinguish it virtually from the silky-haired *Anemone Pulsatilla*, which medicinal variety is of highly valuable modern curative use as a Herbal Simple. The active chemical principles of each plant are "anemonin" and "anemonic acid." A tincture is made (H.) with spirit of wine from the entire plant, collected when in flower. This tincture is remarkably beneficial in disorders of the mucous membranes, alike of the respiratory and of the digestive passages. For mucous indigestion following a heavy or rich meal the tincture of Pulsatilla is almost a specific remedy. Three or four drops thereof should be given at once with a tablespoonful of water, hot or cold, and the same dose may be repeated after an hour if then still needed. For catarrhal affections of the eyes and the ears, as well as for catarrhal diarrhœa, the tincture is very serviceable; also for female monthly difficulties its use is always beneficial and safe. As a medicine it best suits persons of a mild, gentle disposition, and of a lymphatic constitution, especially females; it is less appropriate for quick, excitable, energetic men. Anemonin, or Pulsatilla Camphor, which is the active principle of this plant, is prepared by the chemist, and may be given in doses of from one fiftieth to one tenth of a grain rubbed up with dry sugar of milk. Such a dose (or a drop of the tincture with a tablespoonful of water), given every two or three hours, will soon relieve a swollen testicle; and the tincture still more diluted will ease the bladder difficulties of old men. Furthermore, the tincture, in doses of two or three drops with a spoonful of water, will allay spasmodic cough, as of whooping cough, or bronchitis. The vinegar of Wood Anemone made from the leaves retains all the more acrid properties of the plant, and is put, in France, to many rural domestic purposes. When applied in lotions every night for five or six times consecutively, it will heal indolent ulcers; and its rubefacient effects serve instead of those produced externally by mustard. If a teaspoonful is sprinkled within the palms and its volatile vapours are inhaled through the mouth and nose, this will dispel an incipient catarrh. The name Pulsatilla is a diminutive of the Latin *puls*, a pottage, as made from pulse, and used at sacrificial feasts. The title Anemone signifies "wind-flower." Pliny says this flower never opens but when the wind is blowing. The title has been misapprehended as "an emony." Turner says gardeners call the flowers "emonies"; and Tennyson, in his "Northern Farmer," tells of the dead keeper being found "doon in the woild *enemies* afoor I comed to the plaice." Other names of the plant are Wood Crowfoot, Smell Fox (Hants), and Flawflower. Alfred Austin says, "With windflower honey are my tresses smoothed." It is also called the Passover Flower, because blossoming at Easter; and it belongs to the Ranunculaceous order of plants. The flower of the Wood Anemone tells the approach of night, or of a shower, by curling over its petals like a tent; and it has been said that fairies nestle within, having first pulled the curtains round them. Among the old Romans, to gather the first Anemone of the year was deemed a preservative against fever. The Pasque flower, also named Bluemoney and Easter, or Dane's flower, is of a violet blue, growing in chalky pastures, and less common than the Wood Anemone, but each possesses equally curative virtues.

The seed of the Anemone being very light and downy, is blown away by the first breeze of wind. A ready-witted French senator took advantage of this fact while visiting Bacheliere, a covetous florist, near Paris, who had long held a secret monopoly of certain richly-coloured and splendidly handsome anemones from the East. Vexed to see one man hoard up for himself what ought to be more widely distributed, he walked and talked with the florist in his garden when the anemone plants were in seed. Whilst thus occupied, he let fall his robe, as if by accident, upon the flowers, and so swept off a number of the little feathery seed vessels which clung to his dependent garment, and which he afterwards cultivated at home. The petals of the Pasque flower yield a rich green colour, which is used for staining Easter eggs, this festival having been termed Pask time in old works, from "paske," a crossing-over. The plant is said to grow best with iron in the soil.

ANGELICA (also called MASTER-WORT).

THE wild Angelica grows commonly throughout England in wet places as an umbelliferous plant, with a tall hollow stem, out of which boys like to make pipes. It is purple, furrowed, and downy, bearing white flowers tinged with pink. But the herb is not useful as a simple until cultivated in our gardens, the larger variety being chosen for this purpose, and bearing the name *Archangelica.*

> "Angelica, the happy counterbane,
> Sent down from heaven by some celestial scout,
> As well its name and nature both avow't."

It came to this country from northern latitudes in 1568. The aromatic stems are grown abundantly near London in moist fields for the use of confectioners. These stems, when candied, are sold as a favourite sweetmeat. They are grateful to the feeble stomach, and will relieve flatulence promptly. The roots of the garden Angelica contain plentifully a peculiar resin called "angelicin," which is stimulating to the lungs, and to the skin: they smell pleasantly of musk, being an excellent tonic and carminative. An infusion of the plant may be made by pouring a pint of boiling water on an ounce of the bruised root, and two tablespoonfuls of this should be given three or four times in the day; or the powdered root may be administered in doses of from ten to thirty grains. The infusion will relieve flatulent stomach-ache, and will promote menstruation if retarded. It is also of use as a stimulating bronchial tonic in the catarrh of aged and feeble persons. Angelica, taken in either medicinal form, is said to cause a disgust for spirituous liquors. In high Dutch it is named the root of the Holy Ghost. The fruit is employed for flavouring some cordials, notably *Chartreuse.* If an incision is made in the bark of the stems, and the crown of the root, at the commencement of spring, a resinous gum exudes with a special aromatic flavour as of musk or benzoin, for either of which it can be substituted. Gerard says: "If you do but take a piece of the root, and hold it in your mouth, or chew the same between your teeth, it doth most certainly drive away pestilent aire." Icelanders eat both the stem and the roots raw with butter. These parts of the plant, if wounded, yield a yellow juice which becomes, when dried, a valuable medicine beneficial in chronic rheumatism and gout. Some have said the Archangelica was revealed in a dream by an angel to cure the plague; others aver that it blooms on the day of Michael the Archangel (May 8th, old style), and is therefore a preservative against evil spirits and witchcraft.

ANISEED.

THE Anise (*Pimpinella*), from "bipenella," because of its secondary, feather-like leaflets, belongs to the umbelliferous plants, and is cultivated in our gardens; but its aromatic seeds chiefly come from Germany. The careful housewife will do well always to have a supply of this most useful Simple closely bottled in her store cupboard. The herb is a variety of the Burnet Saxifrage, and yields an essential oil of a fine blue colour. To make the essence of Aniseed one part of the oil should be mixed with four parts of spirit of wine. This oil, by its chemical basis, "anethol," represents the medicinal properties of the plant. It has a special influence on the bronchial tubes to encourage expectoration, particularly with children. For infantile catarrh, after its first feverish stage, Aniseed tea is very useful. It should be made by pouring half-a-pint of boiling water on two teaspoonfuls of the seeds, bruised in a mortar, and given when cold in doses of one, two, or three teaspoonfuls, according to the age of the child. For the relief of flatulent stomach-ache, whether in children or in adults, from five to fifteen drops of the essence may be given on a lump of sugar, or mixed with two dessertspoonfuls of hot water. Gerard says: "The Aniseed helpeth the yeoxing, or hicket (hiccough), and should be given to young children to eat which are like to have the falling sickness, or to such as have it by patrimony or succession." The odd literary mistake has been sometimes made of regarding Aniseed as a plural noun: thus, in "The Englishman's Doctor," it is said, "Some anny seeds be sweet, and some bitter." An old epithet of the Anise was, *Solamen intestinorum*—"The comforter of the bowels." The Germans have an almost superstitious belief in the medicinal virtues of Aniseed, and all their ordinary household bread is plentifully flavoured with the whole seeds. The mustaceœ, or spiced cakes of the Romans, introduced at the close of a rich entertainment, to prevent indigestion, consisted of meal, with anise, cummin, and other aromatics used for staying putrescence or fermentation within the intestines. Such a cake was commonly brought in at the end of a marriage feast; and hence the bridecake of modern times has taken its origin, though the result of eating this is rather to provoke dyspepsia than to prevent it. Formerly, in the East, these seeds were in use as part payment of taxes: "Ye pay tithe of mint, anise [dill ?], and cummin!" The oil destroys lice and the itch insect, for which purpose it may be mixed with lard or spermaceti as an ointment. The seed has been used for smoking, so as to promote expectoration.

Besides containing the volatile oil, Aniseed yields phosphates, malates, gum, and a resin. The leaves, if applied externally, will help to remove freckles; and, "Let me tell you this," says a practical writer of the present day, "if you are suffering from bronchitis, with attacks of spasmodic asthma, just send for a bottle of the liqueur called 'Anisette,' and take a dram of it with a little water. You will find it an immediate palliative; you will cease barking like Cerberus; you will be soothed, and go to sleep."—*Experto crede!* "I have been bronchitic and asthmatic for twenty years, and have never known an alleviative so immediately efficacious as 'Anisette.'"

For the restlessness of languid digestion, a dose of essence of Aniseed in hot water at bedtime is much to be commended. In the Paregoric Elixir, or "Compound Tincture of Camphor," prescribed as a sedative cordial by doctors (and containing some opium), the oil of Anise is also included—thirty drops in a pint of the tincture. This oil is of capital service as a bait for mice.

APPLE.

THE term "Apple" was applied by the ancients indiscriminately to almost every kind of round fleshy fruit, such as the thornapple, the pineapple, and the love-apple. Paris gave to Venus a golden apple; Atalanta lost her classic race by staying to pick up an apple; the fruit of the Hesperides, guarded by a sleepless dragon, were golden apples; and through the same fruit befell "man's first disobedience," bringing "death into the world and all our woe" (concerning which the old Hebrew myth runs that the apple of Eden, as the first fermentable fruit known to mankind, was the beginner of intoxicating drinks, which led to the knowledge of good and evil).

Nothing need be said here about the Apple as an esculent; we have only to deal with this eminently English, and most serviceable fruit in its curative and remedial aspects. Chemically, the Apple is composed of vegetable fibre, albumen, sugar, gum, chlorophyll, malic acid, gallic acid, lime, and much water. Furthermore, German analysts say that the Apple contains a larger percentage of phosphorus than any other fruit or vegetable. This phosphorus is specially adapted for renewing the essential nervous "lethicin" of the brain and spinal cord. Old Scandinavian traditions represent the Apple as the food of the gods, who, when they felt themselves growing feeble and infirm, resorted to this fruit for renewing their powers of mind and body. Also the acids of the Apple are of signal use for men of sedentary habits, whose livers are sluggish of action; they help to eliminate from the body noxious matters, which, if retained, would make the brain heavy and dull, or produce jaundice, or skin eruptions, or other allied troubles. Some experience of this sort has led to the custom of our taking Apple sauce with roast pork, roast goose, and similar rich dishes. The malic acid of ripe Apples, raw or cooked, will neutralize the chalky matter engendered in gouty subjects, particularly from an excess of meat eating. A good, ripe, raw Apple is one of the easiest of vegetable substances for the stomach to deal with, the whole process of its digestion being completed in eighty-five minutes. Furthermore, a certain aromatic principle is possessed by the Apple, on which its peculiar flavour depends, this being a fragrant essential oil—the valerianate of amyl—in a small but appreciable quantity. It can be made artificially by the chemist, and used for imparting the flavour of apples to sweetmeats and confectionery. Gerard found that "the pulp of roasted Apples, mixed in a wine quart of faire water, and laboured together until it comes to be as Apples and ale—which we call lambswool (Celtic, 'the day of Apple fruit')—never faileth in certain diseases of the raines, which myself hath often proved, and gained thereby both crownes and credit." Also, "The paring of an Apple cut somewhat thick, and the inside whereof is laid to hot, burning or running eyes at night when the party goes to bed, and is tied or bound to the same, doth help the trouble very speedily, and, contrary to expectation, an excellent secret." A poultice made of rotten Apples is commonly used in Lincolnshire for the cure of weak, or rheumatic eyes. Likewise in the *Hotel des Invalides*, at Paris, an Apple poultice is employed for inflamed eyes, the apple being roasted, and its pulp applied over the eyes without any intervening substance To obviate constipation two or three Apples taken at night, whether baked or raw, are admirably efficient. It was said long ago: "They do easily and speedily pass through the belly, therefore they do mollify the belly," and for this reason a modern maxim teaches that :—

"To eat an Apple going to bed
Will make the doctor beg his bread."

There was concocted in Gerard's day an ointment with the pulpe of Apples, and swine's grease, and rose-water, which was used to beautifie the face, and to take away the roughnesse of the skin, and which was called in the shops "pomatum," from the apples, "poma," whereof it was prepared. As varieties of the Apple, mention is made in documents of the twelfth century, of the pearmain, and the costard, from the latter of which has come the word costardmonger, as at first a dealer in this fruit, and now applied to our costermonger. Caracioli, an Italian writer, declared that the only ripe fruit he met with in Britain was a *baked* apple. The juices of Apples are matured and lose their rawness by keeping the fruit a certain time. These juices, together with those of the pear, the peach, the plum, and other such fruits, if taken without adding cane sugar, diminish acidity in the stomach rather than provoke it: they become converted chemically into alkaline carbonates, which correct sour fermentation. It is said in Devonshire that apples shrump up if picked when the moon is on the wane. From the bark of the stem and root of the apple, pear and plum trees, a glucoside is to be obtained in small crystals, which possesses the peculiar property of producing artificial diabetes in animals to whom it is given.

The juice of a sour Apple, if rubbed on warts first pared away to the quick, will serve to cure them. The wild "Scrab," or Crab Apple, armed with thorns, grows in our fields and hedgerows, furnishing verjuice, which is rich in tannin, and a most useful application for old sprains. In the United States of America an infusion of appletree bark is given with benefit during intermittent, remittent, and bilious fevers. We likewise prescribe Apple water as a grateful cooling drink for feverish patients. Francatelli directs that it should be made thus: "Slice up thinly three or four Apples without peeling them, and boil them in a very clean saucepan, with a quart of water and a little sugar until the slices of apple become soft; the apple water must then be strained through a piece of muslin, or clean rag, into a jug, and drank when cold." If desired, a small piece of the yellow rind of a lemon may be added, just enough to give it a flavour.

About the year 1562 a certain rector of St. Ives, in Cornwall, the Rev. Mr. Attwell, practised physic with milk and Apples so successfully in many diseases, and so spread his reputation, that numerous sufferers came to him from all the neighbouring counties. In Germany ripe Apples are applied to warts for removing them, by reason of the earthy salts, particularly the magnesia, of the fruit. It is a fact, though not generally known, that magnesia, as occurring in ordinary Epsom salts, will cure obstinate warts, and the disposition thereto. Just a few grains, from three to six, not enough to produce any sensible medicinal effect, taken once a day for three or four weeks, will surely dispel a crop of warts. Old cheese ameliorates Apples if eaten when crude, probably by reason of the volatile alkali, or ammonia of the cheese neutralizing the acids of the Apple. Many persons make a practice of eating cheese with Apple pie. The "core" of an Apple is so named from the French word, *cœur*, "heart."

The juice of the cultivated Apple made by fermentation into cider, which means literally "strong drink," was pronounced by John Evelyn, in his *Pomona*, 1729, to be "in a word the most wholesome drink in Europe, as specially sovereign against the scorbute, the stone, spleen, and what not." This beverage contains alcohol (on the average a little over five per cent.), gum, sugar, mineral matters, and several acids, among which the malic predominates. As an habitual drink, if sweet, it is apt to provoke acid fermentation with a gouty subject, and to develop rheumatism. Nevertheless, Dr. Nash, of Worcester, attributed to cider great virtues in leading to longevity; and a Herefordshire vicar bears witness to its superlative merits thus:—

> "All the Gallic wines are not so boon
> As hearty cider;—that strong son of wood
> In fullest tides refines and purges blood;
> Becomes a known Bethesda, whence arise
> Full certain cures for spittall maladies:
> Death slowly can the citadel invade;
> A draught of this bedulls his scythe, and spade."

Medical testimony goes to show that in countries where cider—not of the sweet sort—is the common beverage, stone, or calculus, is unknown; and a series of enquiries among the doctors of Normandy, a great Apple country, where cider is the principal, if not the sole drink, brought to light the fact that not a single case had been met with there in forty years. Cider Apples were introduced by the Normans; and the beverage began to be brewed in 1284. The Hereford orchards were first planted "tempore" Charles I.

A chance case of stone in the bladder if admitted into a Devonshire or a Herefordshire Hospital, is regarded by the surgeons there as a sort of professional curiosity, probably imported from a distance. So that it may be fairly surmised that the habitual use of natural unsweetened cider keeps held in solution materials which are otherwise liable to be separated in a solid form by the kidneys.

Pippins are apples which have been raised from pips;

a codling is an apple which requires to be "coddled," stewed, or lightly boiled, being yet sour and unfit for eating whilst raw. The John Apple, or Apple John, ripens on St. John's Day, December 27th. It keeps sound for two years, but becomes very shrunken. Sir John Falstaff says (*Henry IV.*, iii. 3) "Withered like an old Apple John." The squab pie, famous in Cornwall, contains apples and onions allied with mutton.

"Of wheaten walls erect your paste:
Let the round mass extend its breast;
Next slice your apples picked so fresh;
Let the fat sheep supply its flesh:
Then add an onion's pungent juice—
A sprinkling—be not too profuse!
Well mixt, these nice ingredients—sure!
May gratify an epicure."

In America, "Apple Slump" is a pie consisting of apples, molasses, and bread crumbs baked in a tin pan. This is known to New Englanders as "Pan Dowdy." An agreeable bread was at one time made by an ingenious Frenchman which consisted of one third of apples boiled, and two-thirds of wheaten flour.

It was through the falling of an apple in the garden of Mrs. Conduitt at Woolthorpe, near Grantham, Sir Isaac Newton was led to discover the great law of gravitation which regulates the whole universe. Again, it was an apple the patriot William Tell shot from the head of his own bright boy with one arrow, whilst reserving a second for the heart of a tyrant. Dr. Prior says the word Apple took its origin from the Sanskrit, *Ap.*,—"water," and *P'hal*,—"fruit," meaning "water fruit," or "juice fruit"; and with this the Latin name *Pomum*—from *Poto*, "to drink"—precisely agrees; if which be so, our apple must have come originally from the East long ages back.

The term "Apple-pie order" is derived from the French phrase, *à plis*, "in plaits," folded in regular plaits; or, perhaps, from *cap à pied*, "armed from head to foot," in perfect order. Likewise the "Apple-pie bed" is so called from the French *à plis*, or it may be from the Apple turnover of Devon and Cornwall, as made with the paste turned over on itself.

The botanical name of an apple tree is Pyrus Malus, of which schoolboys are wont to make ingenious uses by playing on the latter word. Malo, I had rather be; Malo, in an Apple tree; Malo, than a wicked man; Malo, in adversity. Or, again, *Mea mater mala est sus*, which bears the easy translation, "My mother is a wicked old sow"; but the intentional reading of which signifies "Run, mother! the sow is eating the apples." The term "Adam's Apple," which is applied to the most prominent part of a person's throat in front is based on the superstition that a piece of the forbidden fruit stuck in Adam's throat, and caused this lump to remain.

ARUM—THE COMMON.

THE "lords and ladies" (*arum maculatum*) so well known to every rustic as common throughout Spring in almost every hedge row, has acquired its name from the colour of its erect pointed spike enclosed within the curled hood of an upright arrow-shaped leaf. This is purple or cream hued, according to the accredited sex of the plant. It bears further the titles of Cuckoo Pint, Wake Robin, Parson in the Pulpit, Rampe, Starchwort, Arrowroot, Gethsemane, Bloody Fingers, Snake's Meat, Adam and Eve, Calfsfoot, Aaron, and Priest's Pintle. The red spots on its glossy emerald arrow-head leaves, are attributed to the dropping of our Saviour's blood on the plant whilst growing at the foot of the cross. Several of the above appellations bear reference to the stimulating effects of the herb on the sexual organs. Its tuberous root has been found to contain a particular volatile acrid principle which exercises distinct medicinal effects, though these are altogether dissipated if the roots are subjected to heat by boiling or baking. When tasted, the fresh juice causes an acrid burning irritation of the mouth and throat; also, if swallowed it will produce a red raw state of the palate and tongue, with cracked lips. The leaves, when applied externally to a delicate skin will blister it. Accordingly a tincture made (H.) from the plant and its root proves curative in diluted doses for a chronic sore throat, with swollen mucous membrane, and vocal hoarseness, such as is often known as "Clergyman's Sore Throat," and likewise for a feverish sore mouth, as well as for an irresistible tendency to sleepiness, and heaviness after a full meal. From five to ten drops of the tincture, third decimal strength, should be given with a tablespoonful of cold water to an adult three times a day. An ointment made by stewing the fresh sliced root with lard serves efficiently for the cure of ringworm.

The fresh juice yields malate of lime, whilst the plant contains gum, sugar, starch and fat. The name Arum is derived from the Hebrew *jaron*, "a dart," in allusion to the shape of the leaves like spear heads; or, as some think, from *aur*, "fire," because of the acrid juice. The adjective *maculatum* refers to the dark spots or patches which are seen on the smooth shining leaves of the plant. These leaves have sometimes proved fatal to children who have mistaken them for sorrel. The brilliant scarlet coral-like berries which are found set closely about the erect spike of the arum in the autumn are known to country lads as adder's meat—a name corrupted from the Anglo-Saxon *attor*, "poison," as originally applied to these berries, though it is remarkable that pheasants can eat them with impunity.

In Queen Elizabeth's time the Arum was known as starch-wort because the roots were then used for supplying pure white starch to stiffen the ruffs and frills worn at that time by gallants and ladies. This was obtained by boiling or baking the roots, and thus dispelling their acridity. When dried and powdered the root constitutes the French cosmetic, "Cypress Powder." Recently a patented drug, "Tonga," has obtained considerable notoriety for curing obstinate neuralgia of the head and face—this turning out to be the dried scraped stem of an aroid (or arum) called Raphidophora Vitiensis, belonging to the Fiji Islands. Acting on the knowledge of which fact some recent experimenters have tried the fresh juice expressed from our common Arum Maculatum in a severe case of neuralgia which could be relieved previously only by Tonga: and it was found that this juice in doses of a teaspoonful gave similar relief. The British Domestic Herbal, of Sydenham's time, describes a case of alarming dropsy, with great constitutional exhaustion treated most successfully with a medicine composed of Arum and Angelica, which cured in about three weeks. The "English Passion Flower" and "Portland Sago" are other names given to the Arum Maculatum.

ASPARAGUS.

THE Asparagus, belonging to the Lily order of plants, occurs wild on the coasts of Essex, Suffolk, and Cornwall. It is there a more prickly plant than the cultivated vegetable which we grow for the sake of the tender, edible shoots. The Greeks and Romans valued it for their tables, and boiled it so quickly that *velocius quam asparagi coquuntur*—"faster than asparagus is cooked"—was a proverb with them, to which our "done in a jiffy" closely corresponds. The shoots, whether wild or cultivated, are succulent, and contain wax, albumen, acetate of potash, phosphate of potash, mannite, a green resin, and a fixed principle named "asparagin." This asparagin stimulates the kidneys, and imparts a peculiar, strong smell to the urine after taking the shoots; at the same time, the green resin with which the asparagin is combined, exercises gently sedative effects on the heart, calming palpitation, or nervous excitement of that organ. Though not producing actual sugar in the urine, asparagus forms and excretes a substance therein which answers to the reactions used by physicians for detecting sugar, except the fermentation test. It may fairly be given in diabetes with a promise of useful results. In Russia it is a domestic medicine for the arrest of flooding.

Asparagin also bears the chemical name of "althein," and occurs in crystals, which may be reduced to powder, and which may likewise be got from the roots of marsh mallow, and liquorice. One grain of this given three times a day is of service for relieving dropsy from disease of the heart. Likewise, a medicinal tincture is made (H.) from the whole plant, of which eight or ten drops given with a tablespoonful of water three times a day will also allay urinary irritation, whilst serving to do good against rheumatic gout. A syrup of asparagus is employed medicinally in France: and at Aix-les-Bains it forms part of the cure for rheumatic patients to eat Asparagus. The roots of Asparagus contain diuretic virtues more abundantly than the shoots. An infusion made from these roots will assist against jaundice, and congestive torpor of the liver. The shrubby stalks of the plant bear red, coral-like berries which, when ripe, yield grape sugar, and spargancin. Though generally thought to branch out into feathery leaves, these are only ramified stalks substituted by the plant when growing on an arid sandy soil, where no moisture could be got for the maintenance of leaves. The berries are attractive to small birds, who swallow them whole, and afterwards void the seeds, to germinate when thus scattered about. Thus there is some valid reason for the vulgar corruption of the title Asparagus into Sparrow-grass, or Grass. Botanically the plant is a lily which has seen better days. In the United States of America, Asparagus is thought to be undeniably sedative, and a palliative in all heart affections attended with excited action of the pulse. The water in which asparagus has been boiled, if drunk, though somewhat disagreeable, is beneficial against rheumatism. The cellular tissue of the plant furnishes a substance similar to sago. In Venice, the wild asparagus is served at table, but it is strong in flavour and less succulent than the cultivated sort. Mortimer Collins makes Sir Clare, one of his characters in *Clarisse* say: "Liebig, or some other scientist maintains that asparagin—the alkaloid in asparagus—develops *form* in the human brain : so, if you get hold of an artistic child, and give him plenty of asparagus, he will grow into a second Raffaelle !"

Gerard calls the plant "Sperage," "which is easily concocted when eaten, and doth gently loose the belly." Our name, "Asparagus," is derived from a Greek word signifying "the tearer," in allusion to the spikes of some species ; or perhaps from the Persian "Spurgas," a shoot.

John Evelyn, in his *Book of Salads*, derives the term Asparagus in easy fashion, *ab asperitate*, "from the sharpness of the plant." "Nothing," says he, "next to flesh is more nourishing; but in this country we overboil them, and dispel their volatile salts: the water should boil before they are put in." He tells of asparagus raised at Battersea in a natural, sweet, and well-cultivated soil, sixteen of which (each one weighing about four ounces) were made a present to his wife, showing what "solum, cœlum, and industry will effect." The Asparagus first came into use as a food about 200 B.C., in the time of the elder Cato, and Augustus was very partial to it. The wild Asparagus was called Lybicum, and by the Athenians, Horminium. Roman cooks used to dry the shoots, and when required these were thrown into hot water, and boiled for a few minutes to make them look fresh and green. Gerard advises that asparagus should be sodden in flesh broth, and eaten; or boiled in fair water, seasoned with oil, pepper, and vinegar, being served up as a salad. Our ancestors in Tudor times ate the whole of the stalks with spoons. Swift's patron, Sir William Temple, who had been British Minister at the Hague, brought the art of Asparagus culture from Holland; and when William III. visited Sir William at Moor Park, where young Jonathan was domiciled as Secretary, his Majesty is said to have taught the future Dean of St. Patrick's how to eat asparagus in the Dutch style. Swift afterwards at his own table refused a second helping of the vegetable to a guest until the stalks had been devoured, alleging that "King William always ate his stalks." When the large white asparagus first came into vogue, it was known as the "New Vegetable." This was grown with lavish manure and was called Dutch Asparagus. For cooking the stalks should be cut of equal lengths, and boiled standing upwards in a deep saucepan with nearly two inches of the heads out of the water. Then the steam will suffice to cook these tender parts, whilst the hard stalky portions may be boiled long enough to become soft and succulently wholesome. Two sorts of asparagus are now grown—the one an early kind, pinkish white, cultivated in France and the Channel Islands; the other green and English. At Kynance Cove in Cornwall, there is an island called Asparagus Island, from the abundance in which the plant is found there.

In connection with this popular vegetable may be quoted the following riddle :—

> "What killed a queen to love inclined,
> What on a beggar oft we find,
> Show—to ourselves if aptly joined,
> A plant which we in bundles bind."

BALM.

THE herb Balm, or *Melissa*, which is cultivated quite commonly in our cottage gardens, has its origin in the wild, or bastard Balm, growing in our woods, especially in the South of England, and bearing the name of "Mellitis." Each is a labiate plant, and "Bawme," say the Arabians, "makes the heart merry and joyful." The title, "Balm," is an abbreviation of Balsam, which signifies "the chief of sweet-smelling oils;" Hebrew, *Bal smin*, "chief of oils"; and the botanical suffix, *Melissa*, bears reference to the large quantity of honey (*mel*) contained in the flowers of this herb.

When cultivated, it yields from its leaves and tops an essential oil which includes a chemical principle, or "stearopten." "The juice of Balm," as Gerard tells us, "glueth together greene wounds," and the leaves, say both Pliny and Dioscorides, "being applied, do close up woundes without any perill of inflammation." It is now known as a scientific fact that the balsamic oils of aromatic plants make most excellent surgical dressings. They give off ozone, and thus exercise anti-putrescent effects. Moreover, as chemical "hydro-carbons," they contain so little oxygen, that in wounds dressed with the fixed balsamic herbal oils, the atomic germs of disease are starved out. Furthermore, the resinous parts of these balsamic oils, as they dry upon the sore or wound, seal it up, and effectually exclude all noxious air. So the essential oils of balm, peppermint, lavender, and the like, with pine oil, resin of turpentine, and the balsam of benzoin (Friars' Balsam) should serve admirably for ready application on lint or fine rag to cuts and superficial sores. In domestic surgery, the lamentation of Jeremiah falls to the ground: "Is there no balm in Gilead: is there no physician there?" Concerning which "balm of Gilead," it may be here told that it was formerly of great esteem in the East as a medicine, and as a fragrant unguent. It was the true balsam of Judea, which at one time grew nowhere else in the whole world but at Jericho. But when the Turks took the Holy Land, they transplanted this balsam to Grand Cairo, and guarded its shrubs most jealously by Janissaries during the time the balsam was flowing.

In the "Treacle Bible," 1584, Jeremiah viii., *v.* 22, this passage is rendered: "Is there not treacle at Gylead?" Venice treacle, or triacle, was a famous antidote in the middle ages to all animal poisons. It was named *Theriaca* (the Latin word for our present treacle) from the Greek word *Therion*, a small animal, in allusion to the vipers which were added to the triacle by Andromachus, physician to the emperor Nero.

Tea made of our garden balm, by virtue of the volatile oil, will prove restorative, and will promote perspiration if taken hot on the access of a cold or of influenza; also, if used in like manner, it will help effectively to bring on the delayed monthly flow with women. But an infusion of the plant made with cold water, acts better as a remedy for hysterical headache, and as a general nervine stimulant because the volatile aromatic virtues are not dispelled by heat. Formerly, a spirit of balm, combined with lemon peel, nutmeg, and angelica-root, enjoyed a great reputation as a restorative cordial under the name of Carmelite water. Paracelsus thought so highly of balm that he believed it would completely revivify a man, as *primum ens melissæ.* The London Dispensatory of 1696 said: "The essence of balm given in Canary wine every morning will renew youth, strengthen the brain, relieve languishing nature, and prevent baldness." "Balm," adds John Evelyn, "is sovereign for the brain, strengthening the memory, and powerfully chasing away melancholy." In France, women bruise the young shoots of balm, and make them into cakes, with eggs, sugar, and rose water, which they give to mothers in childbed as a strengthener.

It is fabled that the Jew Ahasuerus (who refused a cup of water to our Saviour on His way to Golgotha, and was therefore doomed to wander athirst until Christ should come again) on a Whitsuntide evening, asked for a draught of small beer at the door of a Staffordshire cottager who was far advanced in consumption. He got the drink, and out of gratitude advised the sick man to gather in the garden three leaves of Balm, and to put them into a cup of beer. This was to be repeated every fourth day for twelve days, the refilling of the cup to be continued as often as might be wished; then "the disease shall be cured and thy body altered." So saying, the Jew departed and was never seen there again. But the cottager obeyed the injunction, and at the end of the twelve days had become a sound man.

BARBERRY.

THE Common Barberry (*Berberis*), which gives its name to a special order of plants, grows wild as a shrub in our English copses and hedges, particularly about Essex, being so called from *Berberin*, a pearl oyster, because the leaves are glossy like the inside of an oyster shell. It is remarkable for the light colour of its bark, which is yellow inside, and for its three-forked spines. Provincially it is also termed Pipperidge-bush, from "pepin," a pip, and "rouge," red, as descriptive of its small scarlet juiceless fruit, of which the active chemical principles, as well as of the bark, are "berberin" and "oxyacanthin." The sparingly-produced juice of the berries is cooling and astringent. It was formerly held in high esteem by the Egyptians, when diluted as a drink, in pestilential fevers. The inner, yellow bark, which has been long believed to exercise a medicinal effect on the liver, because of its colour, is a true biliary purgative. An infusion of this bark, made with boiling water, is useful in jaundice from congestive liver, with furred tongue, lowness of spirits, and yellow complexion; also for swollen spleen from malarious exposure. A medicinal tincture (H.) is made of the root-branches and the root-bark, with spirit of wine; and if given three or four times a day in doses of five drops with one tablespoonful of cold water, it will admirably rouse the liver to healthy and more vigorous action. Conversely the tincture when of reduced strength will stay bilious diarrhœa. British farmers dislike the

Barberry shrub because, when it grows in cornfields, the wheat near it is blighted, even to the distance of two or three hundred yards. This is because of a special fungus which is common to the Barberry, and being carried by the wind reproduces itself by its spores destructively on the ears of wheat, the Æcidium Berberidis, which generates Puccinia.

Clusius setteth it down as a wonderful secret which he had from a friend, " that if the yellow bark of Barberry be steeped in white wine for three hours, and be afterwards drank, it will purge one very marvellously."

The berries upon old Barberry shrubs are often stoneless, and this is the best fruit for preserving or for making the jelly. They contain malic and citric acids ; and it is from these berries that the delicious *confitures d'epine vinette*, for which Rouen is famous, are commonly prepared. And the same berries are chosen in England to furnish the kernel for a very nice sugar-plum. The syrup of Barberries will make with water an excellent astringent gargle for raw, irritable sore throat ; likewise the jelly gives famous relief for this catarrhal affection. It is prepared by boiling the berries, when ripe, with an equal weight of sugar, and then straining. For an attack of colic because of gravel in the kidneys, five drops of the tincture on sugar every five minutes will promptly relieve, as likewise when albumen is found by analysis in the urine.

A noted modern nostrum belauds the virtues of the Barberry as specific against bile, heartburn, and the black jaundice, this being a remedy which was "discovered after infinite pains by one who had studied for thirty years by candle light for the good of his countrymen." In Gerard's time at the village of Ivor, near Colebrooke, most of the hedges consisted solely of Barberry bushes.

The following is a good old receipt for making Barberry jam :—Pick the fruit from the stalks, and bake it in an earthen pan ; then press it through a sieve with a wooden spoon. Having mixed equal weights of the prepared fruit, and of powdered sugar, put these together in pots, and cover the mixture up, setting them in a dry place, and having sifted some powdered sugar over the top of each pot. Among the Italians the Barberry bears the name of Holy Thorn, because thought to have formed part of the crown of thorns made for our Saviour.

BARLEY.

HORDEUM Vulgare—common Barley—is chiefly used in Great Britain for brewing and distilling ; but it has dietetic and medicinal virtues which entitle it to be considered among serviceable simples. Roman gladiators who depended for their strength and prowess chiefly on Barley, were called Hordearii. Nevertheless, this cereal is less nourishing than wheat, and when prepared as food is apt to purge ; therefore it is not made into bread, except when wheat is scarce and dear, though in Scotland poor people eat Barley bread. In India Barley meal is made into balls of dough for the oxen and camels. Pearl Barley is prepared in Holland and Germany by first shelling the grain, and then grinding it into round white granules. The ancients fed their horses upon Barley, and we fatten swine on this grain made into meal. Among the Greeks beer was known as barley wine, which was brewed without hops, these dating only from the fourteenth century.

A decoction of barley with gum arabic, one ounce of the gum dissolved in a pint of the hot decoction, is a very useful drink to soothe irritation of the bladder, and of the urinary passages. The chemical constituents of Barley are starch, gluten, albumen, oil, and hordeic acid. From the earliest times it has been employed to prepare drinks for the sick, especially in feverish disorders, and for sore lining membranes of the chest. Honey may be added beneficially to the decoction of barley for bronchial coughs. The French make "Orgeat" of barley boiled in successive waters, and sweetened at length as a cooling drink: though this name is now applied in France to a liqueur concocted from almonds.

BASIL.

THE herb Sweet Basil (*Ocymum Basilicum*) is so called because "the smell thereof is fit for a king's house." It grows commonly in our kitchen gardens, but in England it dies down every year, and the seeds have to be sown annually. Botanically, it is named "basilicon," or royal, probably because used of old in some regal unguent, or bath, or medicine.

This, and the wild Basil, belong to the Labiate order of plants. The leaves of the Sweet Basil, when slightly bruised, exhale a delightful odour; they gave the distinctive flavour to the original Fetter-Lane sausages.

The Wild Basil (*Calamintha clinopodium*) or Basil thyme, or Horse thyme, is a hairy plant growing in bushy places, also about hedges and roadsides, and bearing whorls of purple flowers with a strong odour of cloves. The term *Clinopodium* signifies "bed's-foot flower," because "the branches dooe resemble the foot of a bed." In common with the other labiates, Basil, both the wild and the sweet, furnishes an aromatic volatile camphoraceous oil. On this account it is much employed in France for flavouring soups (especially mock turtle) and sauces; and the dry leaves, in the form of snuff, are used for relieving nervous headaches. A tea, made by pouring boiling water on the garden basil, when green, gently but effectually helps on the retarded monthly flow with women. The Bush Basil is *Ocymum minimum*, of which the leafy tops are used for seasoning, and in salads.

The Sweet Basil has been immortalised by Keats in his tender, pathetic poem of *Isabella and the Pot of Basil*, founded on a story from Boccaccio. She reverently possessed herself of the decapitated head of her lover, Lorenzo, who had been treacherously slain:—

> "She wrapped it up, and for its tomb did choose
> A garden pot, wherein she laid it by,
> And covered it with mould, and o'er it set
> *Sweet Basil*, which her tears kept ever wet."

The herb was used at funerals in Persia. Its seeds were sown by the Romans with maledictions and curses through the belief that the more it was abused the better it would prosper. When desiring a good crop they trod it down with their feet, and prayed the gods it might not vegetate. The Greeks likewise supposed Basil to thrive best when sown with swearing; and this fact explains the French saying, *Semer la Basilic*, as signifying "to slander." It was told in Elizabeth's time that the hand of a fair lady made Basil flourish; and this was then planted in pots as an act of gallantry. "Basil," says John Evelyn, "imparts a grateful flavour to sallets if not too strong, but is somewhat offensive to the eyes." Shenstone, in his *School Mistress's Garden*, tells of "the tufted Basil," and Culpeper quaintly says: "Something is the matter; Basil and Rue will never grow together: no, nor near one another." It is related that a certain advocate of Genoa was once sent as an ambassador to treat for conditions with the Duke of Milan; but the Duke harshly refused to hear the message, or to grant the conditions. Then the Ambassador offered him a handful of Basil. Demanding what this meant, the Duke was told that the properties of the herb were, if gently handled, to give out a pleasant odour; but that, if bruised, and hardly wrung, it would breed scorpions. Moved by this witty answer, the Duke confirmed the conditions, and sent the Ambassador honourably home.

BEAN (*see* Pea and Bean).

BELLADONNA (*see* Night Shade).

BENNET HERB (Avens).

THIS, the *Herba Benedicta*, or Blessed Herb, or Avens (*Geum Urbanum*) is a very common plant of the Rose tribe, in our woods, hedges, and shady places. It has an erect hairy stem, red at the base, with terminal bright yellow drooping flowers. The ordinary name Avens—or Avance, Anancia, Enancia—signifies an antidote, because it was formerly thought to ward off the Devil, and evil spirits, and venomous beasts. Where the root is in a house Satan can do nothing, and flies from it: "therefore" (says Ortus Sanitatis) "it is blessed before all other herbs; and if a man carries the root about him no venomous beast can harm him." The herb is sometimes called Way Bennet, and Wild Rye. Its graceful trefoiled leaf, and the fine golden petals of its flowers, symbolising the five wounds of Christ, were sculptured by the monks of the thirteenth century on their Church architecture. The botanical title of this plant, *Geum*, is got from *Geuo*, "to yield an agreeable fragrance," in allusion to the roots. Hence also has been derived another appellation of the Avens—*Radix Caryophyllata*, or "clove root," because when freshly dug out of the ground the roots smell like cloves. They yield tannin freely, with mucilage, resin, and muriate of lime, together with a heavy volatile oil. The roots are astringent and antiseptic, having been given in infusion for ague, and as an excellent cordial sudorific in chills, or for fresh catarrh. To make this a pint of boiling water should be poured on half an ounce of the dried root, or rather more of the fresh root, sliced. Half a wineglassful will be the dose, or ten grains of the powdered root. An extract is further made. When the petals of the flower fall off, a small round prickly ball is to be seen.

BETONY.

FEW, if any, herbal plants have been more praised for their supposed curative virtues than the Wood Betony (*Stachys Betonica*), belonging to the order of Labiates. By the common people it is often called Bitny. The name *Betonica* is from the Celtic "ben," head, and "tonic," good, in allusion to the usefulness of the herb against infirmities of the head. It is of frequent growth in shady woods and meadows, having aromatic leaves, and spikes (stakoi) of light purple flowers. Formerly it was held in the very highest esteem as a leading herbal simple. The Greeks loudly extolled its good qualities. Pliny, in downright raptures, styled it *ante cunctas laudatissima!* An old Italian proverb ran thus: *Vende la tunica en compra la Betonia*, "Sell your coat, and buy Betony;" whilst modern Italians, when speaking of a most excellent man, say,

"He has as many virtues as Betony"—*He piu virtù che Bettonica.*

In the *Medicina Britannica*, 1666, we read: "I have known the most obstinate headaches cured by daily breakfasting for a month or six weeks on a decoction of Betony, made with new milk, and strained."

Antonius Musa, chief physician to the Emperor Augustus, wrote a book entirely on the virtues of this herb. Meyrick says, inveterate headaches after resisting every other remedy, have been cured by taking daily at breakfast a decoction made from the leaves and tops of the Wood Betony. Culpeper wrote: "This is a precious herb well worth keeping in your house." Gerard tells that "Betony maketh a man have a good appetite to his meat, and is commended against ache of the knuckle bones" (sciatica).

A pinch of the powdered herb will provoke violent sneezing. The dried leaves formed an ingredient in Rowley's British Herb Snuff, which was at one time quite famous against headaches.

And yet, notwithstanding all this concensus of praise from writers of different epochs, it does not appear that the Betony, under chemical analysis and research, shows itself as containing any special medicinal or curative constituents. It only affords the fragrant aromatic principles common to most of the labiate plants.

Parkinson, who enlarged the *Herbal* of Gerard, pronounced the leaves and flowers of Wood Betony, "by their sweet and spicy taste, comfortable both in meate and medicine." Anyhow, Betony tea, made with boiling water poured on the plant, is a safe drink, and likely to prove of benefit against languid nervous headaches; and the dried herb may be smoked as tobacco for relieving the same ailment. To make Betony tea, put two ounces of the herb to a quart of water over the fire, and let this gradually simmer to three half-pints. Give a wine-glassful of the decoction three times a day. A conserve may be made from the flowers for similar purposes. The Poet Laureate, A. Austin, mentions "lye of Betony to soothe the brow." Both this plant, and the *Water Betony*—so called from its similarity of leaf—bear the name of Kernel-wort, from having tubers or kernels attached to the roots, and from being therefore supposed, on the doctrine of signatures, to cure diseased kernels or scrofulous glands in the neck; also to banish piles from the fundament.

But the Water Betony (Figwort) belongs not to the labiates, but to the *Scrophulariaceæ*, or scrofula-curing order of plants. It is called in some counties "brown-wort," and in Yorkshire "bishopsleaves," or, *l'herbe du siége*, which term has a double meaning—in allusion both to the seat in the temple of Cloacina (W.C.) and to the ailments of the lower body in connection therewith, as well as to the more exalted "See" of a Right Reverend Prelate. In old times the Water figwort was famous as a vulnerary, both when used externally, and when taken in decoction. The name "brown-wort" has been got either from the brown colour of the stems and flowers, or, more probably, from its growing abundantly about the "brunnen," or public German fountains. Wasps and bees are fond of the flowers. In former days this herb was relied on for the cure of toothache, and for expelling the particular disembodied spirit, or "mare," which visited our Saxon ancestors during their sleep after supper, being familiarly known to them as the "nightmare." The "Echo" was in like manner thought by the Saxons to be due to a spectre, or mare, which they called the "wood mare." The Water

Betony is said to make one of the ingredients in Count Mattœi's noted remedy, "anti-scrofuloso." The Figwort is named in Somersetshire "crowdy-kit" (the word kit meaning a fiddle), "or fiddlewood," because if two of the stalks are rubbed together, they make a noise like the scraping of the bow on violin strings. In Devonshire, also, the plant is known as "fiddler."

An allied Figwort—which is botanically called *nodosa*, or knotted—is considered, when an ointment is made with it, using the whole plant bruised and treated with unsalted lard, a sovereign remedy against "burnt holes" or gangrenous chicken-pox, such as often attacks the Irish peasantry, who subsist on a meagre and exclusively vegetable diet, being half starved, and pent up in wretched foul hovels. This herb is said to be certainly curative of hydrophobia, by taking every morning whilst fasting a slice of bread and butter on which the powdered knots of the roots have been spread, following it up with two tumblers of fresh spring water. Then let the patient be well clad in woollen garments and made to take a long fast walk until in a profuse perspiration. The treatment should be continued for nine days. Again, the botanical name of a fig, *ficus*, has been commonly applied to a sore or scab appearing on a part of the body where hair is, or to a red sore in the fundament, *i.e.*, to a pile. And the Figwort is so named in allusion to its curative virtues against piles, when the plant is made into an ointment for outward use, and when the tincture is taken internally. It is specially visited by wasps.

BILBERRY (Whortleberry, or Whinberry).

THIS fruit, which belongs to the Cranberry order of plants, grows abundantly throughout England in heathy and mountainous districts. The small-branched shrub bears globular, wax-like flowers, and black berries, which are covered, when quite fresh, with a grey bloom. In the West of England they are popularly called "whorts," and they ripen about the time of St. James' Feast, July 25th. Other names for the fruit are Blueberry, Bulberry, Hurtleberry, and Huckleberry. The title Whinberry has been acquired from its growing on Whins, or Heaths; and Bilberry signifies dark coloured; whence likewise comes Blackwort as distinguished in its aspect from the Cowberry and the Cranberry. By a corruption the original word Myrtleberry has suffered change of its initial M into W. (Whortleberry.) In the middle ages the Myrtleberry was used in medicine and cookery, to which berry the Whortleberry bears a strong resemblance. It is agreeable to the taste, and may be made into tarts, but proves mawkish unless mixed with some more acid fruit.

The Bilberry (*Vaccinium Myrtillus*) is an admirable astringent, and should be included as such among the domestic medicines of the housewife. If some good brandy be poured over two handfuls of the fruit in a bottle, this will make an extract which continually improves by being kept. Obstinate diarrhœa may be cured by giving doses of a tablespoonful of this extract taken with a wineglassful of warm water, and repeated at intervals of two hours whilst needed, even for the more severe cases of dysenteric diarrhœa. The berries contain chemically much tannin. Their stain on the lips may be quickly effaced by sucking at a lemon. In Devonshire they are eaten at table with cream. The Irish call them "frawns." If the first tender leaves are properly gathered and dried, they can scarcely be distinguished from good tea. Moor game live on these berries in the autumn. Their juice will stain paper or linen purple :—

> "Sanguineo splendore rosas vaccinia nigro,
> Induit, et dulci violas ferrugine pingit."
>
> CLAUDIAN.

They are also called in some counties, Blaeberries, Truckleberries, and Blackhearts.

The extract of Bilberry is found to be a very useful application for curing such skin diseases as scaly eczema, and other eczema which is not moist or pustulous ; also for burns and scalds. Some of the extract is to be laid thickly on the cleansed skin with a camel hair brush, and a thin layer of cotton wool to be spread over it, the whole being fastened with a calico or gauze bandage. This should be changed gently once a day.

Another Vaccinium (oxycoccos), the Marsh Whortleberry, or Cranberry, or Fenberry—from growing in fens—is found in peat bogs, chiefly in the North. This is a low plant with straggling wiry stems, and solitary terminal bright red flowers, of which the segments are bent back in a singular manner. Its fruit likewise makes excellent tarts, and forms a considerable article of commerce at Langtown, on the borders of Cumberland. The fruit stalks are crooked at the top, and before the blossom expands they resemble the head and neck of a crane.

BLACKBERRY.

THIS is the well-known fruit of the Common Bramble (*Rubus fructicosus*), which grows in every English hedgerow, and which belongs to the Rose order of plants. It has long been esteemed for its bark and leaves as a capital astringent, these containing much tannin; also for its fruit, which is supplied with malic and citric acids, pectin, and albumen. Blackberries go often by the name of "bumblekites," from "bumble," the cry of the bittern, and kyte, a Scotch word for belly; the name bumblekite being applied, says Dr. Prior, "from the rumbling and bumbling caused in the bellies of children who eat the fruit too greedily." "Rubus" is from the Latin *ruber*, red.

The blackberry has likewise acquired the name of scaldberry, from producing, as some say, the eruption known as scaldhead in children who eat the fruit to excess; or, as others suppose, from the curative effects of the leaves and berries in this malady of the scalp; or, again, from the remedial effects of the leaves when applied externally to scalds.

It has been said that the young shoots, eaten as a salad, will fasten loose teeth. If the leaves are gathered in the Spring and dried, then, when required, a handful of them may be infused in a pint of boiling water, and the infusion, when cool, may be taken, a teacupful at a time, to stay diarrhœa, and for some bleedings. Similarly, if an ounce of the bruised root is boiled in three half-pints of water, down to a pint, a teacupful of this may be given every three or four hours. The decoction is also useful against whooping-cough in its spasmodic stage. The bark contains tannin; and if an ounce of the same be boiled in a pint and a half of water, or of milk, down to a pint, half a teacupful of the decoction may be given every hour or two for staying relaxed bowels. Likewise the fruit, if desiccated in a moderately hot oven, and afterwards reduced to powder (which should be kept in a well corked bottle) will prove an efficacious remedy for dysentery.

Gerard says: "Bramble leaves heal the eyes that hang out, and stay the hæmorrhoides [piles] if they can be laid thereunto." The *London Pharmacopœia* (1696) declared the ripe berries of the bramble to be a great cordial, and to contain a notable restorative spirit. In Cruso's *Treasury of Easy Medicines* (1771), it is directed for old inveterate ulcers: "Take a decoction of blackberry leaves made in wine, and foment the ulcers with this whilst hot each night and morning, which will heal them, however difficult to be cured." The name of the bush is derived from brambel, or brymbyll, signifying prickly; its blossom as well as the fruit, ripe and unripe, in all stages, may be seen on the bush at the same time. With the ancient Greeks Blackberries were a popular remedy for gout.

As soon as blackberries are over-ripe, they become quite indigestible. Country folk say in Somersetshire and Sussex: "The devil goes round on Old Michaelmas Day, October 11th, to spite the Saint, and spits on the blackberries, so that they who eat them after that date fall sick, or have trouble before the year is out." Blackberry wine and blackberry jam are taken for sore throats in many rustic homes. Blackberry jelly is useful for dropsy from feeble ineffective circulation. To make "blackberry cordial," the juice should be expressed from the fresh ripe fruit, adding half a pound of white sugar to each quart thereof, together with half an ounce of both nutmeg and cloves; then boil these together for a short time, and add a little brandy to the mixture when cold.

In Devonshire the peasantry still think that if any one is troubled with "blackheads," *i.e.*, small pimples, or boils, he may be cured by creeping from East to West on the hands and knees nine times beneath an arched bramble bush. This is evidently a relic of an old Dryad superstition when the angry deities who inhabited particular trees had to be appeased before the special diseases which they inflicted could be cured. It is worthy of remark that the Bramble forms the subject of the oldest known apologue. When Jonathan upbraided the men of Shechem for their base ingratitude to his father's house, he related to them the parable of the trees choosing a king, by whom the Bramble was finally elected, after the olive, the fig tree, and the vine had excused themselves from accepting this dignity.

In the Roxburghe Ballad of "The Children in the Wood," occurs the verse—

> "Their pretty lips with Blackberries
> Were all besmeared and dyed;
> And when they saw the darksome night
> They sat them down, and cryed."

The French name for blackberries is *mûres sauvages*, also *mures de haie;* and in some of our provincial districts they are known as "winterpicks," growing on the Blag.

Blackberry wine, which is a trustworthy cordial astringent remedy for looseness of the bowels, may be made thus: Measure your berries, and bruise them, and to every gallon of the fruit add a quart of boiling water. Let the mixture stand for twenty-four hours, occasionally stirring; then strain off the liquid, adding to every gallon a couple of pounds of refined sugar, and keep it in a cask tightly corked till the following October, when it will be ripe and rich.

A noted hair-dye is said to be made by boiling the leaves of the bramble in strong lye, which then imparts permanently to the hair a soft, black colour. Tom Hood, in his humorous way, described a negro funeral as "going a black burying." An American poet graphically tells us :—

> "Earth's full of Heaven,
> And every common bush afire with God !
> But only they who see take off their shoes ;
> The rest sit round it, and—pluck blackberries."

BLUEBELL (Wild Hyacinth).

THIS,—the *Agraphis mutans*,—of the Lily tribe—is so abundant in English woods and pastures, whilst so widely known, and popular with young and old, as to need no description. Hyacinth petals are marked in general with dark spots, resembling in their arrangement the Greek word AI, alas ! because a youth, beloved by Apollo, and killed by an ill-wind, was changed into this flower. But the wild Hyacinth bears no such character on its petals, and is therefore called "non-scriptus." The graceful curl of the petals, not their dark violet colour, has suggested to the poets "hyacinthine locks."

In Walton's *Angler* the Bluebell is mentioned as Culverkeys, the same as "Calverkeys" in Wiltshire. No particular medicinal uses have attached themselves to the wild Hyacinth flower as a herbal simple. The root is round, and was formerly prized for its abundant clammy juice given out when bruised, and employed as starch. Miss Pratt refers to this as poisonous ; and our Poet Laureate teaches :—

> "In the month when earth and sky are one,
> To squeeze the blue bell 'gainst the adder's bite."

When dried and powdered, the root as a styptic is of special virtue to cure the whites of women : in doses of not more than three grains at a time. "There is hardly," says Sir John Hill, "a more powerful remedy." Tennyson has termed the woodland abundance of Hyacinths in full spring time as "The heavens up-breaking through the earth." On the day of St. George, the Patron Saint of England, these wild hyacinths tinge the meadows and pastures with their deep blue colour—an emblem of the ocean empire, over which England assumes the rule.

But the chief charms of the Bluebell are its beauty and early appearance. Now is "the winter past; the rain is over and gone; the flowers appear on the earth; the time for the singing of birds is come; and the voice of the turtle is heard in the land."

"This earth is one great temple, made
For worship everywhere;
The bells are flowers in sun and shade
Which ring the heart to prayer."

"The city bell takes seven days
To reach the townsman's ear;
But he who kneels in Nature's ways,
Has Sabbath all the year."

The Hairbell (*Campanula rotundifolia*) is the Bluebell of Scotland; and nothing rouses a Scot to anger more surely than to exhibit the wild Hyacinth as the true Bluebell.

BOG BEAN (or Marsh-trefoil).

THE Buck-bean, or Bog-bean, which is common enough in stagnant pools, and on our spongy bogs, is the most serviceable of all known herbal tonics. It may be easily recognised growing in water by its large leaves overtopping the surface, each being composed of three leaflets, and resembling the leaf of a Windsor Broad Bean. The flowers when in bud are of a bright rose colour, and when fully blown they have the inner surface of their petals thickly covered with a white fringe, on which account the plant is known also as "white fluff." The name Buckbean is perhaps a corruption of *scorbutus*, scurvy ; this giving it another title, "scurvy bean." And it is termed "goat's bean," perhaps from the French *le bouc*, "a he-goat." The plant flowers for a month and therefore bears the botanical designation, "Menyanthes" (*trifoliata*) from *meen*, "a month," and *anthos*, "a flower." It belongs to the Gentian tribe, each of which is distinguished by a tonic and appetising bitterness of taste. The root of the Bog Bean is the most bitter part, and is therefore selected for medicinal use. It contains a chemical glucoside, "Menyanthin," which consists of glucose and a volatile product, "Menyanthol." For curative purposes druggists supply an infusion of the herb, and a liquid extract in combination with liquorice. These preparations are in moderate doses, strengthening and antiscorbutic; but when given more largely they are purgative and emetic. Gerard says if the plant "be taken with mead, or honied water, it is of use against a cough"; in which respect it is closely allied to the Sundew (another plant of the bogs) for relieving whooping-cough after the first feverish stage, or any similar hacking, spasmodic cough. A tincture is made (H.) from the whole plant with spirit of wine, and this proves most useful for clearing obscuration of the sight, when there is a sense, especially in the open-air, of a white vibrating mist before the eyes ; and therefore it has been given with marked success in early stages of amaurotic paralysis of the retina. The dose should be three or four drops of the tincture with a tablespoonful of cold water three times in the day for a week at a time.

BORAGE.

THE Borage, with its gallant blue flower, is cultivated in our gardens as a pot herb, and is associated in our minds with bees and claret cup. It grows wild in abundance on open plains where the soil is favourable, and it has a long-established reputation for cheering the spirits. Botanically, it is the *Borago officinalis*, this title being a corruption of *cor-ago, i.e., cor*, the heart, *ago*, I stimulate —*quia cordis affectibus medetur*, because it cures weak conditions of the heart. An old Latin adage says: *Borago ego gaudia semper ago*—"I, Borage, bring always courage"; or the name may be derived from the Celtic, *Borrach*, "a noble person." This plant was the Bugloss of the older botanists, and it corresponds to our Common Bugloss, so called from the shape and bristly surface of its leaves, which resemble *bous-glossa*, the tongue of an ox. Chemically, the plant Borage contains potassium and calcium combined with mineral acids. The fresh juice affords thirty per cent., and the dried herb three per cent. of nitrate of potash. The stems and leaves supply much saline mucilage, which, when boiled and cooled, likewise deposits nitre and common salt. These crystals, when ignited, will burn with a succession of small sparkling explosions, to the great delight of the schoolboy. And it is to such saline qualities the wholesome, invigorating effects and the specially refreshing properties of the Borage are supposed to be mainly due. For which reason, the plant, "when taken in sallets," as says an old herbalist, "doth exhilarate, and make the mind glad," almost in the same way as a bracing sojourn by the seaside during an autumn holiday. The flowers possess cordial virtues which are very revivifying, and have been much commended against melancholic depression of the nervous system. Burton, in his

Anatomy of Melancholy (1676), wrote with reference to the frontispiece of that book :—

> "Borage and Hellebore fill two scenes,
> Sovereign plants to purge the veins
> Of melancholy, and cheer the heart
> Of those black fumes which make it smart;
> The best medicine that God e'er made
> For this malady, if well assaid."

"The sprigs of Borage," wrote John Evelyn, "are of known virtue to revive the hypochondriac and cheer the hard student."

According to Dioscorides and Pliny, the Borage was that famous nepenthe of Homer which Polydamas sent to Helen for a token "of such rare virtue that when taken steep'd in wine, if wife and children, father and mother, brother and sister, and all thy dearest friends should die before thy face, thou could'st not grieve, or shed a tear for them." "The bowl of Helen had no other ingredient, as most criticks do conjecture, than this of borage." And it was declared of the herb by another ancient author: *Vinum potatum quo sit macerata buglossa mœrorum cerebri dicunt auferre periti* :—

> "To enliven the sad with the joy of a joke,
> Give them wine with some borage put in it to soak."

The Romans named the Borage *Euphrosynon*, because when put into a cup of wine it made the drinkers of the same merry and glad.

Parkinson says, "The seed of Borage helpeth nurses to have more store of milk, for which purpose its leaves are most conducing." Its saline constituents promote activity of the kidneys, and for this reason the plant is used in France to carry off catarrhs which are feverish. The fresh herb has a cucumber-like odour, and when compounded with lemon and sugar, added to wine and water, it makes a delicious "cool tankard," as a summer drink. "A syrup concocted of the floures," said Gerard, "quieteth the lunatick person, and the leaves eaten raw do engender good blood." Of all nectar-loving insects, bees alone know how to pronounce the "open sesame" of admission to the honey pots of the Borage.

BROOM.

THE Broom, or Link (*Cytisus scoparius*) is a leguminous shrub which is well known as growing abundantly on open places in our rural districts. The prefix "cytisus" is derived from the name of a Greek island where Broom abounded. It formerly bore the name of *Planta Genista*, and gave rise to the historic title, "Plantagenet." A sprig of its golden blossom was borne by Geoffrey of Anjou in his bonnet when going into battle, making him conspicuous throughout the strife. In the *Ingoldsby Legends* it is said of our second King Henry's head-dress :—

"With a great sprig of broom, which he bore as a badge in it,
He was named from this circumstance, Henry Plantagenet."

The stalks of the Broom, and especially the topmost young twigs, are purgative, and act powerfully on the kidneys to increase the flow of urine. They contain chemically an acid principle, "scoparin," and an alkaloid, "sparteine." For medical purposes these terminal twigs are used (whether fresh or dried) to make a decoction which is of great use in dropsy from a weak heart, but it should not be given where congestion of the lungs is present. From half to one ounce by weight of the tops should be boiled down in a pint of water to half this quantity, and a wineglassful may be taken as a dose every four or six hours. For more chronic dropsy, a compound decoction of broom may be given with much benefit. To make this, use broom-tops and dandelion roots, of each half an ounce, boiling them in a pint of water down to half a pint, and towards the last adding half an ounce of bruised juniper berries. When cold, the decoction should be strained and a wineglassful may be had three or four times a day. "Henry the Eighth, a prince of famous memory, was wonte to drinke the distilled water of broome flowers against surfeits and diseases therefrom arising." The flower-buds, pickled in vinegar, are sometimes used as capers; and the roasted seeds have been substituted for coffee. Sheep become stupefied or excited when by chance constrained to eat broom-tops.

The generic name, *Scoparius*, is derived from the Latin word *scopa*, a besom, this signifying "a shrub to sweep with." It has been long represented that witches delight to ride thereon: and in Holland, if a vessel lying in dock has a besom tied to the top of its mast, this advertises it as in search of a new owner. Hence has arisen the saying about a woman when seeking a second husband, *Zij steetk 't dem bezen*, "She hangs out the broom."

There is a tradition in Suffolk and Sussex :—

> "If you sweep the house with Broom in May,
> You'll sweep the head of the house away."

Allied to the Broom, and likewise belonging to the Papilionaceous order of leguminous plants, though not affording any known medicinal principle, the Yellow Gorse *(Ulex)* or Furze grows commonly throughout England on dry exposed plains. It covers these during the flowering season with a gorgeous sheet of yellow blossoms, orange perfumed, and which entirely conceals the rugged brown unsightly branches beneath. Its elastic seed vessels burst with a crackling noise in hot weather, and scatter the seeds on all sides. "Some," says Parkinson, "have used the flowers against the jaundice," but probably only because of their yellow colour. "The seeds," adds Gerard, "are employed in medicines against the stone, and the staying of the laske (*laxitas*, looseness). They are certainly astringent, and contain tannin. In Devonshire the bush is called "Vuzz," and in Sussex "Hawth."

The Gorse is rare in Scotland, thriving best in our cool humid climate. In England it is really never out of blossom, not even after a severe frost, giving rise to the well-known saying "Love is never out of season except when the Furze is out of bloom." It is also known as Fursbush, Furrs and Whins, being crushed and given as fodder to cattle. The tender shoots are protected from being eaten by herbivorous animals in the same way as are the thistles and the holly, by the angles of the leaves having grown together so as to constitute prickles.

"'Twere to cut off an epigram's point,
Or disfurnish a knight of his spurs,
If we foolishly tried to disjoint
Its arms from the lance-bearing Furze."

Linnœus "knelt before it on the sod: and for its beauty thanked his God."

The *Butcher's Broom*, *Ruscus* (*or Bruscus*) *aculeatus*, or prickly, is a plant of the Lily order, which grows chiefly in the South of England, on heathy places and in woods. It bears sharp-pointed, stiff leaves (each of which produces a small solitary flower on its upper surface), and scarlet berries. The shrub is also known as Knee Hulyer, Knee Holly (confused with the Latin *cneorum*), Prickly Pettigrue and Jews' Myrtle. Butchers make besoms of its twigs, with which to sweep their stalls or blocks: and these twigs are called "pungi topi," "prickrats," from being used to preserve meat from rats. Jews buy the same for service during the Feast of Tabernacles; and the boughs have been employed for flogging chilblains. The Butcher's Broom has been claimed by the Earls of Sutherland as the distinguishing badge of their followers and Clan, every Sutherland volunteer wearing a sprig of the bush in his bonnet on field days. This shrub is highly extolled as a free promoter of urine in dropsy and obstructions of the kidneys; a pint of boiling water should be poured on an ounce of the fresh twigs, or on half-an-ounce of the bruised root, to make an infusion, which may be taken as tea. The root is at first sweet to the taste, and afterwards bitter.

BRYONY.

OUR English hedgerows exhibit Bryony of two distinct sorts—the white and the black—which differ much, the one from the other, as to medicinal properties, and which belong to separate orders of plants. The White Bryony is botanically a cucumber, being of common growth at our roadsides, and often called the White Vine; it also bears the name of Tetterberry, from curing a disease of the skin known as tetters. It climbs about with long straggling stalks, which attach themselves by spiral tendrils, and which produce rough, palmated leaves. Insignificant pale-green flowers spring in small clusters from the bottom of these leaves. The round berries are at first green, and afterwards brilliantly red. Chemically, the plant contains "bryonin," a medicinal substance which is intensely bitter; also malate and phosphate of lime, with gum, starch, and sugar.

A tincture is made (H.) from the fresh root collected before the plant flowers, which is found to be of superlative use for the relief of chronic rheumatism (especially when aggravated by moving), and for subduing active congestions of the serous membranes which line the heart-bag, the ribs, the outer coat of the brain, and which cover the bowels. In the treatment of pleurisy, this tincture is invaluable. Four drops should be given in a tablespoonful of cold water every three or four hours. Also for any contused bruising of the skin, and especially for a black eye, to promptly bathe the injured part with a decoction of White Bryony root will speedily subdue the swelling, and will prevent discoloration far better than a piece of raw beef applied outside as the remedy most approved in the Ring.

In France, the White Bryony is deemed so potent and perilous, that its root is named the devil's turnip—*navet du diable.*

Our English plant, the *Bryonia dioica*, purges as actively as colocynth, if too freely administered.

The name Bryony is two thousand years old, and comes from a Greek word *bruein*, "to shoot forth rapidly."

From the incised root of the White Bryony exudes a milky juice which is aperient of action, and which has been commended for epilepsy, as well as for obstructed liver and dropsy; also its tincture for chronic constipation.

The popular herbal drink known as Hop Bitters is said to owe many of its supposed virtues to the bryony root, substituted for the mandrake which it is alleged to contain. The true mandrake is a gruesome herb, which was held in superstitious awe by the Greeks and the Romans. Its root was forked, and bears some resemblance to the legs of a man; for which reason the moneymakers of the past increased the likeness, and attributed supernatural powers to the plant. It was said to grow only beneath a murderer's gibbet, and when torn from the earth by its root to utter a shriek which none might hear and live. From earliest times, in the East, a notion prevailed that the mandrake would remove sterility. With which purpose in view, Rachel said to Leah: "Give me, I pray thee, of thy son's mandrakes' (Genesis xxx. *v.* 14). In later times the Bryony has come into use instead of the true mandrake, and it has continued to form a profitable spurious article with mountebank doctors. In Henry the Eighth's day, ridiculous little images made from Bryony roots, cut into the figure of a man, and with grains of millet inserted into the face as eyes, the same being known as pappettes or mammettes, were accredited with magical powers, and fetched high prices with simple folk. Italian ladies have been known to pay as much as thirty golden ducats for one of these artificial mandrakes. Readers of Thalaba (Southey) will remember the fine scene in which Khawla procures this plant to form part of the waxen figure of the Destroyer. Unscrupulous vendors of the fraudulent articles used to seek out a thriving young Bryony plant, and to open the earth round it. Then being prepared with a mould such as is used for making Plaster of Paris figures, they fixed it close to the root, and fastened it with wire to keep it in place. Afterwards, by filling the earth up to the root they left it to assume the required shape, which was generally accomplished in a single summer.

The medicinal tincture (H.) of White Bryony (*Bryonia alba*) is of special service to persons of dark hair and complexion, with firm fibre of flesh, and of a bilious cross-grained temperament. Also it is of particular use for relieving coughs, and colds of a feverish bronchial sort, caught by exposure to the east wind. On the contrary, the catarrhal troubles of sensitive females, and of young children, are better met by Ipecacuanha :—

"Coughing in a shady grove
Sat my Juliana,
Lozenges I gave my love,
Ipecacuanha—
Full twenty from the lozenge box
The greedy nymph did pick;
Then, sighing sadly, said to me—
My Damon, I am sick."

George Canning.

THYRSIS ET PHYLLIS.

In nemore umbroso Phyllis mea forte sedebat,
Cui mollem exhausit tussis anhela sinum:
Nec mora : de loculo deprompsi pyxida lœvo,
Ipecacuaneos, exhibuique trochos :
Illa quidem imprudens medicatos leniter orbes
Absorpsit numero bisque quaterque decem :
Tum tenero ducens suspiria pectore dixit,
"Thyrsi! Mihi stomachum nausea tristis habet."

The *Black Bryony* (Lady's-seal, or Oxberry), which likewise grows freely in our hedges, is quite a different plant from its nominal congener. It bears the name of *Tamus Vulgaris*, and belongs to the natural order of Yams. It is also called the Wild Hop, and Tetterberry or Tetterwort (in common with the greater Celandine), because curing the skin disease known as tetters ; and further, Blackbindweed. It has smooth heart-shaped leaves, and produces scarlet, elliptical berries larger than those of the White Bryony. A tincture is made (H.) from the root-stock, with spirit of wine, which proves a most useful application to unbroken chilblains, when made into a lotion with water, one part to twenty. The plant is called Black Bryony (*Bryonia nigra*) from its dark leaves and black root. It is not given at all internally, but the acrid pulp of the root has been used as a stimulating plaster.

BUCKTHORN.

THE common Buckthorn grows in our woods and thickets, and used to be popularly known because of the purgative syrup made from its juice and berries. It bears dense branches of small green flowers, followed by the black berries, which purge violently. If gathered before they are ripe they furnish a yellow dye. When ripe, if mixed with gum arabic and lime water, they form the pigment called "Bladder Green." Until late in the present century—*O dura ilia messorum!*—English rustics, when requiring an aperient dose for themselves or their children, had recourse to the syrup of Buckthorn. But its action was so severe, and attended with such painful gripings, that as time went on the medicine was discarded, and it is now employed in this respect almost exclusively by the cattle doctor. Dodœus taught about Buckthorn berries: "They be not meet to be administered but to young and lusty people of the country, which do set more store of their money than their lives." The shrub grows chiefly on chalk, and near brooks. The name Buckthorn is from the German *buxdorn*, boxthorn, hartshorn. In Anglo-Saxon it was Heorotbremble. It is also known as Waythorn, Rainberry Thorn, Highway Thorn and Rhineberries. Each of the berries contains four seeds: and the flesh of birds which eat thereof is said to be purgative. When the juice is given medicinally it causes a bad stomach-ache, with much dryness of the throat: for which reason Sydenham always ordered a basin of soup to be given after it. Chemically the active principle of the Buckthorn is "rhamno-cathartine." Likewise a milder kind of Buckthorn, which is much more useful as a Simple, grows freely in England, the *Rhamnus frangula* or so-called "black berry-bearing Alder," though this appellation is a mistake, because botanically the Alder never bears any berries. This black Buckthorn is a slender shrub, which occurs in our woods and thickets. The juice of its berries is aperient, without being irritating, and is well suited as a laxative for persons of delicate constitution. It possesses the merit of continuing to answer in smaller doses after the patient has become habituated to its use. The berry of the *Rhamnus frangula* may be known by its containing only two seeds. Country people give the bark boiled in ale for jaundice; and this bark is the black dogwood of gunpowder makers. Lately a certain aperient medicine has become highly popular with both doctors and patients in this country, the same being known as Cascara Sagrada. It is really an American Buckthorn, the *Rhamnus Persiana*, and it possesses no true advantage over our black Alder Buckthorn, though the bark of this latter must be used a year old, or it will cause griping A fluid extract of the English mild Buckthorn, or of the American Cascara, is made by our leading druggists, of which from half to one teaspoonful may be given for a dose. This is likewise a tonic to the intestines, and is especially useful for relieving piles. Lozenges also of the Alder Buckthorn are dispensed under the name of "Aperient Fruit Lozenges;" one, or perhaps two, being taken for a dose as required.

There is a Sea Buckthorn, *Hippophœ*, which belongs to a different natural order, *Elœagnaceœ*, a low shrubby tree, growing on sandhills and cliffs, and called also Sallowthorn. The fruit is made (in Tartary) into a pleasant jelly, because of its acid flavour, and used in the Gulf of Bothnia for concocting a fish sauce.

The name signifies "giving light to a horse," being conferred because of a supposed power to cure equine blindness: or it may mean "shining underneath," in allusion to the silvery underside of the leaf.

The old-fashioned Cathartic Buckthorn of our hedges and woods has spinous thorny branchlets, from which its name, *Rhamnus*, is thought to be derived, because the shrub is set with thorns like as the ram. At one time this Buckthorn was a botanical puzzle, even to Royalty, as the following lines assure us :—

"Hicum, peridicum ; all clothed in green;
The King could not tell it, no more could the Queen;
So they sent to consult wise men from the East,
Who said it had horns, though it was not a beast."

BURNET SAXIFRAGE (*see* Pimpernel).

BUTTERCUP.

THE most common Buttercup of our fields (*Ranunculus bulbosus*) needs no detailed description. It belongs to the order termed *Ranunculaceæ*, so-called from the Latin *rana*, a frog, because the several varieties of this genus grow in moist places where frogs abound. Under the general name of Buttercups are included the creeping Ranunculus, of moist meadows ; the *Ranunculus acris*, Hunger Weed, or Meadow Crowfoot, so named from the shape of the leaf (each of these two being also called King Cup), and the *Ranunculus bulbosus* mentioned above. "King-Cob" signifies a resemblance between the unexpanded flowerbud and a stud of gold, such as a king would wear; so likewise the folded calyx is named Goldcup, Goldknob and Cuckoobud. The term Buttercup has become conferred through a mistaken notion that this flower gives butter a yellow colour through the cows feeding on it (which is not the case), or, perhaps, from the polished, oily surface of the petals. The designation really signifies "button cop," or *bouton d'or*, "the batchelor's button"; this terminal syllable, *cup*, being corrupted from the old English word "cop," a head. It really means "button head." The Buttercup generally is known in Wiltshire and the adjoining counties as Crazy, or Crazies, being reckoned by some as an insane plant calculated to produce madness; or as a corruption of Christseye (which was the medieval name of the Marigold).

A burning acridity of taste is the common characteristic of the several varieties of the Buttercup. In its fresh state the ordinary field Buttercup is so acrimonious that by merely pulling up the plant by its root, and carrying it some little distance in the hand, the palm becomes reddened and inflamed. Cows will not eat it unless very hungry, and then the mouth of the animal becomes sore and blistered. The leaves of the Buttercup, when bruised and applied to the skin, produce a blistering of the outer cuticle, with a discharge of a watery fluid, and with heat, redness, and swelling. If these leaves are masticated in the mouth they will induce pains like a stitch between the ribs at the side, with the sharp catchings of neuralgic rheumatism. A medicinal tincture is made (H.) from the bulbous Buttercup with spirit of wine, which will, as a similar, cure *shingles* very expeditiously, both the outbreak of small watery pimples clustered together at the side, and the accompanying sharp pains between the ribs. Also this tincture will promptly relieve neuralgic side-ache, and pleurisy which is of a passive sort. From six to eight drops of the tincture may be taken with a tablespoonful of cold water by an adult three or four times a day for either of the aforesaid purposes. In France, this plant is called "jaunet." Buttercups are most probably the "Cuckoo Buds" immortalised by Shakespeare. The fresh leaves of the Crowfoot (*Ranunculus acris*) formed a part of the famous cancer cure of Mr. Plunkett in 1794. This cure comprised Crowfoot leaves, freshly gathered, and dog's-foot fennel leaves, of each an ounce, with one drachm of white arsenic levigated, and with five scruples of flowers of sulphur, all beaten together into a paste, and dried by the sun in balls, which were then powdered, and, being mixed with yolk of egg, were applied on pieces of pig's bladder. The juice of the common Buttercup (*Bulbosus*), known sometimes as "St. Anthony's Turnip," if applied to the nostrils, will provoke sneezing, and will relieve passive headache in this way. The leaves have been applied as a blister to the wrists in rheumatism, and when infused in boiling water as a poultice over the pit of the stomach as a counter-irritant. For sciatica the tincture of the bulbous buttercup has proved very helpful.

The *Ranunculus flammata*, Spearwort, has been used to produce a slight blistering effect by being put under a limpet shell against the skin of the part to be relieved, until some smarting and burning have been sensibly produced, with incipient vesication of the outermost skin.

The *Ranunculus Sceleratus*, Marsh Crowfoot, or Celery-leaved Buttercup, called in France "*herbe sardonique*," and "*grenouillette d'eau*," when made into a tincture (H.) with spirit of wine, and given in small diluted doses, proves curative of stitch in the side, and of neuralgic pains between the ribs, likewise of pleurisy without feverishness. The dose should be five drops of the third decimal tincture with a spoonful of water every three or four hours. This plant grows commonly at the sides of our pools, and in wet ditches, bearing numerous small yellow flowers, with petals scarcely longer than the calyx.

CABBAGE.

"THE time has come," as the walrus said in *Alice and the Looking Glass*, "to talk of many things"—

"Of shoes, and ships, and sealing-wax; of *Cabbages*, and kings."

The Cabbage, which is fabled to have sprung from the tears of the Spartan lawgiver, Lycurgus, began as the Colewort, and was for six hundred years, according to Pliny and Cato, the only internal remedy used by the Romans. The Ionians had such a veneration for Cabbages that they swore by them, just as the Egyptians did by the onion. With ourselves, the wild Cabbage, growing on our English sea cliffs, is the true Collet, or Colewort, from which have sprung all our varieties of Cabbage—cauliflower, greens, broccoli, etc. No vegetables were grown for the table in England before the time of Henry the Eighth. In the thirteenth century it was the custom to salt vegetables because they were so scarce; and in the sixteenth century a Cabbage from Holland was deemed a choice present.

The whole tribe of Cabbages is named botanically *Brassicaceæ—apo tou brassein*—because they heat, or ferment. By natural order they are cruciferous plants; and all contain much nitrogen, or vegetable albumen, with a considerable quantity of sulphur; hence they tend strongly to putrefaction, and when decomposed their odour is very offensive. Being cut into pieces, and pressed close in a tub with aromatic herbs and salt, so as to undergo an acescent fermentation (which is arrested at that stage), Cabbages form the German *Saurkraut*, which is strongly recommended against scurvy. The white Cabbage is most putrescible; the red most emollient and pectoral. The juice of the red cabbage made into syrup, without any condiments, is useful in chronic coughs, and in bronchial asthma. The leaves of the common white Cabbage, when gently bruised and applied to a blistered surface, will promote a free discharge, as also when laid next the skin in dropsy of the ankles. All the Coleworts are called "Crambe," from *krambos*, dry, because they dispel drunkenness.

"There is," says an old author, "a natural enmitie between the Colewort and the vine, which is such that the vine, if growing near unto it, withereth and perisheth; yea, if wine be poured into the Colewort while it is boiling, it will not be any more boiled, and the colour thereof will be quite altered." The generic term Colewort is derived from *caulis*, a stalk, and *wourte*, as applied to all kinds of herbs that "do serve for the potte." "Good worts," exclaimed Falstaff, catching at Evans' faulty pronunciation of *words*,—"good worts," —"good cabbages." An Irish cure for sore throat is to tie Cabbage leaves round it; and the same remedy is applied in England with hot Cabbage leaves for a swollen face. In the Island of Jersey coarse Cabbages are grown abundantly on patches of roadside ground, and in corners of fields, the stalks of which attain the height of eight, ten, or more feet, and are used for making walking sticks or *cannes en tiges de choux*. These are in great demand on the island, and are largely exported. It may be that a specially tall cabbage of this sort gave rise to the Fairy tale of "Jack and the bean stalk." The word Cabbage bears reference to *caba* (*caput*), a head, as signifying a Colewort which forms a round head. *Kohl rabi*, from *caulo-rapum*, cabbage turnip, is a name given to the *Brassica oleracea.* In 1595 the sum of twenty shillings was paid for six Cabbages and a few carrots, at the port of Hull, by the purveyor to the Clifford family.

The red Cabbage is thought in France to be highly anti-scorbutic; and a syrup is made from it with this purpose in view. The juice of white Cabbage leaves will cure warts.

The *Brassica oleracea* is one of the plants used in Count Mattæi's vaunted nostrum, "anti-scrofuloso." This, the sea Cabbage, with its pale clusters of handsome yellow flowers, is very ornamental to our cliffs. Its leaves, which are conspicuously purple, have a bitter taste when uncooked, but become palatable for boiling if first repeatedly washed; and they are sold at Dover as a market vegetable. These should be boiled in two waters, of which the first will be made laxative, and the second, or thicker decoction, astringent, which fact was known to Hippocrates, who said "*jus caulis solvit cujus substantia stringit.*"

Sir Anthony Ashley brought the Cabbage into English cultivation. It is said a Cabbage is sculptured at his feet on his monument in Wimbourne Minster, Dorset. He imported the Cabbage (Cale) from Cadiz (Cales), where he held a command, and grew rich by seizing other men's possessions, notably by appropriating some jewels entrusted to his care by a lady. Hence he is said to have got more by Cales (Cadiz) than by Cale (Cabbage); and this is, perhaps, the origin of our term "to cabbage." Among tailors, this phrase "to cabbage" is a cant saying which means to filch the cloth when cutting out for a customer. Arbuthnot writes "Your tailor, instead of shreds, cabbages whole yards of cloth." Perhaps the word comes from the French *cabasser*, to put into a basket.

From the seed of the wild Cabbage (Rape, or Navew) rape-seed oil is extracted, and the residue is called rape-cake, or oil-cake.

Some years ago it was customary to bake bread-rolls wrapped in Cabbage leaves, for imparting what was considered an agreeable flavour. John Evelyn said: "In general, Cabbages are thought to allay fumes, and to prevent intoxication; but some will have them noxious to the sight." After all it must be confessed the Cabbage is greatly to be accused for lying undigested in the stomach, and for provoking eructations; which makes one wonder at the veneration the ancients had for it, calling the tribe divine, and swearing *per brassicam*, which was for six hundred years held by the Romans a panacea: though "*Dis crambee thanatos*"—"Death by twice Cabbage"—was a Greek proverb. Gerard says the Greeks called the Cabbage *Amethustos*, not only because it driveth away drunkennesse; but also for that it is like in colour to the pretious stone called the amethyst." The Cabbage was Pompey's best beloved dish. To make a winter salad it is customary in America to choose a firm white Cabbage, and to shred it very fine, serving it with a dressing of plain oil and vinegar. This goes by the name of "slaw," which has a Dutch origin.

The free presence of hydrogen and sulphur causes a very strong and unpleasant smell to pervade the house during the cooking of Cabbages. Nevertheless, this sulphur is a very salutary constituent of the vegetable, most useful in scurvy and scrofula. Partridge and Cabbage suit the patrician table; bacon and Cabbage better please the taste and the requirements of the proletarian. The nitrogen of this and other cruciferous plants serves to make them emit offensive stinks when they lie out of doors and rot.

For the purulent scrofulous ophthalmic inflammation of infants, by cleansing the eyes thoroughly every half-hour with warm water, and then packing the sockets each time with fresh Cabbage leaves cleaned and bruised to a soft pulp, the flow of matter will be increased for a few days, but a cure will be soon effected. Pliny commended the juice of the raw Cabbage with a little honey for sore and inflamed eyes which were moist and weeping, but not for those which were dry and dull.

In Kent and Sussex, when a Cabbage is cut and the stalk left in the ground to produce "greens" for the table, a cottager will carve an × on the top flat surface of the upright stalk, and thus protect it against mischievous garden sprites and demons.

Some half a century ago medical apprentices were taught the art of blood-letting by practising with a lancet on the prominent veins of a Cabbage leaf.

Carlyle said "of all plants the Cabbage grows fastest to completion." His parable of the oak and the Cabbage conveys the lesson that those things which are most richly endowed when they come to perfection, are the slowest in their production and development.

CAPSICUM (CAYENNE).

THE *Capsicum*, or Bird Pepper, or Guinea Pepper, is a native of tropical countries; but it has been cultivated throughout Great Britain as a stove plant for so many years (since the time of Gerard, 1636) as to have become practically indigenous. Moreover, its fruit-pods are so highly useful, whether as a condiment, or as a medicine, that no apology is needed for including it among serviceable Herbal Simples. The Cayenne pepper of our tables is the powdered fruit of Bird Pepper, a variety of the Capsicum plant, and belonging likewise to the order of *Solanums*; whilst the customary "hot" pickle which we take with our cold meats is prepared from another variety of the Capsicum plant called "Chilies." This plant —the Bird Pepper—exercises an important medicinal action, which has only been recently recognized by doctors. The remarkable success which has attended the use of Cayenne pepper as a substitute for alcohol with hard drinkers, and as a valuable drug in *delirium tremens*, has lately led physicians to regard the Capsicum as a highly useful, stimulating, and restorative medicine. For an intemperate person, who really desires to wean himself from taking spirituous liquors, and yet feels to need a substitute at first, a mixture of tincture of Capsicum with tincture of orange peel and water will answer very effectually, the doses being reduced in strength and frequency from day to day. In *delirium tremens*, if the tincture of Capsicum be given in doses of half-a-dram well diluted with water, it will reduce the tremor and agitation in a few hours, inducing presently a calm prolonged sleep. At the same time the skin will become warm, and will perspire naturally; the pulse will fall in quickness, but whilst regaining fulness and volume; and the kidneys, together with the bowels, will act freely.

Chemically the plant furnishes an essential oil with a crystalline principle, "capsicin," of great power. This oil may be taken remedially in doses of from half to one drop rubbed up with some powdered white sugar, and mixed with a wineglassful of hot water.

The medicinal tincture is made with sixteen grains of

the powdered Capsicum to a fluid ounce of spirit of wine; and the dose of this tincture is from five to twenty drops with one or two tablespoonfuls of water. In the smaller doses it serves admirably to relieve pains in the loins when depending on a sluggish inactivity of the kidneys. Unbroken chilblains may be readily cured by rubbing them once a day with a piece of sponge saturated with the tincture of Capsicum until a strong tingling is induced. In the early part of the present century, a medicine of Capsicum with salt was famous for curing severe influenza with putrid sore throat. Two dessert spoonfuls of small red pepper, or three of ordinary cayenne pepper, were beaten together with two of fine salt, into a paste, and with half-a-pint of boiling water added thereto. Then the liquor was strained off when cold, and half-a-pint of very sharp vinegar was mixed with it, a tablespoonful of the united mixture being given to an adult every half, or full hour, diluted with water if too strong. For inflammation of the eyes, with a relaxed state of the membranes covering the eyeballs and lining the lids, the diluted juice of the Capsicum is a sovereign remedy. Again, for toothache from a decayed molar, a small quantity of cayenne pepper introduced into the cavity will often give immediate relief. The tincture or infusion given in small doses has proved useful to determine outwardly the eruption of measles and scarlet fever, when imperfectly developed because of weakness. Also for a scrofulous discharge of matter from the ears, Capsicum tincture, of a weak strength, four drops with a table-spoonful of cold water three times a day, to a child, will prove curative.

A Capsicum ointment, or "Chili paste," scarcely ever fails to relieve chronic rheumatism when rubbed in topically for ten minutes at a time with a gloved hand; and an application afterwards of dry heat will increase the redness and warmth, which persist for some while, and are renewed by walking. This ointment, or paste, is made of the Oleo-resin—Capsicin—half-an-ounce, and Lanolin five ounces, the unguent being melted, and, after adding the Capsicin, letting them be stirred together until cold. The powder or tincture of Capsicum will give energy to a languid digestion, and will correct the flatulency often incidental to a vegetable diet. Again, a gargle containing Capsicum in a proper measure will afford prompt relief in many forms of sore throat, both by its stimulating action, and by virtue of its special affinities (H.); this particularly holds good for a relaxed state of the throat, the uvula, and the tonsils. Cayenne pepper is employed in the adulteration of gin.

The "Peter Piper" of our young memories took pickled pepper by the peck. He must have been a Homœopathic prover with a vengeance; but has left no useful record of his experiments—the more's the pity—for our guidance when prescribing its diluted forms.

CARAWAY.

THE common Caraway is a herb of the umbelliferous order found growing on many waste places in England, though not a true native of Great Britain. Its well-known aromatic seeds should be always at hand in the cupboard of every British housewife. The plant got its name from inhabiting Caria, a province of Asia Minor. It is now cultivated for commerce in Kent and Essex; and the essential oil distilled from the home grown fruit is preferred in this country. The medicinal properties of the Caraway are cordial and comforting to the stomach in colic and in flatulent indigestion; for which troubles a dose of from two to four drops of the essential oil of Caraway may be given on a lump of sugar, or in a teaspoonful of hot water.

For earache, in some districts the country people pound up the crumb of a loaf hot from the oven, together with a handful of bruised Caraway seeds; then wetting the whole with some spirit, they apply it to the affected part. The plant has been long naturalised in England, and was known here in Shakespeare's time, who mentions it in the second part of *Henry IV.* thus: "Come, cousin Silence! we will eat a pippin of last year's graffing, with a dish of Caraways; and then to bed!" The seeds grow numerously in the small flat flowers placed thickly together on each floral plateau, or umbel, and are best known to us in seed cake, and in Caraway comfits. They are really the dried fruit, and possess, when rubbed in a mortar, a warm aromatic taste, with a fragrant spicy smell. Caraway comfits consist of these fruits encrusted with white sugar; but why the wife of a comfit maker should be given to swearing, as Shakespeare avers, it is not easy to see. The young roots of Caraway plants may be sent to table like parsnips; they warm and stimulate a cold languid stomach. These mixed with milk and made into bread, formed the *chara* of Julius Cæsar, eaten by the soldiers of Valerius. Chemically the volatile oil obtained from Caraway seeds consists of "carvol," and a hydro-carbon, "carvene," which is a sort of "camphor." Dioscorides long ago advised the oil for pale-faced girls; and modern ladies have not disregarded the counsel.

From six pounds of the unbruised seeds, four ounces of the pure essential oil can be expressed. In Germany the peasants flavour their cheese, soups, and household bread—jager—with the Caraway; and this is not a modern custom, for an old Latin author says: *Semina carui satis communiter adhibentur ad condiendum panem; et rustici nostrates esitant jusculum e pane, seminibus carui, et cerevisiâ coctum.*

The Russians and Germans make from Caraways a favourite liqueur "Kummel," and the Germans add them as a flavouring condiment to their sawerkraut. In France Caraways enter into the composition of *l'huile de Venus*, and of other renowned cordials.

An ounce of the bruised seeds infused for six hours in a pint of cold water makes a good Caraway julep for infants, from one to three teaspoonfuls for a dose. It "consumeth winde, and is delightful to the stomack; the powdered seed put into a poultice taketh away blacke and blew spots of blows and bruises." "The oil, or seeds of Caraway do sharpen vision, and promote the secretion of milk." Therefore dim-sighted men and nursing mothers may courageously indulge in seed cake!

The name Caraway comes from the Gælic *Caroh*, a ship, because of the shape which the fruit takes. By cultivation the root becomes more succulent, and the fruit larger, whilst more oily, and therefore acquiring an increase of aromatic taste and odour. In Germany the seeds are given for hysterical affections, being finely powdered and mixed with ginger and salt to spread with butter on bread. As a draught for flatulent colic twenty grains of the powdered seeds may be taken with two teaspoonfuls of sugar in a wineglassful of hot water. Caraway-seed cake was formerly a standing institution at the feasts given by farmers to their labourers at the end of wheat sowing. But narcotic effects have been known to follow the chewing of Caraway seeds in a large quantity, such as three ounces at a time.

As regards its stock of honey the Caraway may be termed, like Uriah Heep, and in a double sense, "truly umbel." The diminutive florets on its flat disk are so shallow that lepidopterous and hymenopterous insects, with their long proboses, stand no chance of getting a meal. They fare as poorly as the stork did in the fable, whom the fox invited to dinner served on a soup plate. As Sir John Lubbock has shown, out of fifty-five visitants to the Caraway plant for nectar, one moth, nine bees, twenty-one flies, and twenty-four miscellaneous midges constituted the dinner party.

CHAMOMILE.

No Simple in the whole catalogue of herbal medicines is possessed of a quality more friendly and beneficial to the intestines than "Chamomile flowers." This herb was well known to the Greeks, who thought it had an odour like that of apples, and therefore they named it "Earth Apple," from two of their words, *kamai*—on the ground, and *melon*—an apple. The Spaniards call it *Manzanilla*, from a little apple, and they give the same name to one of their lightest sherries flavoured with this plant. The flowers, or "blows" of the Chamomile belong to the daisy genus, having an outer fringe of white ray florets, with a central yellow disk, in which lies the chief medicinal virtue of the plant. In the cultivated Chamomile the white petals increase, while the yellow centre diminishes; thus it is that the curative properties of the wild Chamomile are the more powerful. The true Chamomile is to be distinguished from the bitter Chamomile (*matricaria chamomilla*) which has weaker properties, and grows erect, with several flowers at a level on the same stalk. The true Chamomile grows prostrate, and produces but one flower (with a convex, not conical, yellow disk) from each stem, whilst its leaves are divided into hair-like segments. The flowers exhale a powerful aromatic smell, and present a peculiar bitter to the taste. When distilled with water they yield a small quantity of most useful essential oil, which, if fresh and good, is always of a bluish colour. It should be green or blue, and not faded to yellow. This oil is a mixture of ethers, among which "chamomilline," or the valerianate of butyl, predominates. Medicinally it serves to lower nervous excitability reflected from some organ in trouble, but remote from the part where the pain is actually felt; so it is very useful for such spasmodic coughs as are due to indigestion; also for distal neuralgia, pains in the head or limbs from the same cause, and for nervous colic of the bowels. The oil may be given in doses of from two to four drops on a lump of sugar, or in a dessert-spoonful of milk. An officinal tincture (*Tinctura anthemidis*) is made from the flowers of the true Chamomile (*Anthemis nobilis*) with rectified spirit of wine. The dose of this is from three to ten drops with a spoonful of water. It serves usefully to correct the summer diarrhœa of children, or that which occurs during teething, when the stools are green, slimy and parti-coloured. The true Chamomile, the bitter Chamomile, and the Feverfew, are most obnoxious to flies and mosquitoes. An infusion of their respective leaves in spirit will, if used as a wash to the face, arms, or any exposed part of the body, protect effectually from an attack by these petty foes, which are quaintly described in an old version of our Bible as "the pestilence that walketh in the darkness, and the bug that destroyeth at noonday." Chamomile tea is an excellent stomachic when taken in moderate doses of half-a-teacupful at a time. It should be made by pouring half-a-pint of boiling water on half-an-ounce of the dried flower heads, and letting this stand for fifteen minutes. A special tincture (H.) of *Chamomilla* is made from the bitter Chamomile (*Matricaria*), which, when given in small doses of three or four drops in a dessertspoonful of cold water every hour, will signally relieve severe neuralgic pains, particularly if they are aggravated at night. Likewise this remedy will quickly cure restlessness and fretfulness in children from teething, and who refuse to be soothed save by being carried about.

The name, *Matricaria*, of the bitter Chamomile is derived from *mater cara*, "beloved mother," because the herb is dedicated to St. Anne, the reputed mother of the Virgin Mary, or from *matrix*, as meaning "the womb." This herb may be known from the true Chamomile because having a large, yellow, conical disk, and no scales on the receptacles.

Chamomile tea is also an excellent drink for giving to aged persons an hour or more before dinner. Francatelli directs that it should be made thus: "Put about thirty flowers into a jug, and pour a pint of boiling water on them; cover up the tea, and when it has stood for about ten minutes pour it off from the flowers into another jug, and sweeten with sugar or honey." A teacupful of this Chamomile tea, into which is stirred a large dessertspoonful of moist sugar, with a little grated ginger added, will answer the purpose now indicated. For outward application, to relieve inflammatory pains, or congestive neuralgia, hot fomentations made of the infused Chamomile "blows" are invaluable. Bags may be loosely stuffed with the flowers, and steeped well in boiling water before being applied. But for internal use the infusion and the extract of the herb are comparatively useless, because much of the volatile essential oil is dissipated by boiling, or by dry heat. This oil made into pills with bread crumbs, and given whilst fasting two hours before a meal, will effectually dispel intestinal worms. True Chamomile flowers may be known from spurious ones (of the Feverfew) which have no bracts on the receptacle when the florets are removed.

It is remarkable that each Chamomile is a plant physician, as nothing contributes so much to the health of a garden as a number of Chamomile herbs dispersed about it. Singularly enough, if another plant is drooping, and apparently dying, in nine cases out of ten it will recover if you place a herb of Chamomile near it.

The stinking Chamomile (*Anthemis cotula*) or Mayweed, grows in cornfields, having a fœtid smell, and often blistering the hand which gathers it. Another name which it bears is "dog's fennel," because of the disagreeable odour, and the leaf resembling fennel. Similar uses may be made of it as with the other Chamomiles, but less effectively. It has solitary flowers with erect stems.

Dr. Schall declares that the Chamomile is not only a preventive of nightmare, but the sole certain remedy for this complaint. As a carminative injection for tiresome flatulence, it has been found eminently beneficial to employ Chamomile flowers boiled in tripe broth, and strained through a cloth, and with a few drops of the oil of Aniseed added to the decoction.

Falstaffe says in *Henry IV.*: "Though Chamomile, the more it is trodden on the faster it grows; yet youth, the more it is wasted the sooner it wears." For coarse feeders and drunkards Chamomile is peculiarly suitable. Its infusion will cut short an attack of delirium tremens in the early stage. Gerard found the oil of the flowers a remedy against all weariness; and quaint old Culpeper reminds us that the Egyptians dedicated the Chamomile to the sun because it cured agues. He slyly adds: "They were like enough to do it, for they were the arrantest apes in their religion I ever read of."

CARROT.

OUR garden Carrot, or Dauke, is a cultivated variety of the *Daucus sylvestris*, or wild carrot, an umbelliferous plant, which groweth of itself in untoiled places, and is called *philtron*, because it serveth for love matters. This wild Carrot may be found abundantly in our fields and on the sea shore; the term Carrot being Celtic, and signifying "red of colour," or perhaps derived from caro, flesh, because this is a fleshy vegetable. Daucus is from the Greek *daio*, to burn, on account of the pungent and stimulating qualities. It is common also on our roadsides, being popularly known as "Bee's nest," because the stems of its flowering head, or umbel, form a concave semi-circle, or nest, which bees, when belated from the hive will use as a dormitory. The small purple flower which grows in the middle of the umbel has been found beneficial for the cure of epilepsy. The juice of the Carrot contains "carotine" in red crystals; also pectin, albumen, and a particular volatile oil, on which the medicinal properties of the root depend. The seeds are warm and aromatic to the taste, whilst they are slightly diuretic. A tea made from the whole plant, and taken each night and morning, is excellent when the lithic acid, or gouty disposition prevails, with the deposit of a brick-dust sediment in the urine on its becoming cool.

The chief virtues of Carrots lie in the strong antiseptic qualities they possess, which prevent all putrescent changes within the body. In Suffolk they were given long since as a secret specific for preserving and restoring the wind of horses, but cows if fed long on them will make bloody urine. Wild Carrots are superior medicinally to those of the cultivated kind. Carrot sugar got from the inspissated juice of the roots may be used at table, and is good for the coughs of consumptive children. The seeds of the wild Carrot were formerly esteemed as a specific remedy for jaundice; and in Savoy the peasants now give an infusion of the roots for the same purpose; whilst this infusion has served to prevent stone in the bladder throughout several years when the patient had been previously subject to frequent attacks.

Carrots boiled sufficiently, and mashed into a pulp, when applied directly to a putrid, indolent sore, will sweeten and heal it. The Carrot poultice was first used by Sulzer for mitigating the pain, and correcting the stench of foul ulcers. Raw scraped Carrot is an excellent plaster for chapped nipples. At Vichy, where derangements of the liver and of the biliary digestion are particularly treated, Carrots in one or another form are served at every meal, whether in soup, or as a vegetable; and considerable efficacy of cure is attributed to them. In the time of Parkinson (1640) the leaves of the Carrot were thought to be so ornamental that ladies wore them as a head-dress instead of feathers. A good British wine may be brewed from the roots of the Carrot; and very tolerable bread may be prepared for travellers from these roots when dried and powdered. Pectic acid can be extracted by the chemist from Carrots, which will solidify plain sugared water into a wholesome appetising jelly. One part of this pectic acid dissolved in a little hot water, and added to make three hundred parts of warm water, is soon converted into a mass of trembling jelly. The yellow core of the Carrot is the part which is difficult of digestion with some persons, not the outer red layer. Before the French Revolution the sale of Carrots and oranges was prohibited in the Dutch markets, because of the unpopular aristocratic colour of these commodities. In one thousand parts of a Carrot there are ninety-five of sugar, and (according to some chemists) only three of starch. In country districts raw Carrots are sometimes given to children for expelling worms, probably because the vegetable matter passes mechanically through the body unchanged, and scours it. "Remember, William," says Sir Hugh Evans in the *Merry Wives of Windsor*, "Focative is *Caret*," "and that" replies Mrs. Quickly, "is a good root."

> "The man in the moon drinks claret,
> But he is a dull Jack-a-dandy;
> Would he know a sheep's head from a Carrot
> He should learn to drink cider and brandy."
> Song of Mad Tom in *Midsummer Night's Dream*.

CELANDINE (Greater, and Lesser).

THIS latter flower is a conspicuous herald of spring, which is strikingly welcome to every one living in the country throughout England, and a stranger to none. The Pile-wort, or lesser Celandine, bespangles all our banks with its brilliant, glossy, golden stars, coming into blossom on or about March 7th, St. Perpetua's day. They are a timely tocsin for five o'clock tea, because punctually at that hour they shut up their showy petals until 9.0 a.m. on the following morning. The well-known little herb, with its heart-shaped leaves, is a Ranunculus, and bears the affix *ficaria* from its curative value in the malady called *ficus*—a "red sore in the fundament" (Littleton, 1684).

The popular title, Pilewort, from *Pila*, a ball, was probably first acquired because, after the doctrine of signatures, the small oval tubercles attached to its stringy roots were supposed to resemble and to cure piles. Nevertheless, it has been since proved practically that the whole plant, when bruised and made into an ointment with fresh lard, is really useful for healing piles; as likewise when applied to the part in the form of a poultice or hot fomentation. "There be those also who thinke that if the herbe be but carried about by one that hath the piles the paine forthwith ceaseth." It has sometimes happened that the small white tubercles collected about the roots of the plant, when washed bare by heavy rains, and lying free on the ground, have given rise to a supposed shower of wheat. After flowering the Pilewort withdraws its substance of leaf and stem into a small rounded tube underground, so as to withstand the heat of summer, and the cold of the subsequent winter.

With the acrid juice of this herb, and of others belonging to the same Ranunculous order, beggars in England used to produce sores about their body for the sake of exciting pity, and getting alms. They afterwards cured these sores by applying fresh mullein leaves to heal them. The lesser Celandine furnishes a golden yellow volatile oil, which is readily converted into anemonic acid.

Wordsworth specially loved this lesser Celandine, and turned his lyre to sing its praises :—

> "There is a flower that shall be mine,
> 'Tis the little Celandine;
> I will sing as doth behove
> Hymns in praise of what I love."

In token of which affectionate regard these flowers have been carved on the white marble of his tomb.

The greater Celandine, or *Cœli donum* (*Chelidonium majus*), though growing freely in our waste places and hedgerows, is, perhaps, scarcely so well known as its diminutive namesake. Yet most persons acquainted with our ordinary rural plants have repeatedly come across this conspicuous herb, which exudes a bright yellow juice when bruised. It has sharply cut vivid leaves of a dull green, with a small blossom of brilliant yellow, and is not altogether unlike a buttercup, though growing to the height of a couple of feet. But this Celandine belongs to the Poppy tribe, whilst the Buttercup is a Ranunculus. The technical name of the greater Celandine (*Chelidonium*) comes from the Greek word *Chelidon*, a swallow, because of an ancient tradition that the bird makes use of this herb to open the eyes of its young, or to restore their sight when it has been lost:—

> "Cæcatis pullis hâc lumina mater hirundo
> (Plinius ut scripsit) quamvis sint eruta, reddit."

The ancients entertained a strong belief that birds are gifted with a knowledge of herbs; the woodpecker, for instance, seeking out the Springwort to remove obstructions, and the linnet making use of the Eyebright to restore its vision.

Queen Elizabeth in the forty-sixth year of her age was attacked with such a grievous toothache that she could obtain no rest by night or day because of the torture she endured. The lords of her council decided on sending for an "outlandish physician" named Penatus, who was famous for curing this agonising pain. He advised that when all was said and done, if the tooth was hollow, it were best to have it drawn; but as Her Majesty could not bring herself to submit to the use of chirurgical instruments, he suggested that the *Chelidonius major*—our greater Celandine—should be put into the tooth, and this stopped with wax, which would so loosen the tooth that in a short time it might be pulled out with the fingers. Aylmer, Bishop of London, tried to encourage the Queen by telling her that though he was an old man, and had not many teeth to spare, she should see a practical experiment made on himself. Thereupon he bade the surgeon who was in attendance extract one of his teeth in Her Majesty's presence.

This plant, the *Chelidonium majus*, is still used in Suffolk for toothache by way of fomentation. It goes also by the name of "Fenugreek" (*Fœnum Græcum*), Yellow Spit, Grecian Hay, and by that of Tetterwort. The root contains chemically "chelidonin" and "sanguinarin."

On the doctrine of signatures the herb, because of its bright orange-coloured juice, was formerly believed to be curative of jaundice. A medicinal tincture (H.) made from the entire plant with spirit of wine is at the present time held in high esteem by many physicians for overcoming torpid conditions of the liver. Eight or ten drops of this tincture, or of the fresh juice of the plant, may be given for a dose three times in the day in sweetened water when bilious yellowness of the skin is present, with itching, and with clayey stools, dark thick urine, constipation, and a pain in the right shoulder; also for neuralgia of the head and face on the right side. It is certainly remarkable that though the fanciful theory of choosing curative plants by their signatures has been long since exploded, yet doctors of to-day select several yellow medicines for treating biliary disorders—to wit, this greater Celandine with its ochreous juice; the Yellow Barberry; the Dandelion;

the Golden Seal (Hydrastis); the Marigold; Orange; Saffron; and Tomato. Animals poisoned by the greater Celandine have developed active and pernicious congestion of the lungs and liver. Clusius found by experience that the juice of the greater Celandine, when squeezed into small green wounds of what sort so ever, wonderfully cured them. "If the juice to the bigness of a pin's head be dropped into the eye in the morning in bed, it takes away outward specks, and stops incipient suffusions." Also if the yellow juice is applied to warts, or to corns, first gently scraped, it will cure them promptly and painlessly. The greater Celandine is by genus closely allied to the horned Poppy which grows so abundantly on our coasts. Its tincture given in small doses proves of considerable service in whooping-cough when very spasmodic.

Curious remedies for this complaint have found rustic favour: in Yorkshire owl broth is considered to be a specific; again in Gloucestershire a roasted mouse is given to be eaten by the patient; and in Staffordshire the child is made to look at the new moon whilst the right hand of the nurse is rubbed up and down its bare belly.

CELERY.

THE Parsleys are botanically named *Selinon*, and by some verbal accident, through the middle letter "n" in this word being changed into "r," making it *Seliron*, or, in the Italian, *Celeri*, our Celery (which is a Parsley) obtained its title. It is a cultivated variety of the common Smallage (*Small ache*) or wild Celery (*Apium graveolens*), which grows abundantly in moist English ditches, or in water. This is an umbelliferous herb, unwholesome as a food, and having a coarse root, with a fetid smell. But, like many others of the same natural order, when transplanted into the garden, and bleached, it becomes aromatic and healthful, making an excellent condimentary vegetable. But more than this, the cultivated Celery may well take rank as a curative Herbal Simple. Dr. Pereira has shown us that it contains sulphur (a known preventive of rheumatism) as freely as do the cruciferous plants, Mustard, and the Cresses. In 1879, Mr. Gibson Ward, then President of the Vegetarian Society, wrote some letters to the *Times*, which commanded much attention, about Celery as a food and a medicament. "Celery," said he, "when cooked, is a very fine dish, both as a nutriment and as a purifier of the blood. I will not attempt to enumerate all the marvellous cures I have made with Celery, lest medical men should be worrying me *en masse.* Let me fearlessly say that rheumatism is impossible on this diet; and yet English doctors in 1876 allowed rheumatism to kill three thousand six hundred and forty human beings, every death being as unnecessary as is a dirty face."

The seeds of our Sweet Celery are carminative, and act on the kidneys. An admirable tincture is made from these seeds, when bruised, with spirit of wine; of which a teaspoonful may be taken three times a day, with a spoonful or two of water. The root of the Wild Celery, Smallage, or Marsh Parsley, was reckoned, by the ancients, one of the five great aperient roots, and was employed in their diet drinks. The Great Parsley is the Large Age, or Large Ache; as a strange inconsistency the Romans adorned the heads of their guests, and the tombs of their dead with crowns of the Smallage. Our cultivated Celery is a capital instance of the fact that most of the poisonous plants can, by human ingenuity, be so altered in character as to become eminently serviceable for food or medicine. Thus, the Wild Celery, which is certainly poisonous when growing exposed to daylight, becomes most palatable, and even beneficial, by having its edible leaf stalks earthed up and bleached during their time of cultivation.

Dr. Pereira says the digestibility of Celery is increased by its maceration in vinegar. As taken at table, Celery possesses certain qualities which tend to soothe nervous irritability, and to relieve sick headaches. "This herb Celery [Sellery] is for its high and grateful taste," says John Evelyn, in his *Acetaria*, "ever placed in the middle of the grand sallet at our great men's tables, and our Prætor's feasts, as the grace of the whole board." It contains some sugar and a volatile odorous principle, which in the wild plant smells and tastes strongly and disagreeably. The characteristic odour and flavour of the cultivated plant are due to this essential oil, which has now become of modified strength and qualities; also when freshly cut it affords albumen, starch, mucilage, and mineral matter. Why Celery accompanies cheese at the end of dinner it is not easy to see. This is as much a puzzle as why sucking pig and prune sauce should be taken in combination,—of which delicacies James Bloomfield Rush, the Norwich murderer, desired that plenty should be served for his supper the night before he was hanged, on April 20th, 1849.

CENTAURY.

Of all the bitter appetising herbs which grow in our fields and hedgerows, and which serve as excellent simple tonics, the Centaury, particularly its white flowered variety, belonging to the Gentian order of plants, is the most efficacious. It shares in an abundant measure the restorative antiseptic virtues of the Field Gentian and the Buckbean. There are four wild varieties of the Centaury, square stemmed, and each bearing flat tufts of flowers which are more or less rose coloured. The ancients named this bitter plant the Gall of the Earth, and it is now known as Christ's Ladder, or Felwort.

Though growing commonly in dry pastures, in woods, and on chalky cliffs, yet the Centaury cannot be reared in a garden. Of old its tribe was called "Chironia," after Chiron, the Greek Centaur, well skilled in herbal physic; and most probably the name of our English plant was thus originated. But the Germans call the Centaury *Tausendgulden kraut*—"the herb of a thousand florins,"—either because of its high medicinal value, or as a corruption of *Centum aureum*, "a hundred golden sovereigns." Centaury has become popularly reduced in Worcestershire to Centre of the Sun. Its generic adjective "erythrœa" signifies red. The flowers open only in fine weather, and not after twelve o'clock (noon) in the day. Chemically the herb contains erythrocentaurin—a bitter principle of compound character,—together with the usual herbal constituents, but with scarcely any tannin. The tops of the Centaury, especially of that *flore albo*—with the light coloured petals—are given in infusion, or in powder, or when made into an extract. For languid digestion, with heartburn after food, and a want of appetite, the infusion prepared with cold water, an ounce of the herb to a pint, is best; but for muscular rheumatism the infusion should be made with boiling water. A wineglassful of either will be the proper dose, two or three times a day.

CHERRY.

THE wild Cherry (*Cerasus*), which occurs of two distinct kinds, has by budding and grafting begotten most of our finest garden fruits of its genus. The name *Cerasus* was derived from Kerasous, a city of Cappadocia, where the fruit was plentiful. According to Pliny, Cherries were first brought to Rome by Lucullus after his great victory over Mithridates, 89 B.C. The cultivated Cherry disappeared in this country during the Saxon period, and was not re-introduced until the reign of Henry VIII. The *Cerasus sylvestris* is a wild Cherry tree rising to the height of thirty or forty feet, and producing innumerable small globose fruits; whilst the *Cerasus vulgaris*, another wild Cherry, is a mere shrub, called *Cerevisier* in France, of which the fruit is sour and bitter. Cherry stones have been found in the primitive lake dwellings of Western Switzerland. There is a tradition that Christ gave a Cherry to St. Peter, admonishing him not to despise little things. In the time of Charles the First, Herrick, the clergyman poet, wrote a simple song, to which our well-known pretty "Cherry Ripe" has been adapted :—

> "Cherry ripe! ripe! I cry,
> Full and fair ones! come, and buy!
> If so be you ask me where
> They do grow: I answer there
> Where my Julia's lips do smile,
> There's the land: a cherry isle."

"Cherries on the ryse" (or, on twigs) was well known as a London street cry in the fifteenth century; but these were probably the fruit of the wild Cherry, or Gean tree. In France soup made from Cherries, and taken with bread, is the common sustenance of the wood cutters and charcoal burners of the forest during the winter. The French distil from Cherries a liqueur named *Eau de Cerises*, or, in German, *Kirschwasser*; whilst the Italians prepare from a Cherry called *Marusca* the liqueur noted as *Marasquin*. Cherries termed as Mazzards are grown in Devon and Cornwall. A gum exudes from the bark of the Cherry tree which is equal in value to gum arabic. A caravan going from Ethiopia to Egypt, says Husselquist, and a garrison of more than two hundred men during a siege which lasted two months, were kept alive with no other food than this gum, "which they sucked often and slowly." It is known chemically as "cerasin," and differs from gum acacia in being less soluble.

The leaves of the tree and the kernels of the fruit contain a basis of prussic acid.

The American wild Cherry (*Prunus virginiana*) yields from its bark a larger quantity of the prussic acid principle, which is sedative to the nervous centres, and also some considerable tannin. As an infusion, or syrup, or vegetable extract, it will allay nervous palpitation of the heart, and will quiet the irritative hectic cough of consumption, whilst tending to ameliorate the impaired digestion. Its preparations can be readily had from our leading druggists, and are found to be highly useful. A teaspoonful of the syrup, with one or two tablespoonfuls of cold water, is a dose for an adult every three or four hours. The oozing of the gum-tears from the trunk and boughs is due to the operation of a minute parasitic fungus. Helena, in the *Midsummer Night's Dream*, paints a charming picture of the close affection between Hermia and herself—

"So we grew together
Like to a double Cherry—seeming parted,
But yet a union in partition:
Two lovely berries moulded on one stem."

CHERVIL, or BEAKED PARSLEY.

"THERE is found," writes Parkinson, "during June and July, in almost every English hedge, a certain plant called *Chærophyllum*, in show very like unto Hemlockes, of a good and pleasant smell and taste, which have caused us to term it 'Sweet Chervill.'" And in modern times this plant has taken rank as a pot herb in our gardens, though its virtues and uses are not sufficiently known. "The root is great, thick and long, exceedingly sweet in smell, and tasting like unto anise seeds. This root is much used among the Dutch people in a kind of loblolly or hotchpot, which they do eat, calling it *warmus*. The seeds taken as a salad whilst they are yet green, exceed all other salads by many degrees in pleasantness of taste, sweetness of smell, and wholesomeness for the cold and feeble stomach." In common with other camphoraceous and strongly aromatic herbs, by reason of its volatile oil and its terebinthine properties, the *Scandix*, or Sweet Chervil, was entitled to make one of the choice spices used for composing the holy oil with which the sacred vessels of the Tabernacle were anointed by Moses. It belongs to the particular group of umbelliferous plants which is endowed with balsamic gums, and with carminative essences appealing powerfully to the sense of smell.

The herb Chervil was in the mind of Roman Catullus when discoursing sweet verses of old to his friend Fabullus:—

"Nam unguentum dabo quod meæ puellæ
Donârunt veneres, cupidinesque.
Quod tu quum olfacies deo rogabis
Totum ut te faciat. Fabulle! nasum."

"I will give you a perfume my damsels gave me,
Sweet daughters of Venus, sad hoydens are ye!
Which the moment you smell will incite you to pray
My Fabullus! to live as 'all nose' from that day."

Evelyn taught (1565) that "the tender tops of Cherville should never be wanting in our sallets, being exceeding wholesome, and chearing the spirits; also that the roots boiled and cold are to be much commended for aged persons." But in 1745 several Dutch soldiers were poisoned by eating the rough wild Chervil, from which the cultivated sweet variety is to be distinguished by its having its stems swollen beneath the joints—much as our blue-blooded patricians are signalised by gouty knuckles and bunioned feet.

The botanical name of the Sweet Chervil (*Chærophyllum*) signifies a plant which rejoices the heart—*Kairei-phyllum.* "The roots," said an old writer, "are very good for old people that are dull and without courage; they gladden and comfort the spirits, and do increase their lusty strength." The juice is slightly aperient, and abundantly lacteal when mixed with goat's milk, or in gruel. Physicians formerly held this herb in high esteem, as capable of curing most chronic disorders connected with the urinary passages, and gravel. Some have even asserted that if these distempers will not yield to a constant use of Chervil, they will be scarcely curable by any other medicine. The Wild Chervil will "help to dissolve any tumours or swellings in all parts of the body speedily, if applied to the place, as also to take away the spots and marks in the flesh and skin, of congealed blood by blows or bruises." The feathery leaves of Chervil, which are of a bright emerald hue in the spring, become of a rich purple in the autumn, just as the objectionably carroty locks of Tittlebat Titmouse, in *Ten Thousand a Year*, became vividly green under "Cyanochaitanthropopoion," and were afterwards strangely empurpled by "Tetragmenon abracadabra," at nine and sixpence the bottle.

CHESTNUTS (Horse, and Sweet).

EVER since 1633 the *Horse Chestnut* tree has grown and flourished in England, having been brought at first from the mountains of Northern Asia. For the most part it is rather known and admired for its wealth of shade, its large handsome floral spikes of creamy, pink-tinted blossom, and its white, soft wood, than supposed to exercise useful medicinal properties. But none the less is this tree remarkable for the curative virtues contained in its large nuts of mahogany polish, its broad palmate leaves, and its smooth silvery bark. These virtues have been discovered and made public especially by physicians and chemists of the homœopathic school. From the large digitated leaves an extract is made which has proved of service in whooping-cough, and of which from one-third to half a teaspoonful may be given for a dose. On the Continent the bark is held in estimation for cutting short attacks of intermittent fever and ague by acting in the same way as Peruvian bark, though it is much more astringent. But the nuts are chiefly to be regarded as the medicinal belongings of the Horse Chestnut tree; and their bodily sphere of action is the rectum, or lower bowel, in cases of piles, and of obstinate constipation. Their use is particularly indicated when the bottom of the back gives out on walking, with aching and a sense of weariness in that region. Likewise, signal relief is found to be wrought by the same remedy when the throat is duskily red and dry, in conjunction with costiveness, and piles. A tincture is made (H.) from the ripe nuts with spirit of wine, for the purposes described above, or the nuts themselves are finely powdered and given in that form. These nuts are starchy, and contain so much potash, that they may be used when boiled for washing purposes.

In France and Switzerland they are employed for cleansing wool and bleaching linen, on account of their "saponin." Botanically, the Horse Chestnut is named *Æsculus hippocastanea*—the first word coming from *esca*, food; and the second from *hippos*, a horse; and *Castana*, the city, so called. The epithet "horse" does not imply any remedial use in diseases of that animal, but rather the size and coarseness of this species as compared with the Sweet Spanish Chestnut. In the same way we talk of the horse radish, the horse daisy, and the horse leech. In Turkey the fruit is given to horses touched or broken in the wind, but in this country horses will not eat it. Nevertheless, Horse Chestnuts may be used for fattening cattle, particularly sheep, the nuts being cut up, and mixed with oats, or beans. Their bitterness can be removed by first washing the Chestnuts in lime water. Medicinally, the ripe nut of this tree is employed, being collected in September or October, and deprived of its shell. The odour of the flowers is powerful and peculiar. No chemical analysis of them, or of the nuts, has been made, but they are found to contain tannin freely. Rich-coloured, of a reddish brown, and glossy, these nuts have given their name to a certain shade of mellow dark auburn hair. Rosalind, in *As You Like It*, says "Orlando's locks are of a good colour: I' faith your Chestnut was ever the only colour."

Of the Horse Chestnut tincture, two or three drops, with a spoonful of water, taken before meals and at bedtime, will cure almost any simple case of piles in a week. Also, carrying a Horse Chestnut about the person, is said to obviate giddiness, and to prevent piles.

Taken altogether, the Horse Chestnut, for its splendour of blossom, and wealth of umbrageous leaf, its polished mahogany fruit, and its special medicinal virtues, is *facile princeps* the belle of our English trees. But, like many a ball-room beauty, when the time comes for putting aside the gay leafy attire, it is sadly untidy, and makes a great litter of its cast-off clothing.

It has been ingeniously suggested that the cicatrix of the leaf resembles a horse-shoe, with all its nails evenly placed.

The Sweet Spanish Chestnut tree is grown much less commonly in this country, and its fruit affords only material for food, without possessing medicinal properties; though, in the United States of America, an infusion of the leaves is thought to be useful for staying the paroxysms of whooping-cough. Of all known nuts, this (the Sweet Chestnut, Stover Nut, or Meat Nut) is the most farinaceous and least oily; hence it is more easy of digestion than any other. To mountaineers it is invaluable, so that on the Apennines and the Pyrenees the Chestnut harvest is the event of the year. The Italian Chestnut-cakes, called *necci*, contain forty per cent. of nutritious matter soluble in cold water; and Chestnut flour, when properly prepared, is a capital food for children.

To be harvested the Chestnuts are spread on a frame of lattice-work overhead, and a fire is kept burning underneath. When dry the fruit is boiled, or steamed, or roasted, or ground into a kind of flour, with which puddings are made, or an excellent kind of bread is produced. The ripe Chestnut possesses a fine creamy flavour, and when roasted it becomes almost aromatic. A good way to cook Chestnuts is to boil them for twenty minutes, and then place them for five minutes more in a Dutch oven.

It was about the fruit of the Spanish tree Shakespeare

said: "A woman's tongue gives not half so great a blow to the ear as will a Chestnut in a farmer's fire." In the United States of America an old time-worn story, or oft repeated tale, is called in banter a "Chestnut," and a stale joker is told "not to rattle the Chestnuts."

For convalescents, after a long serious illness, the French make a chocolate of sweet Chestnuts, which is highly restorative. The nuts are first cooked in *eau de vie* until their shells and the pellicle of the kernels can be peeled off; then they are beaten into a pulp together with sufficient milk and sugar, with some cinnamon added. The mixture is afterwards boiled with more milk, and frothed up in a chocolate pot.

CHICKWEED.

CHICKWEED—called *Alsine* or *Stellaria media*, a floral star of middle magnitude—belongs to the Clove-pink order of plants, and, despite the most severe weather, grows with us all the year round, in waste places by the roadsides, and as a garden weed. It is easily known by its fresh-looking, juicy, verdant little leaves, and by its tiny white star-like flowers; also by a line of small stiff hairs, which runs up one side of the stalk like a vegetable hog-mane, and when it reaches a pair of leaves immediately shifts its position, and runs up higher on the opposite side.

The fact of our finding Chickweed (and Groundsel) in England, as well as on the mainland of Europe, affords a proof that Britain, when repeopled after the great Ice age, must have been united somewhere to the Continent; and its having lasted from earliest times throughout Europe, North America, and Siberia, seems to show that this modest plant must be possessed of some universal utility which has enabled it to hold its own until now in the great evolutionary struggle. It grows wild all over the earth, and serves as food for small birds, such as finches, linnets, and other feathered songsters of the woods. Moreover, we read in the old herbal of Turner: *Qui alunt aviculas caveis inclusas hoc solent illas si quando cibos fastigiant recreare*—or, as Gerard translates this: "Little birds in cages are refreshed with Chickweed when they loath their meat."

The Chickweed is termed *Alsine—quia lucos, vel alsous amat*—because it loves to grow in shady places This small herb abounds with the earthy salts of potash, which are admirable against scurvy when thus found in nature's laboratory, and a continued deprivation from which always proves disastrous to mankind. "The water of Chickweed," says an old writer, "is given to children for their fits, and its juice is used for their gripes." When boiled, the plant may be eaten instead of Spinach. Its fresh juice if rubbed on warts, first pared to the quick, will presently cause them to fall off.

Fresh Chickweed juice, as proved medicinally in 1893, produced sharp rheumatic pains and stitches in the head and eyes, with a general feeling of being bruised; also pressure about the liver and soreness there, with sensations of burning, and of bilious indigestion. Subsequently, the herb, when given in quite small doses of tincture, or fresh juice, or infusion, has been found by its affinity to remove the train of symptoms just described, and to act most reliably in curing obstinate rheumatism allied therewith. Furthermore, a poultice prepared from the fresh green juicy leaves, is emollient and cooling, whilst an ointment made from them with hog's lard, is manifestly healing.

When rain is impending, the flowers remain closed;

and the plant teaches an exemplary matrimonial lesson, seeing that at night its leaves approach one another in loving pairs, and sleep with the tender buds protected between them. Culpeper says: "Chickweed is a fine, soft, pleasing herb, under the dominion of the moon, and good for many things." Parkinson orders thus: "To make a salve fit to heal sore legs, boil a handful of Chickweed with a handful of red rose leaves in a pint of the oil of trotters or sheep's feet, and anoint the grieved places therewith against a fire each evening and morning; then bind some of the herb, if ye will, to the sore, and so shall ye find help, if God will."

CHRISTMAS ROSE—BLACK HELLEBORE.

THIS well-known plant, a native of Southern Europe, and belonging to the Ranunculus order, is grown commonly in our gardens for the sake of its showy white flowers, conspicuous in winter, from December to February. The root has been famous since time immemorial as a remedy for insanity. From its abundant growth in the Grecian island of Anticyra arose the proverb: *Naviget Anticyram*—"Take a voyage to Anticyra," as applied by way of advice to a man who has lost his reason.

When fresh the root is very acrid, and will blister the skin. If dried and given as powder it will cause vomiting and purging, also provoking sneezing when smelt, and inducing the monthly flow of a woman. This root contains a chemical glucoside—"helleborin," which, if given in full doses, stimulates the kidneys to such an excess that their function becomes temporarily paralyzed. It therefore happens that a medicinal tincture (H.) made from the fresh root collected at Christmas, just before the plant would flower, when taken in small doses, will promptly relieve dropsy, especially a sudden dropsical swelling of the skin, with passive venous congestion of the kidneys, as in scrofulous children.

A former method of administering the root was by sticking a particularly sweet apple full of its fibres, and roasting this under hot embers; then the fibres were withdrawn, and the apple was eaten by the patient.

Taken by mischance in any quantity the root is highly poisonous: one ounce of a watery decoction has caused death in eight hours, with vomiting, giddiness, insensibility, and palsy. Passive dropsy in children after scarlet fever may be effectually cured by small doses of the tincture, third decimal strength.

The name Hellebore, as applied to the plant, comes from the Greek *Elein*—to injure, and *Bora*—fodder. It is also known as *Melampodium*, being thus designated because Melampus, a physician in the Peloponnesus (B.C. 1530) watched the effect on his goats when they had eaten the leaves, and cured therewith the insane daughters of Prœtus, King of Argos.

It was famous among the Egyptian and Greek doctors of old as the most effectual remedy for the diseases of mania, epilepsy, apoplexy, dropsy, and gout. The tincture is very useful in mental stupor, with functional impairment of the hearing and sight; likewise for strumous water on the brain.

The original reputation of this herb was acquired because of its purgative properties, which enabled it to carry off black bile which was causing insanity.

No tannin is contained in the root. A few drops of the juice obtained therefrom, if dropped warm into the ear each night and morning, will cure singing and noises in the ears. A proper dose of the powdered root is from five to ten grains. Snuff made with this powder has cured night blindness, as among the French prisoners at Norman Cross in 1806. The Gauls used to rub the points of their hunting spears with Hellebore, believing that the game they killed was thus rendered more tender. Hahnemann said that at least one third of the cases of insanity occurring in lunatic asylums may be cured by this and the white Hellebore (an allied plant) in such small doses as of the tincture twelfth dilution, given in the patient's drink.

A bastard Hellebore, which is *fœtidus*, or, "stinking," and is known to rustics as Bearsfoot, because of its digitate leaves, grows frequently near houses in this country, though a doubtful native. The sepals of its flowers are purple, and the leaves are evergreen; the petals are green and leaf-like, whilst the nectaries are large and tubular, often containing small flies. The nectar is reputed to be poisonous. Again, this plant bears the names Pegroots, Oxheel, Oxheal, and Setterwort, because used for "settering" cattle. A piece of the root is inserted as a seton (so-called from *seta*—a hank of silk) into the dewlap, and this is termed "pegging," or, "settering," for the benefit of diseased lungs. "The root," says Gerard, consists of many small black strings, involved or wrapped one within another very intricately." The smell of the fresh plant is extremely fetid, and, when taken, it will purge, or provoke vomiting. The leaves are very useful for expelling worms. Dr. Woodville says their juice made into a syrup, with coarse sugar, is almost the only vermifuge he had used against round worms for three years past. "If these leaves be dried in an oven after the bread is drawne out, and the powder thereof be taken in a figge, or raisin, or strewed upon a piece of bread spread with honey, and eaten, it killeth worms in children exceedingly." A decoction made with one drachm of the green leaves, or about fifteen grains of the dried leaves in powder, is the usual dose for a child between four and six years of age; but a larger dose will provoke sickness, or diarrhœa. The medicine should be repeated on two or three consecutive mornings; and it will be found that the second dose acts more powerfully than the first, "never failing to expel round worms by stool, if there be any lodged in the alimentary tube."

CLOVER.

In this country we possess about twenty species of the trefoil, or Clover, which is a plant so well known in its general features by its abundance in every field and on every grass plot, as not to need any detailed description. The special variety endowed with medicinal and curative virtues, is the Meadow Clover (*Trifolium pratense*), or red clover, called by some, Cocksheads, and familiar to children as Suckles, or Honey-suckles, because of the abundant nectar in the long tubes of its corollæ. Other names for it are Bee-bread, and Smere. An extract of this red clover is now confidently said to have the power of healing scrofulous sores, and of curing cancer. The *New York Tribune* of September, 1884, related a case of indisputable cancer of the breast of six years' standing, with an open fetid sore, which had penetrated the chest-wall between the ribs, and which was radically healed by a prolonged internal use of the extract of red clover. Four years afterwards, in September, 1888, "the breast was found to be restored to its normal condition, all but a small place the size of half a dollar, which will in every probability become absorbed like the rest, so that the patient is considered by her physicians to be absolutely cured."

The likelihood is that whatever virtue the red clover can boast for counteracting a scrofulous disposition, and as antidotal to cancer, resides in its highly-elaborated lime, silica, and other earthy salts. Moreover, this experience is not new. Sir Spencer Wells, twenty years ago, recorded some cases of confirmed cancer cured by taking powdered and triturated oyster shells; whilst egg shells similarly reduced to a fine dust have proved equally efficacious. It is remarkable that if the moorlands in the North of England, and in some parts of Ireland, are turned up for the first time, and strewed with lime, white clover springs up there in abundance.

Again, a syrup is made from the flowers of the red clover, which has a trustworthy reputation for curing whooping-cough, and of which a teaspoonful may be taken three or four times in the day. Also stress is laid on the healing of skin eruptions in children, by a decoction of the purple and white meadow trefoils.

The word clover is a corruption of the Latin *clava* a club; and the "clubs" on our playing cards are representations of clover leaves; whilst in France the same black suit is called *trefle.*

A conventional trefoil is figured on our coins, both Irish and English, this plant being the National Badge of Ireland. Its charm has been ever supposed there as an unfailing protection against evil influences, as is attested by the spray in the workman's cap, and in the bosom of the cotter's wife.

The clover trefoil is in some measure a sensitive plant; "its leaves," said Pliny, "do start up as if afraid of an assault when tempestuous weather is at hand."

The phrase, "living in clover," alludes to cattle being put to feed in rich pasturage.

A sworn foe to the purple clover cultivated by farmers, is the Dodder (*Cuscuta trifolii*), a destructive vegetable parasite which strangles the plants in a crafty fashion, and which goes by the name of "hellweed," or "devil's guts." It lies in ambush like a pigmy field octopus, with deadly suckers for draining the sap of its victims. These it mats together in its wiry, sinuous coils, and chokes relentlessly by the acre. Nevertheless, the petty garotter—like a toad, "ugly and venomous, wears yet a precious jewel in its head." "If boiled," says Hill, "with a little ginger, the dodder in decoction works briskly as a purge. Also, the thievish herb, when bruised and applied externally to scrofulous tumours, is an excellent remedy."

The word "dodder" signifies the plural of "dodd," a bunch of threads. The parasite is sometimes called "Red tangle" and "Lady's laces."

Its botanical name *Cuscuta* comes from the Greek *Kassuo*—to sew together. If the piece of land infested with it is closely mown (and the cut material carried away unshaken), being next covered with deal saw-dust, on which a ten per cent. solution of sulphate of iron is freely poured, then by combining with the tannin contained in the stems of the Dodder, this will serve to kill the parasite without doing any injury to the clover or lucerne. Although a parasite the plant springs every year from seed. It is a remedy for swooning or fainting fits.

The Sweet Clover (or yellow Melilot), when prepared as a tincture (H.), with spirit of wine, and given as a medicine in material doses, causes, in sensitive persons, a severe headache, sometimes with a determination of blood to the head, and bleeding from the nose. When administered, on the principle of curative affinity, in much smaller doses, it is singularly beneficial against nervous headaches, with oppression of the brain, acting helpfully within five minutes. Dr. Hughes (Brighton) writes: "I value this medicine much in nervous headaches, and I always carry it in my pocket-case—as the mother tincture—which I generally administer *by olfaction*." For epilepsy, it is said in the United States of America to be "the one grand master-remedy," by giving a drop of the tincture every five minutes during the attack, and five drops five times a day in water, for some weeks afterwards.

The Melilot (from *mel*, honey, and *lotus*, because much liked by bees) is known as Plaster Clover from its use since Galen's time in plasters for dispersing tumours. Continental physicians still employ the same made of melilot, wax, resin, and olive oil. The plant contains, "Coumarin" in common with the Sweet Woodruff, and the Tonquin Bean. Other names for it are "Harts' Clover," because deer delight to feed on it, and "King's Clover," or "Corona Regis," because "the yellow floures doe crown the top of the stalkes as with a chaplet of gold." It is an herbaceous plant common in waste places, and having light green leaves; when dried it smells like Woodruff, or new hay.

CLUB MOSS.

THOUGH not generally thought worth more than a passing notice, or to possess any claims of a medicinal sort, yet the Club Moss, which is of common growth in Great Britain on heaths and hilly pastures, exerts by its spores very remarkable curative effects, and therefore it should be favourably regarded as a Herbal Simple. It is exclusively due to homœopathic provings and practice, that the *Lycopodium clavatum* (Club Moss) takes an important position amongst the most curative vegetable remedies of the present day.

The word *lycopodium* means "wolf's claw," because of the claw-like ends to the trailing stems of this moss; and the word *clavatum* signifies that its inflorescence resembles a club. The spores of Club Moss constitute a fine pale-yellow, dusty powder which is unctuous, tasteless, inodorous, and only medicinal when pounded in an agate mortar until the individual spores, or nuts, are fractured.

By being thus triturated, the nuts give out their contents, which are shown to be oil globules, wherein the curative virtues of the moss reside. Sugar of milk is then rubbed up for two hours or more with the broken spores, so as to compose a medicinal powder, which is afterwards to be further diluted; or a tincture is made from the fractured spores, with spirit of ether, which will develop their specific medicinal properties. The Club Moss, thus prepared, has been experimentally taken by provers in varying material doses; and is found through its toxical affinities in this way to be remarkably useful for chronic mucous indigestion and mal-nutrition, attended with sallow complexion, slow, difficult digestion, flatulence, waterbrash, heartburn, decay of bodily strength, and mental depression. It is said that whenever a fan-like movement of the wings of the nostrils can be observed during the breathing, the whole group of symptoms thus detailed is *specially* curable by Club Moss.

As a dose of the triturated powder, reduced to a weaker dilution, ten grains may be taken twice a day mixed with a dessertspoonful of water ; or of the tincture largely reduced in strength, ten drops twice a day in like manner. Chemically, the oil globules extracted from the spores contain "alumina" and "phosphoric acid." The diluted powder has proved practically beneficial for reducing the swelling and for diminishing the pulsation of aneurism when affecting a main blood-vessel of the heart.

In Cornwall the Club Moss is considered good against most diseases of the eyes, provided it be gathered on the third day of the moon when first seen ; being shown the knife whilst the gatherer repeats these words :—

> "As Christ healed the issue of blood,
> Do thou cut what thou cuttest for good."

"Then at sundown the Club Moss should be cut by the operator whilst kneeling, and with carefully washed hands. It is to be tenderly wrapped in a fair white cloth, and afterwards boiled in water procured from the spring nearest the spot where it grew," and the liquor is to be applied as a fomentation; or the Club Moss may be "made into an ointment with butter from the milk of a new cow." Such superstitious customs had without doubt a Druidic origin, and they identify the Club Moss with the Selago, or golden herb, "Cloth of Gold" of the Druids. This was reputed to confer the power of understanding the language of birds and beasts, and was intimately connected with some of their mysterious rites; though by others it is thought to have been a sort of Hedge Hyssop (*Gratiola*).

The Common Lycopodium bears in some districts the name of "Robin Hood's hatband." Its unmoistenable powder from the spores is a capital absorbing application to weeping, raw surfaces. At the shops, this powder of the Club Moss spores is sold as "witch meal," or "vegetable sulphur." For trade purposes it is obtained from the ears of a Wolfsfoot Moss, the *Lycopodium clavatum*, which grows in the forests of Russia and Finland. The powder is yellow of colour, dust-like and smooth to the touch. Half a drachm of it given during July in any proper vehicle has been esteemed "a noble remedy to cure stone in the bladder." Being mixed with black pepper, it was recognized by the College of Physicians in 1721 as a medicine of singular value for preventing and curing hydrophobia. Dr. Mead, who had repeated experience of its worth, declared that he never knew it to fail when combined with cold bathing.

Club Moss powder ignites with a flicker, and is used for stage lightning. It is the *Blitzmehl*, or lightning-meal of the Germans, who give it in doses of from fifteen to twenty grains for the cure of epilepsy in children.

When the "Mortal Struggle" was produced (see *Nicholas Nickleby*) by Mr. Vincent Crummles at Portsmouth, with the aid of Miss Snevelicci, and the Infant Phenomenon, lurid lightning was much in request to astonish the natives; and this was sufficiently well simulated by igniting, with a sudden flash and a hiss, highly inflammable spores of the Club Moss projected against burning tow within a hollow cone, producing weird scenic effects.

COLTSFOOT.

THE Coltsfoot, which grows abundantly throughout England in places of moist, heavy soil, especially along the sides of our raised railway banks, has been justly termed "nature's best berb for the lungs, and her most eminent thoracic." Its seeds are supposed to have lain dormant from primitive times, where our railway cuttings now upturn them and set them growing anew; and the rotting foliage of the primeval herb by retaining its juices, is thought to have promoted the development and growth of our common earthworm.

The botanical name of Coltsfoot is *Tussilago farfara*, signifying *tussis ago*, "I drive away a cold"; and *farfar*, the white poplar tree, which has a similar leaf. It is one of the Composite order, and the older authors named this plant, *Filius ante patrem*—"the son before the father," because the flowers appear and wither before the leaves are produced. These flowers, at the very beginning of Spring, stud the banks with gay, golden. leafless blossoms, each growing on a stiff scaly stalk, and resembling a dandelion in miniature. The leaves, which follow later on, are made often into cigars, or are smoked as British herbal tobacco, being mixed for this purpose with the dried leaves and flowers of the eyebright, buckbean, betony, thyme, and lavender, to which some persons add rose leaves, and chamomile flowers. All these are rubbed together by the hands into a coarse powder, Coltsfoot forming quite one-half of the same; and this powder may be very beneficially smoked for asthma, or for spasmodic bronchial cough. Linnoeus said, "*Et adhuc hodie plebs in Sueciâ instar tabaci contra tussim fugit*"—"Even to-day the Swiss people cure their coughs with Coltsfoot employed like tobacco." When the flowers are fully blown and fall off, the seeds with their "clock" form a beautiful head of white flossy silk, and if this flies away when there is no wind it is said to be a sure sign of coming rain. The Goldfinch often lines her nest with the soft pappus of the Coltsfoot. In Paris the Coltsfoot flower is painted on the doorposts of an apothecary's house.

From earliest times, the plant has been found helpful in maladies of the chest. Hippocrates advised it with honey for "ulcerations of the lungs." Dioscorides, Pliny, and Galen, severally commended the use of its smoke, conducted into the mouth through a funnel or reed, for giving ease to cough and difficult breathing; they named it *breechion*, from *brecx*, a cough.

In taste, the leaves are harsh, bitter, and mucilaginous. They appear late in March, being green above, with an under-surface which is white, and cottony. Sussex peasants esteem the white down of the leaves as a most valuable medicine.

All parts of the plant contain chemically tannin, with a special bitter principle, and free mucilage; so that the herb is to be considered emollient, demulcent, and tonic. Dr. Cullen employed a decoction of the leaves with much benefit in scrofula, where the use of sea water had failed. And Dr. Fuller tells about a girl cured of twelve scrofulous sores, by drinking daily, for four months, as much as she could of Coltsfoot tea, made so strong from the leaves as to be sweet and glutinous. A modern decoction is prepared from the herb with boiling water poured on the leaves, and with liquorice root and honey added.

But, "hark! I hear the pancake bell," said Poor Richard in his almanack, 1684; alluding to pancakes then made with Coltsfoot, like tansies, and fried with saged butter.

A century later it was still the fashion to treat consumptive young women with quaint remedies. Mrs. Delaney writes in 1758, "Does Mary cough in the night? two or three snails boiled in her barley water may be of great service to her."

Again, the confectioner provides Coltsfoot rock, concocted in fluted sticks of a brown colour, as a sweetmeat, and flavoured with some essential oil—as aniseed, or dill—these sticks being well beloved by most schoolboys. The dried leaves, when soaked out in warm water, will serve as an excellent emollient poultice.

A certain preparation, called "Essence of Coltsfoot," found great favour with our grandsires for treating their colds. This consisted of Balsam of Tolu and Friar's Balsam in equal parts, together with double the quantity of Spirit of Wine. It did not really contain a trace of Coltsfoot, and the nostrum was provocative of inflammation, because of the spirit in excess. Dr. Paris said: "And this, forsooth, is a pectoral for coughs! If a patient with a catarrh should recover whilst using such a remedy, I should certainly designate it a lucky escape, rather than a skilful cure." Gerard wrote about Coltsfoot: "The fume of the dried leaves, burned upon coles, effectually helpeth those that fetch their winde thicke, and breaketh without peril the impostumes of the brest"; also "the green leaves do heal the hot inflammation called Saint Anthony's fire."

The names of the herb—Coltsfoot, and Horsehoof—are derived from the shape of the leaf. It is likewise known as Asses' foot, and Cough wort; also as Foal's foot, and Bull's foot, Hoofs, and (in Yorkshire) Cleats.

To make an infusion or decoction of the plant for a confirmed cough, or for chronic bronchitis, pour a pint of boiling water on an ounce of the dried leaves and flowers, and take half a teacupful of it when cold three or four times in the day. The silky down of the seedheads is used in the Highlands for stuffing pillows, and the presence of coal is said to be indicated by an abundant growth of the herb.

Another species, the Butter bur (*Tussilago petasites*),

is named from *petasus*, an umbrella, or a broad covering for the head. It produces the largest leaves of any plant in Great Britain, which sometimes measure three feet in breadth. This plant was thought to be of great use in the time of the plague, and thus got the names of Pestilent wort, Plague flower and Bog Rhubarb. Both it, and the Coltsfoot, are specific remedies (H.) for severe and obstinate neuralgia in the small of the back, and the loins, a medicinal tincture being prepared from each herb.

COMFREY.

THE Comfrey of our river banks, and moist watery places, is the *Consound*, or Knit-back, or Bone-set, and Blackwort of country folk; and the old *Symphytum* of Dioscorides. It has derived these names from the consolidating and vulnerary qualities attributed to the plant, from *confirmo*, to strengthen together, or the French, *comfrie*. This herb is of the Borage tribe, and is conspicuous by its height of from one to two feet, its large rough leaves, which provoke itching when handled, and its drooping white or purple flowers growing on short stalks. Chemically, the most important part of the plant is its "mucilage." This contains tannin, asparagin, sugar, and starch granules. The roots are sweet, sticky, and without any odour. "*Quia tanta præstantia est*," says Pliny, "*ut si carnes duræ coquuntur conglutinet addita; unde nomen!*"—"and the roots be so glutinative that they will solder or glew together meat that is chopt in pieces, seething in a pot, and make it into one lump: the same bruysed, and lay'd in the manner of a plaister, doth heale all fresh and green wounds." These roots are very brittle, and the least bit of them will start growing afresh.

The whole plant, beaten to a cataplasm, and applied hot as a poultice, has always been deemed excellent for soothing pain in any tender, inflamed or suppurating part. It was formerly applied to raw indolent ulcers as a glutinous astringent, and most useful vulnerary. Pauli recommended it for broken bones, and externally for wounds of the nerves, tendons, and arteries. More recently surgeons have declared that the powdered root (which, when broken, is white within, and full of a slimy juice), if dissolved in water to a mucilage, is far from contemptible for bleedings, fractures, and luxations, whilst it hastens the callus of bones under repair. Its strong decoction has been found very useful in Germany for tanning leather. The leaves were formerly employed for giving a flavour to cakes and panada.

A modern medicinal tincture (H.) is made from the root-stock with spirit of wine; and ten drops of this should be taken three or four times a day with a tablespoonful of cold water. French nurses treat cracked nipples by applying a hollow section of the fresh root over the sore caruncle; and a decoction of the root made by boiling from two to four drachms in a pint of water, is given for bleedings from the lungs or bladder.

The name *Consound*, owned by the Common Comfrey, was given likewise to the daisy and the bugle, in the middle ages. "It joyeth," says Gerard, "in watery ditches, in fat and fruitful meadows." A solve concocted from the fresh herb will certainly tend to promote the healing of bruised and broken parts, suggesting as an appropriate motto for the salve box: "Behold how good and pleasant a thing it is to dwell together in unity! It is like the precious ointment which ran down Aaron's beard." Some foreknowledge of the Comfrey perhaps inspired the Prophet Isaiah to predict that after a time "the heart should rejoice and the bones flourish like a herb." The Poet Laureate tells of

> "This, the Consound,
> Whereby the lungs are easéd of their grief."

About a century ago, the *Prickly Comfrey*—a variety of our Consound—was naturalised in this country from the Caucasus, and has since proved itself amazingly productive to farmers, as, when cultivated, it will grow six crops in the year; and the plant is both preventive and curative of foot and mouth disease in cattle. It bears flowers of a rich blue colour.

From our Common Comfrey a sort of glue is got in Angora, which is used for spinning the famous fleeces of that country. Mr. Cockayne relates that the locksman at Teddington informed him how the bone of his little finger being broken, was grinding and gruuching so sadly for two months, that sometimes he felt quite wrong in his head. One day he saw a doctor go by, and told him about the distress. The doctor said: "You see that Comfrey growing there? Take a piece of its root, and champ it, and put it about your finger, and wrap it up." The man did so, and in four days his finger was well.

CORIANDER.

CORIANDER comfits, sold by the confectioner as admirably warming to the stomach, and corrective of flatulence, consist of small aromatic seeds coated with white sugar. These are produced by the Coriander, an umbelliferous herb cultivated in England from early times for medicinal and culinary uses, though introduced at first from the Mediterranean. It has now become wild as an escape, growing freely in our fields and waste places. Farmers produce it, especially about Essex, under the name of Col, the crops being mown down when ripe, and the fruits being then thrashed out to procure the seeds. The generic name has been derived from *koros*, a bug; alluding to the stinking odour of the bruised leaves, though these, when dried, are fragrant, and pleasant of smell. In some countries, as Egypt and Peru, they are taken in soups. The seeds are cordial, but become narcotic if used too freely. When distilled with water they yield a yellow essential oil of a very aromatic and strong odour.

Coriander water was formerly much esteemed as a carminative for windy colic. Being so aromatic and comfortably stimulating, the fruit is commended for aiding the digestion of savoury pastry, and to correct the griping tendencies of such medicines as senna and rhubarb. It contains malic acid, tannin, the special volatile oil of the herb, and some fatty matter.

Distillers of gin make use of this fruit, and veterinary surgeons employ it as a drug for cattle and horses. Alston says, "The green herb—seeds and all—stinks intolerably of bugs"; and Hoffman admonishes, "*Si largius sumptura fuerit semen non sine periculo e suâ sede et statu demovet, et qui sumpsere varia dictu pudenda blaterant.*" The fruits are blended with curry powder, and are chosen to flavour several liquors. By the Chinese a power of conferring immortality is thought to be possessed by the seeds. From a passage in the Book of Numbers where manna is likened to Coriander seed, it would seem that this seed was familiar to the Israelites and used by them for domestic purposes. Robert Turner says when taken in wine it stimulates the animal passions.

COWSLIP.

OUR English pastures and meadows, especially where the soil is of blue lias clay, become brilliantly gay, "with gaudy cowslips drest," quite early in the spring. But it is a mistake to suppose that these flowers are a favourite food with cows, who, in fact, never eat them if they can help it. The name Cowslip is really derived, says Dr. Prior, from the Flemish words, *kous loppe*, meaning "hose flap," a humble part of woollen nether garments. But Skeat thinks it arose from the fact that the plant was supposed to spring up where a patch of cow dung had fallen.

Originally, the Mullein—which has large, oval, woolly leaves—and the Cowslip were included under one common Latin name, *Verbascum;* for which reason the attributes of the Mullein still remain accredited by mistake to the second plant. Former medical writers called the Cowslip *herba paralysis*, or, "palsywort," because of its supposed efficacy in relieving paralysis. The whole plant is known to be gently narcotic and somniferous. Pope praised the herb and its flowers on account of their sedative qualities:—

> "For want of rest,
> Lettuce and Cowslip wine—*Probatum est.*"

Whilst Coleridge makes his *Christabel* declare with reference to the fragrant brew concocted from its petals, with lemons and sugar:—

> "It is a wine of virtuous powers,
> My mother made it of wild flowers."

Physicians for the last two centuries have used the powdered roots of the Cowslip (and the Primrose) for wakefulness, hysterical attacks, and muscular rheumatism: and the cowslip root was named of old both *radix paralyseos*, and *radix arthritica*. This root, and the flowers, have an odour of anise, which is due to their containing some volatile oil identical with mannite. Their more acrid principle is "saponin." Hill tells us that when boiled in ale, the roots are taken by country persons for giddiness, with no little success. "They be likewise in great request among those that use to hunt after goats and roebucks on high mountains, for the strengthening of the head when they pass by fearful precipices and steep places, in following their game, so that giddiness and swimming of the brain may not seize upon them." The dose of the dried and powdered flowers is from fifteen to twenty grains. A syrup of a fine yellow colour may also be made from the petals, which answers the same purposes. Three pounds of the fresh blossoms should be infused in five pints of boiling water, and then simmered down to a proper consistence with sugar.

Herbals of the Elizabethan date, say that an ointment made from cowslip flowers "taketh away the spots and wrinkles of the skin, and doth add beauty exceedingly, as divers ladies, gentlewomen, and she citizens—whether wives or widows—know well enough."

The tiny people were then supposed to be fond of nestling in the drooping bells of Cowslips, and hence the flowers were called fairy cups; and, in accordance with the doctrine of signatures, they were thought effective for removing freckles from the face.

> "In their gold coats spots you see,
> These be rubies: fairy favours.
> In these freckles live their savours."

The cluster of blossoms on a single stalk sometimes bears the name of "lady's keys" or "St. Peter's wort," either because it resembles a bunch of keys as St.

Peter's badge, or because as *primula veris* it unlocks the treasures of spring.

Cowslip flowers are frequently done up by playful children into balls, which they call tisty tosty, or simply a tosty. For this purpose the umbels of blossoms fully blown are strung closely together, and tied into a firm ball.

The leaves were at one time eaten in salad, and mixed with other herbs to stuff meat, whilst the flowers were made into a delicate conserve.

Yorkshire people call this plant the Cowstripling; and in Devonshire, where it is scarcely to be found, because of the red marl, it has come about that the foxglove goes by the name of Cowslip. Again, in some provincial districts, the Cowslip is known as Petty Mullein, and in others as Paigle (Palsywort). The old English proverb, "As blake as a paigle," means, "As yellow as a cowslip."

One word may be said here in medicinal favour of the poor cow, whose association with the flower now under discussion has been so unceremoniously disproved. The breath and smell of this sweet-odoured animal are thought in Flintshire to be good against consumption. Henderson tells of a blacksmith's apprentice who was restored to health when far advanced in a decline, by taking the milk of cows fed in a kirkyard. In the south of Hampshire, a useful plaster of fresh cow-dung is applied to open wounds. And even in its evolutionary development, the homely animal reads us a lesson; for *Dat Deus immiti cornua curta bovi*, says the Latin proverb—"Savage cattle have only short horns." So was it in "the House that Jack built," where the fretful creature that tossed the dog had but one horn, and this grew crumpled.

CRESSES.

THE Cress of the herbalist is a noun of multitude: it comprises several sorts, differing in kind but possessing the common properties of wholesomeness and pungency. Here "order in variety we see"; and here, "though all things differ, all agree." The name is thought by some to be derived from the Latin verb *crescere*, to grow fast.

Each kind of Cress belongs to the Cruciferous genus of plants; whence comes, perhaps, the common name The several varieties of Cress are stimulating and antiscorbutic, whilst each contains a particular essential principle, of acrid flavour, and of sharp biting qualities. The whole tribe is termed *lepidium*, or "siliquose," scaly, with reference to the shape of the seed-pouches. It includes "Land Cress (formerly dedicated to St. Barbara); Broad-leaved Cress (or the Poor-man's pepper); Penny Cress (*thlapsus*); Garden, or Town Cress; and the well known edible Water Cress." Formerly the Greeks attached much value to the whole order of Cresses, which they thought very beneficial to the brain. A favourite maxim with them was, "Eat Cresses, and get wit."

In England these plants have long been cultivated as a source of profit; whence arose the saying that a graceless fellow is not worth a "kurse" or cress—in German, *kers.* Thus Chaucer speaks about a character in the *Canterbury Tales*, "Of paramours ne fraught he not a kers." But some writers have referred this saying rather to the wild cherry or kerse, making it of the same significance as our common phrase, "Not worth a fig."

As Curative Herbal Simples we need only consider the Garden or Town Cress, and the Water Cress: whilst regarding the other varieties rather as condiments, and salad herbs to be taken by way of pleasant wholesome appetisers at table. These aromatic herbs were employed to season the homely dishes of our forefathers, before commerce had brought the spices of the East at a cheap rate to our doors; and Cresses were held in common favour by peasants for such a purpose. The black, or white pepper of to-day, was then so costly that "to promise a saint yearly a pound of it was considered a liberal bequest." And therefore the leaves of wild Cresses were eaten as a substitute for giving pungency to the food. Remarkable among these was the *Dittander Sativus*, a species found chiefly near the sea, with foliage so hot and acrid, that the plant then went by the name of "Poor-man's Pepper," or "Pepper Wort." Pliny said, "It is of the number of scorching and blistering Simples." "This herbe," says Lyte, "is fondly and unlearnedly called in English Dittany. It were better in following the Dutchmen to name it Pepperwort."

The *Garden Cress*, called *Sativum* (from *satum*, a pasture), is the sort commonly coupled with the herb Mustard in our familiar "Mustard and Cress." It has been grown in England since the middle of the sixteenth century, and its other name *Town* Cress refers to its cultivation in "tounes," or enclosures. It was also known as Passerage; from *passer*, to drive away—rage, or madness, because of its reputed power to expel hydrophobia. "This Garden Cress," said Wm. Coles in his *Paradise of Plants*, 1650, "being green, and therefore more qualified by reason of its humidity, is eaten by country people, either alone with butter, or with lettice and purslane, in sallets, or otherwise."

It contains sulphur, and a special ardent volatile medicinal oil. The small leaves combined with those of our white garden Mustard are excellent against rheumatism and gout. Likewise it is a preventive of scurvy by reason of its mineral salts. In which salutary respects the twin plants, Mustard and Cress, are happily consorted, and well play a capital common part, like the "two single gentlemen rolled into one" of George Colman, the younger.

The *Water Cress (Nasturtium officinale)* is among cresses, to use an American simile, the "finest toad in the puddle." This is because of its superlative medicinal worth, and its great popularity at table. Early writers called the herb "Shamrock," and common folk now-a-days term it the "Stertion." Zenophon advised the Persians to feed their children on Water-cresses *(kardamon esthie)* that they might grow in stature and have active minds.

The Latin name *Nasturtium* was given to the Watercress because of its volatile pungency when bruised and smelt; from *nasus*, a nose, and *tortus*, turned away, it being so to say, "a herb that wriths or twists the nose." For the same reason it is called *Nasitord* in France. When bruised its leaves affect the eyes and nose almost like mustard. They have been usefully applied to the scald head and tetters of children. In New Zealand the stems grow as thick as a man's wrist, and nearly choke some of the rivers. Like an oyster, the Water-cress is in proper season only when there is an "r" in the month.

According to an analysis made recently in the School of Pharmacy at Paris, the Water-cress contains a sulpho-nitrogenous oil, iodine, iron, phosphates, potash, certain other earthy salts, a bitter extract, and water. Its volatile oil which is rich in nitrogen and sulphur (problematical) is the sulpho-cyanide of allyl. Anyhow there is much sulphur possessed by the whole plant in one form or another, together with a considerable quantity of mineral matter. Thus the popular plant is so constituted as to be particularly curative of scrofulous affections, especially in the spring time, when the bodily humours are on the ferment. Dr. King Chambers writes (*Diet in Health and Disease*), "I feel sure that the infertility, pallor, fetid breath, and bad teeth which characterise some of our town populations are to a great extent due to their inability to get fresh antiscorbutic vegetables as articles of diet: therefore I regard the Water-cress seller as one of the saviours of her country." Culpeper said pithily long ago: "They that will live in health may eat Water-cress if they please; and if they won't, I cannot help it."

The scrofula to which the Water-cress and its allied plants are antidotal, got its name from *scrofa*, "a burrowing pig," signifying the radical destruction of important glands in the body by this undermining constitutional disease. Possibly the quaint lines which nurses have long been given to repeat for the amusement of babies while fondling their infantine fingers bear a hidden meaning which pointedly imports the scrofulous taint. This nursery distich, as we remember, personates the fingers one by one as five little fabulous pigs:—the first small piggy doesn't feel well; and the second one threatens the doctor to tell; the third little pig has to linger at home; and the fourth small porker of meat has none; then the fifth little pig, with a querulous note, cries "weak, weak, weak" from its poor little throat.

"Œgrotat multis doloribus porculus ille:
Ille rogat fratri medicum proferre salutem:
Debilis ille domi mansit vetitus abire;
Carnem digessit nunquam miser porculus ille;
'Eheu!' ter repetens, 'eheu!' perporculus, 'eheu!'
Vires exiguas luget plorante susurro."

On account of its medicinal constituents the herb has been deservedly extolled as a specific remedy for tubercular consumption of the lungs. Haller says: "We have seen patients in deep declines cured by living almost entirely on this plant;" and it forms the chief ingredient of the *Sirop Antiscorbutique* given so successfully by the French faculty in scrofula and other allied diseases. Its active principles are at their best when the plant is in flower; and the amount of essential oil increases according to the quantity of sunlight which the leaves obtain, the proportion of iron being determined according to the quality of the water, and the measure of phosphates by the supply of dressing afforded. The leaves remain green when grown in the shade, but become of a purple brown because of their iron when exposed to the sun. The expressed juice, which contains the peculiar taste and pungency of the herb, may be taken in doses of from one to two fluid ounces at each of the three principal meals, and it should always be had fresh. When combined with the juice of Scurvy grass and of Seville oranges it makes the popular antiscorbutic medicine known as "Spring juices."

A Watér-cress cataplasm applied cold in a single layer, and with a pinch of salt sprinkled thereupon makes a most useful poultice to heal foul scrofulous ulcers; and will also help to resolve glandular swellings.

Water-cresses squeezed and laid against warts were said by the Saxon leeches to work a certain cure on these excrescences. In France the Water-cress is dipped in oil and vinegar to be eaten at table with chicken or a steak. The Englishman takes it at his morning or evening meal, with bread and butter, or at dinner in a salad. It loses some of its pungent flavour and of its curative qualities when cultivated; and therefore it is more appetising and useful when freshly gathered from natural streams. But these streams ought to be free from contamination by sewage matter, or any drainage which might convey the germs of fever, or other blood poison: for, as we are admonished, the Water-cress plant acts as a brush in impure running brooks to detain around its stalks and leaves any dirty disease-bringing flocculi.

Some of our leading druggists now make for medicinal use a liquid extract of the *Nasturtium officinale*, and a spirituous juice (or *succus*) of the plant. These preparations are of marked service in scorbutic cases, where weakness exists without wasting, and often with spongy gums, or some skin eruption. They are best when taken with lemon juice.

The leaf of the unwholesome Water parsnep, or Fool's Cress, resembles that of the Water-cress, and grows near it not infrequently: but the leaves of the true Water-cress never embrace the stem of the plant as do the leaf stalks of its injurious imitators. Herrick the joyous poet of "dull Devonshire" dearly loved the Water-cress, and its kindred herbs. He piously and pleasantly made them the subject of a quaint grace before meat:—

> "Lord, I confess too when I dine
> The pulse is Thine:
> And all those other bits that be
> There placed by Thee:
> The wurts, the perslane, and the mess
> of Water-cress."

The true *Nasturtium* (*Tropæolum majus*), or *greater Indian Cress* grows and is cultivated in our flower gardens as a brilliant ornamental creeper. It was brought from Peru to France in 1684, and was called *La grande Capucine*, whilst the botanical title *tropæolum*, a trophy, was conferred because of its shield-like leaves, and its flowers resembling a golden helmet. An old English name for the same plant was Yellow Lark'sheels.

Two years later it was introduced into England. This partakes of the sensible and useful qualities of the other cresses. The fresh plant and the dark yellow flowers have an odour like that of the Water-cress, and its bruised leaves emit a pungent smell. An infusion made with water will bring out the antiscorbutic virtues of the plant which are specially aromatic, and cordial. The flowers make a pretty and palatable addition to salads, and the nuts or capsules (which resemble the "cheeses" of Mallow) are esteemed as a pickle, or as a substitute for Capers. Invalids have often preferred this plant to the Scurvy grass as an antiscorbutic remedy. In the warm summer months the flowers have been observed about the time of sunset to give out sparks, as of an electrical kind, which were first noticed by a daughter of Linnœus.

The *Water-cress* is justly popular with persons who drink freely overnight, for its power of dissipating the fumes of the liquor, and of clearing away lethargic inaptitude for work in the morning: also for dispelling the tremors, and the foul taste induced by excessive tobacco smoking.

Closely allied thereto is another cruciferous plant, the Scurvy grass (*Cochleare*), named also "Spoonwort" from its leaves resembling in shape the bowl of an old-fashioned spoon. This is thought to be the famous *Herba Britannica* of the ancients. Our great navigators have borne testimony to its never failing use in scurvy, and, though often growing many miles from the sea, yet the taste of the herb is always found to be salt. If eaten in its fresh state, as a salad, it is the most effectual of all the antiscorbutic plants, the leaves being admirable also to cure swollen and spongy gums. It grows along the muddy banks of the Avon, likewise in Wales, and is found in Cumberland, more commonly near the coast; and again on the mountains of Scotland. It may be readily cultivated in the garden for medicinal use.

The Cuckoo flower, or "Ladies' Smock" (Cardamine) from *Cardia damao*, "I strengthen the heart," is another wholesome Cress with the same sensible properties as the Water-cress, only in an inferior degree, while the strong pungency of its flavour prevents it from being equally popular. This plant bears also the names of "Lucy Locket," and "Smell Smocks." In Cornwall the flowering tops have been employed for the cure of epilepsy throughout several generations with singular success; though the use of the leaves only for this purpose has caused disappointment. From one to three drams of these flowering tops are to be taken two or three times a day.

By the Rev. Mr. Gregor (1793) and by his descendants this remedy was given for inveterate epilepsy with much benefit. Lady Holt, and her sister Lady Bracebridge, of Aston Hall, Warwickshire, were long famous for curing severe cases of the same infirmity by administering this herb. They gave the powdered heads of the flowers when in full bloom—twelve grains three times a day for many weeks together.

Sir George Baker in 1767 read a paper before the London College of Physicians on the value of these flowers in convulsive disorders. He related five cures of St. Vitus' dance, spasmodic convulsions, and spasmodic asthma. Formerly the flowers were admitted into the

London Pharmacopœia. The herb was named Ladies' Smock in honour of the Virgin Mary, because it comes first into flower about Lady Day, being abundant with its delicate lilac blossoms in our moist meadows and marshes:

> "Lady Smocks all silver white
> Do paint the meadows with delight."

This plant is also named "Milk Maids," "Bread and Milk," and "Mayflower." Gerard says "it flowers in April and May when the Cuckoo doth begin to sing her pleasant notes without stammering." One of his characters is made by the Poet Laureate to—

> "Steep for Danewulf leaves of Lady Smock,
> For they keep strong the heart."

"And so much," as says William Cole, herbalist, in his *Paradise of Plants*, 1650, "for such Plants as cure the Scurvy."

CUMIN.

CUMIN *(Cuminum cyminum)* is not half sufficiently known, or esteemed as a domestic condiment of medicinal value, and culinary uses; whilst withal of ready access as one of our commonest importations from Malta and Sicily for flavouring purposes, and veterinary preparations. It is an umbelliferous plant, and large quantities of its seeds are brought every year to England. The herb has been cultivated in the East from early days, being called "Cuminum" by the Greeks in classic times. The seeds possess a strong aromatic odour with a penetrating and bitter taste; when distilled they yield a pungent powerful essential oil. The older herbalists esteemed them superior in comforting carminative qualities to those of the fennel or caraway. They are eminently useful to correct the flatulence of languid digestion, serving also to relieve dyspeptic headache, to allay colic of the bowels, and to promote the monthly flow of women.

In Holland and Switzerland they are employed for flavouring cheese; whilst in Germany they are added to bread as a condiment.

Here the seeds are introduced in the making of curry powder, and are compounded to form a stimulating liniment; likewise a warming plaster for quickening the sluggish congestions of indolent parts. The odorous volatile oil of the fruit contains the hydro-carbons "Cymol," and "Cuminol," which are redolent of lemon and caraway odours. A dose of the seeds is from fifteen to thirty grains. Cumin symbolised cupidity among the Greeks: wherefore Marcus Antoninus was so nick-named because of his avarice; and misers were jocularly said to have eaten Cumin.

The herb was thought to specially confer the gift of retention, preventing the theft of any object which contained it, and holding the thief in custody within the invaded house; also keeping fowls and pigeons from straying, and lovers from proving fickle. If a swain was going off as a soldier, or to work a long way from his home, his sweetheart would give him a loaf seasoned with Cumin, or a cup of wine in which some of the herb had been mixed.

The ancients were acquainted with the power of Cumin to cause the human countenance to become pallid; and as a medicine the herb is well calculated to cure such pallor of the face when occurring as an illness. Partridges and pigeons are extremely fond of the seeds: respecting the scriptural use of which in the payment of taxes we are reminded (Luke xi. *v.* 42)—"Ye pay tithe of mint, and anise, and cummin." It has been discovered by Grisar that Cumin oil exercises a special action which gives it importance as a medicine. This is to signally depress nervous reflex excitability when administered in full doses, as of from two to eight drops of the oil on sugar. And when the aim is to stimulate such reflex sensibility as impaired by disease, small diluted doses of the oil serve admirably to promote this purpose.

CURRANTS.

THE original Currants in times past were small grapes, grown in Greece at Zante, near Corinth, and hence termed Corinthians; then they became Corantes, and eventually Currants. But, as an old Roman proverb pertinently said: *Non cuivis homini contingit adire Corinthum,* "It was not for everyone to visit fashionable Corinth." And therefore the name of Currants became transferred in the Epirus to certain small fruit of the Gooseberry order which closely resembled the grapes of Zante, but were identical rather with the Currants of our modern kitchen gardens, such as we now use for making puddings, pies, jams, and jellies. The bushes which produce this fruit grow wild in the Northern parts of Great Britain, and belong to the Saxifrage order of plants. The wild Red Currant bears small berries which are intensely acid. In modern Italy basketsful are gathered in the woods of the Apennines, and the Alps.

Currants are not mentioned in former Greek or Roman literature, nor do they seem to have been cultivated by the Anglo-Saxons, or the Normans. Our several sorts of Currants afford a striking illustration of the mode which their parent bushes have learnt to adopt so as to attract by their highly coloured fruits the birds which shall disperse their seeds. These colours are not developed until the seed is ripe for germination; because if birds devoured them prematurely the seed would fall inert. But simultaneously come the ripeness and the soft sweet pulp, and the rich colouring, so that the birds may be attracted to eat the fruit, and spread the seed in their droppings. Zeuxis, a famous Sicilian painter four hundred years before Christ, depicted currants and grapes with such fidelity that birds came and tried to peck them out from his canvas.

White Currants are the most simple in kind; and the Red are a step in advance. If equal parts of either fruit and of sugar are put over the fire, the liquid which separates spontaneously will make a very agreeable jelly because of the "pectin" with which it is chemically furnished. Nitric acid will convert this pectin into oxalic acid, or salts of sorrel. The juice of Red Currants also contains malic and citric acids, which are cooling and wholesome. In the Northern counties this red Currant is called Wineberry, or Garnetberry, from its rich ruddy colour, and transparency. Its sweetened juice is a favourable drink in Paris, being preferred there to the syrup of *orgeat* (almonds). When made into a jelly with sugar the juice of red Currants is excellent in fevers, and acts as an anti-putrescent; as likewise if taken at table with venison, or hare, or other "high" meats. This fruit especially suits persons of sanguine temperament. Both red and white Currants are without doubt trustworthy remedies in most forms of obstinate visceral obstruction, and they correct impurities of the blood, being certainly antiseptic.

The black Currant is found growing wild in England, for the most part by the edges of brooks, and in moist grounds, from mid-Scotland southwards. Throughout Sussex and Kent the shrub is called "Gazles" as corrupted from the French *Groseilles* (Gooseberries). The fruit is cooling, laxative, and anodyne. Its thickened juice concocted over the fire, with, or without sugar, formed a "rob" of Old English times. The black Currant is often named by our peasantry "Squinancy," or "Quinsyberry," because a jelly prepared therefrom has been long employed for sore throat and quinsy. The leaf glands of its young leaves secrete from their under surface a fragrant odorous fluid. Therefore if newly gathered, and infused for a moment in very hot water and then dried, the leaves make an excellent substitute for tea; also these fresh leaves when applied to a gouty part will assuage pain, and inflammation. They are used to impart the flavour of brandy to common spirit. Bergius called the leaf, *mundans, pellens, et diuretica.* Botanically the black Currant, *Ribes nigrum*, belongs to the Saxifrage tribe, this generic term Ribes being applied to all fresh currants, as of Arabian origin, and signifying acidity. Grocers' currants come from the Morea, being small grapes dried in the sun, and put in heaps to cake together. Then they are dug out with a crow-bar, and trodden into casks for exportation. Our national plum pudding can no more be made without these currants than "little Tom Tucker who sang for his supper, could cut his bread without any knife, or could find himself married without any wife." Former cooks made an odd use of grocers' currants, according to King, a poet of the middle ages, who says:—

> "They buttered currants on fat veal bestowed,
> And rumps of beef with virgin honey strewed."

On the kitchen Currant a riddling rhyme was long ago to be found in the *Children's Book of Conundrums* :—

> " Higgledy-piggledy, here I lie
> Picked and plucked, and put in a pie;
> My first is snapping, snarling, growling;
> My second noisy, ramping, prowling."

Eccles cakes are delicious Currant sandwiches which are very popular in Manchester.

Black Currant jelly should not be made with too much sugar, else its medicinal virtues will be impaired. A teaspoonful of this jelly may be given three or four times in the day to a child with thrush. In Russia the leaves of the black Currant are employed to fabricate brandy made with a coarse spirit. These leaves and the fruit are often combined by our herbalists with the seeds of the wild carrot for stimulating the kidneys in passive dropsy. A medicinal wine is also brewed from the fruit together with honey. In this country we use a decoction of the leaf, or of the bark as a gargle. In Siberia black Currants grow as large as hazel nuts.

Both the black and the red Currants afford a pleasant home-made wine. *Ex eo optimum vinum fieri potest non deterius vinis retioribus viteis*, wrote Haller in 1750. White Currants, however, yield the best wine, and this may be improved by keeping, even for twenty years. Dr. Thornton says: "I have used old wine of white Currants for calculous affections, and it has surpassed all expectation."

A delicate jelly is made from the red Currant at Bas-le-duc; and a well-known nursery rhyme tells of the tempting qualities of "cherry pie, and currant wine." A rob of black Currant jam is taken in Scotland with whiskey toddy. Shakespeare in the *Winter's Tale* makes Antolycus, the shrewd "picker-up of unconsidered trifles" talk of buying for the sheep-shearing feast "three pounds of sugar, five pounds of currants, and rice." In France a cordial called *Liqueur de cassis* is made from black Currants; and a refreshing drink, *Eau de groseilles*, from the red.

Some forty years ago, at the time of the Crimean war a patriotic song in praise of the French flag was most popular in our streets, and had for its refrain, "Hurrah for the Red, White, and Blue!" So valuable for food and physics are our tricoloured Currants that the same argot may be justly paraphrased in their favour, with a well-merited eulogium of "Hurrah for the White, Red, and Black!"

DAFFODIL.

THE yellow Daffodil, which is such a favourite flower of our early Spring because of its large size, and showy yellow colour, grows commonly in English woods, fields, and orchards. Its popular names, Daffodowndilly, Daffodily, and Affodily, bear reference to the Asphodel, with which blossom of the ancient Greeks this is identical. It further owns the botanical name of Narcissus (pseudo-narcissus)—not after the classical youth who met with his death through vainly trying to embrace his image reflected in a clear stream because of its exquisite beauty, and who is fabled to have been therefore changed into the flower—but by reason of the narcotic properties which the plant possesses, as signified by the Greek word, *Narkao*, "to benumb." Pliny described it as a *Narce narcissum dictum, non a fabuloso puero.* An extract of the bulbs when applied to open wounds has produced staggering, numbness of the whole nervous system, and paralysis of the heart. Socrates called this plant the "Chaplet of the Infernal Gods," because of its narcotic effects. Nevertheless, the roots of the asphodel were thought by the ancient Greeks to be edible, and they were therefore laid in tombs as food for the dead. Lucian tells us that Charon, the ferryman who rowed the souls of the departed over the river Styx, said: "I know why Mercury keeps us waiting here so long. Down in these regions there is nothing to be had but asphodel, and oblations, in the midst of mist and darkness; whereas up in heaven he finds it all bright and clear, with ambrosia there, and nectar in plenty."

In the Middle Ages the roots of the Daffodil were called *Cibi regis*, "food for a king"; but his Majesty must have had a disturbed night after partaking thereof, as they are highly stimulating to the kidneys: indeed, there is strong reason for supposing that these roots have a prior claim to those of the dandelion for lectimingous fame, (*lectus*, "the bed"; *mingo*, to "irrigate").

The brilliant yellow blossom of the Daffodil possesses, as is well known, a bell-shaped crown in the midst of its petals, which is strikingly characteristic. The flower-stalk is hollow, bearing on its summit a membranous sheath, which envelops a single flower of an unpleasant odour. But the Jonquil, which is a cultivated variety of the Daffodil, having white petals with a yellow crown, yields a delicious perfume, which modern chemistry can closely imitate by a hydrocarbon compound. If "naphthalin," a product of coal tar oil, has but the smallest particle of its scent diffused in a room, the special aroma of jonquil and narcissus is at once perceived.

When the flowers of the Daffodil are dried in the sun, if a decoction of them is made, from fifteen to thirty grains will prove emetic like that of Ipecacuanha. From five to six ounces of boiling water should be poured on this quantity of the dried flowers, and should stand for twenty minutes. It will then serve most usefully for relieving the congestive bronchial catarrh of children, being sweetened, and given one third at a time every ten or fifteen minutes until it provokes vomiting. It is also beneficial in this way, but when given less often, for epidemic dysentery.

The chemical principles of the Daffodil have not been investigated; but a yellow volatile oil of disagreeable odour, and a brown colouring matter, have been got from the flowers.

The Arabians commended this oil to be applied for curing baldness, and for stimulating the sexual organs.

Herrick alludes in his *Hesperides* to the Daffodil as portentous of death:—

" When a Daffodil I see
Hanging down its head towards me,
Guess I may what I must be—
First I shall decline my head;
Secondly, I shall be dead;
Lastly, safely buriëd."

Daffodils, popularly known in this country as Lent Lilies, are called by the French *Pauvres filles de Sainte Clare.* The name *Junquillo* is the Spanish diminutive of *Junco,* "the rush," and is given to the jonquil because of its slender rush-like stem. From its fragrant flowers a sweet-smelling yellow oil is obtained.

The medicinal influence of the Daffodil on the nervous system has led to giving its flowers and its bulb for hysterical affections, and even epilepsy, with benefit.

DAISY.

OUR English Daisy is a composite flower which is called in the glossaries "gowan," or Yellow flower. Botanically it is named *Bellis perennis*, probably from *bellis*, "in fields of battle," because of its fame in healing the wounds of soldiers; and *perennis* as implying that though "the rose has but a summer reign, the daisy never dies." The flower is likewise known as "Bainwort," "beloved by children," and "the lesser Consound." The whole plant has been carefully and exhaustively proved for curative purposes; and a medicinal tincture (H.) is now made from it with spirit of wine. Gerard says: "Daisies do mitigate all kinds of pain, especially in the joints, and gout proceeding from a hot humour, if stamped with new butter and applied upon the pained place." And, "The leaves of Daisies used among pot-herbs do make the belly soluble." Pliny tells us the Daisy was used in his time with Mugwort as a resolvent to scrofulous tumours.

The leaves are acrid and pungent, being ungrateful to cattle, and even rejected by geese. These and the flowers, when chewed experimentally, have provoked giddiness and pains in the arms as if from coming boils: also a development of boils, "dark, fiery, and very sore," on the back of the neck, and outside the jaws. For preventing, or aborting these same distressing formations when they begin to occur spontaneously, the tincture of Daisies should be taken in doses of five drops three times a day in water. Likewise this medicine should be given curatively on the principle of affinity between it and the symptoms induced in provers who have taken the same in material toxic doses, "when the brain is muddled, the sight dim, the spirits soon depressed, the temper irritable, the skin pimply, the heart apt to flutter, and the whole aspect careworn; as if from early excesses." Then the infusion of the plant in tablespoonful doses, or the diluted tincture, will answer admirably to renovate and re-establish the health and strength of the sufferer.

The flowers and leaves are found to afford a considerable quantity of oil and of ammoniacal salts. The root was named *Consolida minima* by older physicians. Fabricius speaks of its efficacy in curing wounds and contusions. A decoction of the leaves and flowers was given internally, and the bruised herb blended with lard was applied outside. "The leaves stamped do take away bruises and swellings, whereupon, it was called in old time Bruisewort." If eaten as a spring salad, or boiled like spinach, the leaves are pungent, and slightly laxative.

Being a diminutive plant with roots to correspond, the Daisy, on the doctrine of signatures, was formerly thought to arrest the bodily growth if taken with this view. Therefore its roots boiled in broth were given to young puppies so as to keep them of a small size. For the same reason the fairy Milkah fed her foster child on this plant, "that his height might not exceed that of a pigmy":—

"She robbed dwarf elders of their fragrant fruit,
And fed him early with the daisy-root,
Whence through his veins the powerful juices ran,
And formed the beauteous miniature of man."

"Daisy-roots and cream" were prescribed by the fairy godmothers of our childhood to stay the stature of those gawky youngsters who were shooting up into an ungainly development like "ill weeds growing apace."

Daisies were said of old to be under the dominion of Venus, and later on they were dedicated to St. Margaret of Cortona. Therefore they were reputed good for the special illnesses of females. It is remarkable there is no

Greek word for this plant, or flower. Ossian the Gaelic poet feigns that the Daisy, whose white investments figure innocence, was first "sown above a baby's grave by the dimpled hands of infantine angels."

During mediæval times the Daisy was worn by knights at a tournament as an emblem of fidelity. In his poem the *Flower and the Leaf*, Chaucer, who was ever loud in his praises of the "Eye of Day"—"empresse and floure of floures all," thus pursues his theme :—

> "And at the laste there began anon
> A lady for to sing right womanly
> A bargaret in praising the Daisie :
> For—as methought among her notës sweet,
> She said, '*Si doucet est la Margarete.*'"

The French name *Marguerite* is derived from a supposed resemblance of the Daisy to a pearl ; and in Germany this flower is known as the Meadow Pearl. Likewise the Greek word for a pearl is *Margaritos.*

A saying goes that it is not Spring until a person can put his foot on twelve of these flowers. In the cultivated red Daisies used for bordering our gardens, the yellow central boss of each compound flower has given place to strap-shaped florets like the outer rays, and without pollen, so that the entire flower consists of this purple inflorescence. But such aristocratic culture has made the blossom unproductive of seed. Like many a proud and belted Earl, each of the pampered and richly coloured Daisies pays the penalty of its privileged luxuriance by a disability from perpetuating its species.

The Moon Daisy, or Oxeye Daisy (*Leucanthemum Crysanthemum*), St. John's flower, belonging to the same tribe of plants, grows commonly with an erect stem about two feet high, in dry pastures and roads, bearing large solitary flowers, which are balsamic and make a useful infusion for relieving chronic coughs, and for bronchial catarrhs. Boiled with some of the leaves and stalks they form, if sweetened with honey, or barley sugar, an excellent posset drink for the same purpose. In America the root is employed successfully for checking the night sweats of pulmonary consumption, a fluid extract thereof being made for this object, the dose of which is from fifteen to sixty drops in water.

The Moon Daisy is named Maudlin-wort from St. Mary Magdalene, and bears its lunar name from the Grecian goddess of the moon, Artemis, who particularly governed the female health. Similarly, our bright little Daisy, "the constellated flower that never sets," owns the name Herb Margaret. The Moon Daisy is also called Bull Daisy, Gipsies' Daisy, Goldings, Midsummer Daisy, Mace Flinwort, and Espilawn. Its young leaves are sometimes used as a flavouring in soups and stews. The flower was compared to the representation of a full moon, and was formerly dedicated to the Isis of the Egyptians. Tom Hood wrote of a traveller estranged far from his native shores, and walking despondently in a distant land:—

> "When lo! he starts with glad surprise,
> Home thoughts come rushing o'er him,
> For, modest, wee, and crimson-tipped
> A flower he sees before him.
> With eager haste he stoops him down,
> His eyes with moisture hazy;
> And as he plucks the simple bloom
> He murmurs, 'Lawk, a Daisy'"!

DANDELION.

OWING to long years of particular evolutionary sagacity in developing winged seeds to be wafted from the silky pappus of its ripe flowerheads over wide areas of land, the Dandelion exhibits its handsome golden flowers in every field and on every ground plot throughout the whole of our country. They are to be distinguished from the numerous hawkweeds, by having the outermost leaves of their exterior cup bent downwards whilst the stalk is coloured and shining. The plant-leaves have jagged edges which resemble the angular jaw of a lion fully supplied with teeth; or, some writers say, the herb has been named from the heraldic lion which is vividly yellow, with teeth of gold—in fact, a dandy lion! Again, the flower closely resembles the sun, which a lion represents. It is called by some Blowball, Time Table, and Milk "Gowan" (or golden).

> "How like a prodigal does Nature seem,
> When thou with all thy gold so common art."

In some of our provinces the herb is known as Wiggers, and Swinesnout; whilst again in Devon and Cornwall it is called the Dashelflower. Botanically it belongs to the composite order, and is named *Taraxacum Leontodon*, or eatable, and lion-toothed. This latter when Latinised is *dens leonis*, and in French *dent de lion.* The title Taraxacum is an Arabian corruption of the Greek *trogimon*, "edible"; or it may have been derived from the Greek *taraxos*, "disorder," and *akos*, "remedy." It once happened that a plague of insects destroyed the harvest in the island of Minorca, so that the inhabitants had to eat the wild produce of the country; and many of them then subsisted for some while entirely on this plant. The Dandelion, which is a wild sort of Succory, was known to Arabian physicians, since Avicenna of the eleventh century mentions it as *taraxacon.* It is found throughout Europe, Asia, and North America; possessing a root which abounds with milky juice, and this varying in character according to the time of year in which the plant is gathered.

During the winter the sap is thick, sweet, and albuminous ; but in summer time it is bitter and acrid. Frost causes the bitterness to diminish, and sweetness to take its place ; but after the frost this bitterness returns, and is intensified. The root is at its best for yielding juice about November. Chemically the active ingredients of the herb are taraxacin, and taraxacerine, with inulin (a sort of sugar), gluten, gum, albumen, potash, and an odorous resin, which is commonly supposed to stimulate the liver, and the biliary organs. Probably this reputed virtue was assigned at first to the plant largely on the doctrine of signatures, because of its bright yellow flowers of a bilious hue. But skilled medical provers who have experimentally tested the toxical effects of the Dandelion plant have found it to produce, when taken in excess, troublesome indigestion, characterised by a tongue coated with a white skin which peels off in patches, leaving a raw surface, whilst the kidneys become unusually active, with profuse night sweats, and an itching nettle rash. For these several symptoms when occurring of themselves, a combination of the decoction, and the medicinal tincture will be invariably curative.

To make a decoction of the root, one part of this dried, and sliced, should be gently boiled for fifteen minutes in twenty parts of water, and strained off when cool. It may be sweetened with brown sugar, or honey, if unpalatable when taken alone, several teacupfuls being given during the day. Dandelion roots as collected for the market are often adulterated with those of the common Hawkbit (*Leontodon hispidus*) ; but these are more tough and do not give out any milky juice.

The tops of the roots dug out of the ground, with the tufts of the leaves remaining thereon, and blanched by being covered in the earth as they grow, if gathered in the spring, are justly esteemed as an excellent vernal salad. It was with this homely fare the good wise Hecate entertained Theseus, as we read in Evelyn's *Acetaria*. Bergius says he has seen intractable cases of liver congestion cured, after many other remedies had failed, by the patients taking daily for some months, a broth made from Dandelion roots stewed in boiling water, with leaves of Sorrel, and the yelk of an egg; though (he adds) they swallowed at the same time cream of tartar to keep their bodies open.

Incidentally with respect to the yelk of an egg, as prescribed here, it is an established fact that patients have been cured of obstinate jaundice by taking a raw egg on one or more mornings while fasting. Dr. Paris tells us a special oil is to be extracted from the yelks (only) of hard boiled eggs, roasted in pieces in a frying pan until the oil begins to exude, and then pressed hard. Fifty eggs well fried will yield about five ounces of this oil, which is acrid, and so enduringly liquid that watch-makers use it for lubricating the axles and pivots of their most delicate wheels. Old eggs furnish the oil most abundantly, and it certainly acts as a very useful medicine for an obstructed liver. Furthermore the shell, when finely triturated, has served by its potentialised lime to cure some forms of cancer. Sweet are the uses of adversity! even such as befell the egg symbolised by Humpty-Dumpty:—

> " Humptius in muro requievit Dumptius alto,
> Humptius e muro Dumptius—heu! cecidit!
> Sed non Regis equi, Reginæ exercitus omnis
> Humpti, te, Dumpti, restituere loco."

The medicinal tincture of Dandelion is made from the entire plant, gathered in summer, employing proof spirit which dissolves also the resinous parts not soluble in water. From ten to fifteen drops of this tincture may be taken with a spoonful of water three times in the day.

Of the freshly prepared juice, which should not be kept long as it quickly ferments, from two to three teaspoonfuls are a proper dose. The leaves when tender and white in the spring are taken on the Continent in salads, or they are blanched, and eaten with bread and butter. Parkinson says: "Whoso is drawing towards a consumption, or ready to fall into a cachexy, shall find a wonderful help from the use thereof, for some time together." Officially, according to the London College, are prepared from the fresh dried roots collected in the autumn, a decoction (one ounce to a pint of boiling water), a juice, a fresh extract, and an inspissated liquid extract.

Because of its tendency to provoke involuntary urination at night, the Dandelion has acquired a vulgar suggestive appellation which expresses this fact in most homely terms: *quasi herba lectiminga, et urinaria dicitur:* and this not only in our vernacular, but in most of the European tongues: *quia plus lotii in vesicam derivat quam puerulis retineatur præsertim inter dormiendum, eoque tunc imprudentes et inviti stragula permingunt.*

At Gottingen, the roots are roasted and used instead of coffee by the poorer folk; and in Derbyshire the juice of the stalk is applied to remove warts. The flower of the Dandelion when fully blown is named Priest's Crown (*Caput monachi*), from the resemblance of its naked receptacle after the winged seeds have been all blown away, to the smooth shorn head of a Roman cleric. So Hurdis sings in his poem *The Village Curate* :—

"The Dandelion this :
A college youth that flashes for a day
All gold : anon he doffs his gaudy suit,
Touched by the magic hand of Bishop grave,
And all at once by commutation strange
Becomes a reverend priest : and then how sleek!
How full of grace! with silvery wig at first
So nicely trimmed, which presently grows bald.
But let me tell you, in the pompous globe
Which rounds the Dandelion's head is fitly couched
Divinity most rare."

Boys gather the flower when ripe, and blow away the ball of its silky seed vessels at the crown, to learn the time of day, thus sportively making :—

"Dandelion with globe of down
The school-boy's clock in every town."

DATE.

DATES are the most wholesome and nourishing of all our imported fruits. Children especially appreciate their luscious sweetness, as afforded by an abundant sugar which is easily digested, and which quickly repairs waste of heat and fat. With such a view, likewise, doctors now advise dates for consumptive patients; also because they soothe an irritable chest, and promote expectoration; whilst, furthermore, they prevent costiveness. Dates are the fruit of the Date palm (*Phœnix dactylifera*), or, Tree of Life.

In old English Bibles of the sixteenth century, the name Date-tree is constantly given to the Palm, and the fruit thereof was the first found by the Israelites when wandering in the Wilderness.

Oriental writers have attributed to this tree a certain semi-human consciousness. The name *Phœnix* was bestowed on the Date palm because a young shoot springs always from the withered stump of an old decayed Date tree, taking the place of the dead parent; and the specific term *Dactylifera* refers to a fancied resemblance between clusters of the fruit and the human fingers.

The Date palm is remarkably fond of water, and will not thrive unless growing near it, so that the Arabs say: "In order to flourish, its feet must be in the water, and its head in the fire (of a hot sun)." Travellers across the desert, when seeing palm Dates in the horizon, know that wells of water will be found near at hand: at the same time they sustain themselves with Date jam.

In some parts of the East this Date palm is thought to have been the tree of the forbidden fruit in the Garden of Eden. It is mystically represented as the tree of life in the sculptured foliage of early French churches, and on the primitive mosaics found in the apses of Roman Basilicas. Branches of this tree are carried about in Catholic countries on Palm Sunday. Formerly Dates were sent to England and elsewhere packed in mats from the Persian gulf; but now they arrive in clean boxes, neatly laid, and free from duty; so that a wholesome, sustaining, and palatable meal may be had for one penny, if they are eaten with bread.

The Egyptian Dates are superior, being succulent and luscious when new, but apt to become somewhat hard after Christmas.

The Dates, however, which surpass all others in their general excellence, are grown with great care at Tafilat, two or three hundred miles inland from Morocco, a region to which Europeans seldom penetrate.

These Dates travel in small packages by camel, rail, and steamer, being of the best quality, and highly valued. Their exportation is prohibited by the African authorities at Tafilat, unless the fruit crop has been large enough to allow thereof after gathering the harvest with much religious ceremony.

Dates of a second quality are brought from Tunis, being intermixed with fragments of stalk and branch; whilst the inferior sorts come in the form of a cake, or paste (*adjoue!*), being pressed into baskets. In this shape they were tolerably common with us in Tudor times, and were then used for medicinal purposes. Strutt mentions a grocer's bill delivered in 1581, in which occurs the item of six pounds of dates supplied at a funeral for two shillings; and we read that in 1821 the best kind of dates cost five shillings a pound.

If taken as a portable refection by jurymen and others who may be kept from their customary food Dates will prevent exhaustion, and will serve to keep active the energies of mind and body. The fruit should be selected when large and soft, being moist, and of a reddish yellow colour outside, and not much wrinkled, whilst having within a white membrane between the flesh and the stone.

Beads for rosaries are made in Barbary from Date stones turned in a lathe; or when soaked in water for a couple of days the stones may be given to cattle as a nutritious food, being first ground in a mill. The fodder being astringent will serve by its tannin, which is abundant, to cure or prevent looseness.

In a clever parody on Bret Harte's "Heathen Chinee," an undergraduate is detected in having primed himself before examination thus:—

"Inscribed on his cuffs were the Furies, and Fates,
With a delicate map of the Dorian States:
Whilst they found in his palms, which were hollow,
What are common in Palms—namely, Dates."

Again, a conserve is prepared by the Egyptians from unripe Dates whole with sugar. The soft stones are edible: and this jam, though tasteless, is very nourishing. The Arabs say that Adam when driven out of Paradise took with him three things—the Date, chief of all fruits, the Myrtle, and an ear of Wheat.

Another Palm—the *Sagus*, or, *Cycus revoluta*,—which grows naturally in Japan and the East Indian Islands, being also cultivated in English hot-houses, yields by its gummy pith our highly nutritious sago. This when cooked is one of the best and most sustaining foods for children and infirm old persons. The Indians reserve their finest sago for the aged and afflicted. A fecula is washed from the abundant pith, which is chemically a starch, very demulcent, and more digestible than that of rice. It never ferments in the stomach, and is very suitable for hectic persons. By the Arabs the pith of the Date-bearing Palm is eaten in like manner. The simple wholesome virtues of this domestic substance have been told of from childhood in the well-known nursery rhyme, which has been playfully rendered into Latin and French:—

"There was an old man of Iago
Whom they kept upon nothing but sago;
Oh! how he did jump when the doctor said plump:
'To a roast leg of mutton you may go.'"

"Jamdudum senior quidam de rure Tobagus
Invito mad das carpserat ore dapes;
Sed medicus tandem non injucunda locutus:
'Assœ' dixit 'oves sunt tibi cœna, senex.'"

"J'ai entendu parler d'un veillard de Tobag
Qui ne mangea longtemps que du ris et du sague;
Mais enfin le medecin lui dit ces mots:
'Allez vous en, mon ami, au gigot.'"

DILL.

CORDIAL waters distilled from the fragrant herb called Dill are, as every mother and monthly nurse well know, a sovereign remedy for wind in the infant; whilst they serve equally well to correct flatulence in the grown up "gourmet." This highly scented plant (*Anethum graveolens*) is of Asiatic origin, growing wild also in some parts of England, and commonly cultivated in our gardens for kitchen or medicinal uses.

It "hath a little stalk of a cubit high, round, and joyned, whereupon do grow leaves very finely cut, like to those of Fennel, but much smaller." The herb is of the umbelliferous order, and its fruit chemically furnishes "anethol," a volatile empyreumatic oil similar to that contained in the Anise, and Caraway. Virgil speaks of the Dill in his *Second Eclogue* as the *bene olens anethum*, "a pleasant and fragrant plant." Its seeds were formerly directed to be used by the *Pharmacopœias* of London and Edinburgh. Forestus extols them for allaying sickness and hiccough. Gerard says: "Dill stayeth the yeox, or hicquet, as Dioscorides has taught."

The name *Anethum* was a radical Greek term (*aitho*—to burn), and the herb is still called Anet in some of our country districts. The pungent essential oil which it yields consists of a hydrocarbon, "carvene," together with an oxygenated oil. It is a "gallant expeller of the wind, and provoker of the terms." "Limbs that are swollen and cold if rubbed with the oil of Dill are much eased, if not cured thereby."

A dose of the essential oil if given for flatulent indigestion should be from two to four drops, on sugar, or with a tablespoonful of milk. Of the distilled water sweetened, one or two teaspoonfuls may be given to an infant.

The name Dill is derived from the Saxon verb *dilla*, to lull, because of its tranquillizing properties, and its causing children to sleep. This word occurs in the vocabulary of Oelfric, Archbishop of Canterbury, tenth century. Dioscorides gave the oil got from the flowers for rheumatic pains, and sciatica; also a carminative water distilled from the fruit, for increasing the milk of wet nurses, and for appeasing the windy belly-aches of babies. He teaches that a teaspoonful of the bruised seeds if boiled in water and taken hot with bread soaked therein, wonderfully helps such as are languishing from hardened excrements, even though they may have vomited up their fæces.

The plant is largely grown in the East Indies, where it is known as *Soyah*. Its fruit and leaves are used for flavouring pickles, and its water is given to parturient women.

Drayton speaks of the Dill as a magic ingredient in love potions; and the weird gipsy, Meg Merrilies, crooned a cradle song at the birth of Harry Bertram in which it was said :—

> "Trefoil, vervain, John's wort, *Dill*,
> Hinder witches of their will."

DOCK.

The term Dock is botanically a noun of multitude, meaning originally a bundle of hemp, and corresponding to a similar word signifying a flock. It became in early times applied to a wide-spread tribe of broad-leaved wayside weeds. They all belong to the botanical order of *Polygonaceæ*, or "many kneed" plants, because, like the wife of Yankee Doodle, famous in song, they are "double-jointed;" though he, poor man! expecting to find Mistress Doodle doubly active in her household duties, was, as the rhyme says, "disappointed." The name "Dock" was first applied to the *Arctium Lappa*, or Bur-dock, so called because of its seed-vessels becoming frequently entangled by their small hooked spines in the wool of sheep passing along by the hedge-rows. Then the title got to include other broad-leaved herbs, all of the Sorrel kind, and used in pottage, or in medicine.

Of the Docks which are here recognized, some are cultivated, such as Garden Rhubarb, and the Monk's Rhubarb, or herb Patience, an excellent pot herb; whilst others grow wild in meadows, and by river sides, such as the round-leafed Dock (*Rumex obtusifolius*), the sharp-pointed Dock (*Rumex acutus*), the sour Dock (*Rumex acetosus*), the great water Dock (*Rumex hydrolapathum*), and the bloody-veined Dock (*Rumex sanguineus*).

All these resemble our garden rhubarb more or less in their general characteristics, and in possessing much tannin. Most of them chemically furnish "rumicin," or crysophanic acid, which is highly useful in several chronic diseases of the skin among scrofulous patients. The generic name of several Docks is *rumex*, from the Hebrew *rumach*, a "spear"; others are called *lapathum*, from the Greek verb *lapazein*, to cleanse, because they act medicinally as purgatives.

The common wayside Dock (*Rumex obtusifolius*) is the most ordinary of all the Docks, being large and spreading, and so coarse that cattle refuse to eat it. The leaves are often applied as a rustic remedy to burns and scalds, and are used for dressing blisters. Likewise a popular cure for nettle stings is to rub them with a Dock leaf, saying at the same time:—

"Out nettle: in Dock;
Dock shall have a new smock."

or :—

> "Nettle out : Dock in ;
> Dock remove the nettle sting."

A tea made from the root was formerly given for the cure of boils, and the plant is frequently called Butter-dock, because its leaves are put into use for wrapping up butter. This Dock will not thrive in poor worthless soil; but its broad foliage serves to lodge the destructive turnip fly. The root when dried may be added to tooth powder.

It was under the broad leaf of a roadside Dock that Hop o' My Thumb, famous in nursery lore, sought refuge from a storm, and was unfortunately swallowed whilst still beneath the leaf by a passing hungry cow.

The herb Patience, or Monk's Rhubarb (*Rumex alpinus*), a Griselda among herbs, may be given with admirable effect in pottage, as a domestic aperient, "loosening the belly, helping the jaundice, and dispersing the tympany." This grows wild in some parts, by roadsides, and near cottages, but is not common except as a cultivated herb in the kitchen-garden, known as "Patience-dock." It is a remarkable fact that the toughest flesh-meat, if boiled with the herb, or with other kindred docks, will become quite tender. The name Patience, or Passions, was probably from the Italian *Lapazio*, a corruption of *Lapathum*, which was mistaken for *la passio*, the passion of Christ.

Our *Garden Rhubarb* is a true Dock, and belongs to the "many-kneed," buckwheat order of plants. Its brilliant colouring is due to varying states of its natural pigment (*chlorophyll*), in combination with oxygen. For culinary purposes the stalk, or petiole of the broad leaf, is used. Its chief nutrient property is glucose, which is identical with grape-sugar. The agreeable taste and odour of the plant are not brought out until the leaf stalks are cooked. It came originally from the Volga, and has been grown in this country since 1573. The sour taste of the stalks is due to oxalic acid, or rather to the acid oxalate of potash. This combines with the lime elaborated in the system of a gouty person (having an "oxalic acid" disposition), and makes insoluble and injurious products which have to be thrown off by the kidneys as oxalate crystals, with much attendant irritation of the general system. Sorrel (*Rumex acetosus*) acts with such a person in just the same way, because of the acid oxalate of potash which it contains.

Garden Rhubarb also possesses albumen, gum, and mineral matters, with a small quantity of some volatile essence. The proportion of nutritive substance to the water and vegetable fibre is very small. As an article of food it is objectionable for gouty persons liable to the passage of highly coloured urine, which deposits lithates and urates as crystals after it has cooled; and this especially holds good if hard water, which contains lime, is drunk at the same time.

The round-leaved Dock, and the sharp-pointed Dock, together with the bloody-veined Dock (which is very conspicuous because of its veins and petioles abounding in a blood-coloured juice), make respectively with their astringent roots a useful infusion against bleedings and fluxes; also with their leaves a decoction curative of several chronic skin diseases.

The *Rumex acetosus* (Sour Dock, or Sorrel), though likely to disagree with gouty persons, nevertheless supplies its leaves as the chief constituent of the *Soupe aux herbes*, which a French lady will order for herself after a long and tiring journey. Its title is derived as some think, from *struma*, because curative thereof. This Dock further bears the names of Sour sabs, Sour grabs, Soursuds, Soursauce, Cuckoo sorrow, and Greensauce. Because of their acidity the leaves make a capital dressing with stewed lamb, veal, or sweetbread. Country people beat the herb to a mash, and take it mixed with vinegar and sugar as a green sauce with cold meat. When boiled by itself without water it serves as an excellent accompaniment to roast goose or pork instead of apple sauce. The root of Sorrel when dried has the singular property of imparting a fine red colour to boiling water, and it is therefore used by the French for making barley water look like red wine when they wish to avoid giving anything of a vinous character to the sick. In Ireland Sorrel leaves are eaten with fish, and with other alkalescent foods. Because corrective of scrofulous deposits, Sorrel is specially beneficial towards the cure of scurvy. Applied externally the bruised leaves will purify foul ulcers. Says John Evelyn in his noted *Acetaria* (1720), "Sorrel sharpens the appetite, assuages heat, cools the liver and strengthens the heart; it is an antiscorbutic, resisting putrefaction, and in the making of sallets imparts a grateful quickness to the rest as supplying the want of oranges and lemons. Together with salt it gives both the name and the relish to sallets from the sapidity which renders not plants and herbs only, but men themselves, and their conversations pleasant and agreeable. But of this enough, and perhaps too much! lest while I write of salts and sallets I appear myself *insipid.*"

The Wood Sorrel (*Oxalis acetosella*) is a distinct plant from the Dock Sorrel, and is not one of the *Polygonaceæ*, but a geranium, having a triple leaf which is often employed to symbolise the Trinity. Painters of old

11

placed it in the foreground of their pictures when representing the crucifixion. The leaves are sharply acid through oxalate of potash, commonly called "Salts of Lemon," which is quite a misleading name in its apparent innocence as applied to so strong a poison. The petals are bluish coloured, veined with purple. Formerly, on account of its grateful acidity, a conserve was ordered by the London College to be made from the leaves and petals of Wood Sorrel, with sugar and orange peel, and it was called *Conserva lujulæ.*

The Burdock (*Arctium lappa*) grows very commonly in our waste places, with wavy leaves, and round heads of purple flowers, and hooked scales. From the seeds a medicinal tincture (H.) is made, and a fluid extract, of which from ten to thirty drops, given three times a day, with two tablespoonfuls of cold water, will materially benefit certain chronic skin diseases (such as psoriasis), if taken steadily for several weeks, or months. Dr. Reiter of Pittsburg, U.S.A., says the Burdock seed has proved in his hands almost a specific for psoriasis and for obstinate syphilis. The tincture is of special curative value for treating that depressed state of the general health which is associated with milky phosphates in the urine, and much nervous debility. Eight or ten drops of the reduced tincture should be given in water three times a day.

The root in decoction is an excellent remedy for other skin diseases of the scaly, itching, vesicular, pimply and ulcerative characters. Many persons think it superior to Sarsaparilla. The burs of this Dock are sometimes called "Cocklebuttons," or "Cucklebuttons," and "Beggarsbuttons." Its Anglo-Saxon name was "Fox's clote."

Boys throw them into the air at dusk to catch bats, which dart at the Bur in mistake for a moth or fly;

then becoming entangled with the thorny spines they fall helplessly to the ground. Of the botanical names, *Arctium* is derived from *arktos*, a bear, in allusion to the roughness of the burs; and *Lappa* is from *labein*, to seize. Other appellations of the herb are Clot-bur (from sticking to clouts, or clothes), Clithe, Hurbur, and Hardock. The leaves when applied externally are highly resolvent for tumours, bruises, and gouty swellings. In the *Philadelphia Recorder* for January, 1893, a striking case is given of a fallen womb cured after twenty years' duration by a decoction of Burdock roots. The liquid extract acts as an admirable remedy in some forms (strumous) of longstanding indigestion. The roots contain starch; and the ashes of the plant burnt when green yield carbonate of potash abundantly, with nitre, and inulin.

The Yellow Curled Dock (*Rumex crispus*), so called because its leaves are crisped at their edges, grows freely in our roadside ditches, and waste places, as a common plant; and a medicinal tincture which is very useful (H.) is made from it before it flowers. This is of particular service for giving relief to an irritable tickling cough of the upper air-tubes, and the throat, when these passages are rough and sore, and sensitive to the cold atmosphere, with a dry cough occurring in paroxysms. It is likewise excellent for dispelling any obstinate itching of the skin, in which respect it was singularly beneficial against the contagious army-itch which prevailed during the last American war. It acts like Sarsaparilla chiefly, for curing scrofulous skin affections and glandular swellings. To be applied externally an ointment may be made by boiling the root in vinegar until the fibre is softened, and by then mixing the pulp with lard (to which some sulphur is added at times). In all such cases of a scrofulous sort from five to ten drops of the tincture should be given two or three times a day with a spoonful of cold water.

Rumicin is the active principle of the Yellow Curled Dock; and from the root, containing chrysarobin, a dried extract is prepared officinally, of which from one to four grains may be given for a dose in a pill. This is useful for relieving a congested liver, as well as for scrofulous skin diseases.

"Huds," or the great Water Dock (*Rumex hydrolapathum*) is of frequent growth on our river banks, bearing numerous green flowers in leafless whorls, and being identical with the famous *Herba Britannica* of Pliny. This name does not denote British origin, but is derived from three Teuton words, *brit*, to tighten: *tan*, a tooth; and *ica*, loose; thus expressing its power of bracing up loose teeth and spongy gums. Swedish ladies employ the powdered root as a dentifrice; and gargles prepared therefrom are excellent for sore throat and relaxed uvula. The *fresh* root must be used, as it quickly turns yellow and brown in the air. The green leaves make a capital application for ulcers of the legs. They possess considerable acidity, and are laxative. Horace was aware of this fact, as we learn by his *Sermonum*, *Libr*. ii., *Satir* 4:—

> "Si dura morabitur alvus,
> Mytulus, et viles pellent, obstantia conchæ,
> Et Lapathi brevis herba, sed albo non sine Coo."

ELDER.

"'ARN,' or the common Elder," says Gerard, "groweth everywhere; and it is planted about cony burrows, for the shadow of the conies." Formerly it was much cultivated near our English cottages, because supposed to afford protection against witches. Hence it is that the Elder tree may be so often seen immediately near old village houses. It acquired its name from the Saxon word *eller* or *kindler*, because its hollow branches were made into tubes to blow through for brightening up a dull fire. By the Greeks it was called *Aktee.* The botanical name of the Elder is *Sambucus nigra*, from *sambukee*, a sackbut, because the young branches, with their pith removed, were brought into requisition for making the pipes of this; and other musical instruments.

It was probably introduced as a medicinal plant at the time of the Monasteries. The adjective term *nigra* refers to the colour of the berries. These are without odour, rather acid, and sweetish to the taste. The French put layers of the flowers among apples, to which they impart an agreeable odour and flavour like muscatel. A tract on *Elder and Juniper Berries, showing how useful they may be in our Coffee Houses*, is published with the *Natural History of Coffee*, 1682. Elder flowers are fatal to turkeys.

Hippocrates gave the bark as a purgative; and from his time the whole tree has possessed a medicinal celebrity, whilst its fame in the hands of the herbalist is immemorial. German writers have declared it contains within itself a magazine of physic, and a complete chest of medicaments.

The leaves when bruised, if worn in the hat, or rubbed on the face, will prevent flies from settling on the person. Likewise turnips, cabbages, fruit trees, or corn, if whipped with the branches and green leaves of Elder, will gain an immunity from all depredations of blight; but moths are fond of the blossom.

Dried Elder flowers have a dull yellow colour, being

shrivelled, and possessing a sweet faint smell, unlike the repulsive odour of the fresh leaves and bark. They have a somewhat bitter, gummy taste, and are sold in entire cymes, with the stalks. An open space now seen in Malvern Chase was formerly called Eldersfield, from the abundance of Elder trees which grew there. "The flowers were noted," says Mr. Symonds, "for eye ointments, and the berries for honey rob and black pigments. Mary of Eldersfield, the daughter of Bolingbroke, was famous for her knowledge of herb pharmacy, and for the efficacy of her nostrums."

Chemically the flowers contain a yellow, odorous, buttery oil, with tannin, and malates of potash and lime, whilst the berries furnish viburnic acid. On expression they yield a fine purple juice, which proves a useful laxative, and a resolvent in recent colds. Anointed on the hair they make it black.

A medicinal tincture (H.) is made from the fresh inner bark of the young branches. This, when given in toxical quantities, will induce profuse sweating, and will cause asthmatic symptoms to present themselves. When used in a diluted form it is highly beneficial for relieving the same symptoms, if they come on as an attack of illness, particularly for the spurious croup of children, which wakes them at night with a suffocative cough and wheezing. A dose of four or five drops, if given at once, and perhaps repeated in fifteen minutes, will straightway prove of singular service.

Sir Thomas Browne said that in his day the Elder had become a famous medicine for quinsies, sore throats, and strangulations.

The inspissated juice or "rob" extracted from the crushed berries, and simmered with white sugar, is cordial, aperient, and diuretic. This has long been a popular English remedy, taken hot at bed-time, when a cold is caught. One or two tablespoonfuls are mixed with a tumblerful of very hot water. It promotes perspiration, and is demulcent to the chest. Five pounds of the fresh berries are to be used with one pound of loaf sugar, and the juice should be evaporated to the thickness of honey.

"The recent rob of the Elder spread thick upon a slice of bread and eaten before other dishes," says Dr. Blochwich, 1760, "is our wives' domestic medicine, which they use likewise in their infants and children whose bellies are stop't longer than ordinary; for this juice is most pleasant and familiar to children; or to loosen the belly drink a draught of the wine at your breakfast, or use the conserve of the buds."

Also a capital wine, which may well pass for Frontignac, is commonly made from the fresh berries, with raisins, sugar, and spices. When well brewed, and three years' old, it constitutes English port. "A cup of mulled Elder wine, served with nutmeg and sippets of toast, just before going to bed on a cold wintry night, is "a thing," as Cobbet said, "to be run for." The juice of Elder root, if taken in a dose of one or two tablespoonfuls when fasting, acts as a strong aperient, being "the most excellent purger of watery humours in the world, and very singular against dropsy, if taken once in the week."

John Evelyn, in his *Sylva* (1729), said of the Elder: "If the medicinal properties of its leaves, bark, and berries, were fully known, I cannot tell what our countrymen could ail, for which he might not fetch a remedy from every hedge, either for sickness or wounds." "The buds boiled in water gruel have effected wonders in a fever," "and an extract composed of the berries greatly assists longevity. Indeed,"—so famous is the story of Neander—"this is a catholicum against all infirmities whatever." "The leaves, though somewhat rank of smell, are otherwise, as indeed is the entire shrub, of a very sovereign virtue. The spring-buds are excellently wholesome in pottage; and small ale, in which Elder flowers have been infused, are esteemed by many so salubrious, that this is to be had in most of the eating houses about our town."

"It were likewise profitable for the scabby if they made a sallet of those young buds, who in the beginning of the spring doe bud forth together with those outbreakings and pustules of the skin, which by the singular favour of nature is contemporaneous; these being sometimes macerated a little in hot water, together with oyle, salt, and vinegar, and sometimes eaten. It purgeth the belly, and freeth the blood from salt and serous humours" (1760). Further, "there be nothing more excellent to ease the pains of the hæmorrhoids than a fomentation made of the flowers of the Elder and *Verbusie*, or Honeysuckle, in water or milk, for in a short time it easeth the greatest pain."

If the green leaves are warmed between two hot tiles, and applied to the forehead, they will promptly relieve nervous headache. In Germany the Elder is regarded with much respect. From its leaves a fever drink is made; from its berries a sour preserve, and a wonder-working electuary; whilst the moon-shaped clusters of its aromatic flowers, being somewhat narcotic, are of service in baking small cakes.

The Romans made use of the black Elder juice as a hair dye. From the flowers a fragrant water is now distilled as a perfume; and a gently stimulating ointment is prepared with lard for dressing burns and scalds. Another ointment, concocted from the green berries, with camphor and lard, is ordered by the London College as curative of piles. "The leaves of Elder boiled soft, and with a little linseed oil added thereto, if then laid upon a piece of scarlet or red cloth, and applied to piles as hot as this can be suffered, being removed when cold, and replaced by one such cloth after another upon the diseased part by the space of an hour, and in the end some bound to the place, and the patient put warm to bed. This hath not yet failed at the first dressing to cure the disease, but if the patient be dressed twice, it must needs cure them if the first fail." The Elder was named *Eldrun* and *Burtre* by the Anglo-Saxons. It is now called *Bourtree* in Scotland, from the central pith in the younger branches which children bore out so as to make pop guns:—

> "Bour tree—Bour tree: crooked rung,
> Never straight, and never strong;
> Ever bush, and never tree
> Since our Lord was nailed on thee."

The Elder is specially abundant in Kent around Folkestone. By the Gauls it was called "Scovies," and by the Britons "Iscaw."

This is the tree upon which the legend represents Judas as having hanged himself, or of which the cross was made at the crucifixion. In *Pier's Plowman's Vision* it is said:—

> "Judas he japed with Jewen silver,
> And sithen an eller hanged hymselve."

Gerard says "the gelly of the Elder, otherwise called Jew's ear, taketh away inflammations of the mouth and throat if they be washed therewith, and doth in like manner help the uvula." He refers here to a fungus which grows often from the trunk of the Elder, and the shape of which resembles the human ear. Alluding to this fungus, and to the supposed fact that the berries of the Elder are poisonous to peacocks, a quaint old rhyme runs thus:—

> "For the coughe take Judas' eare,
> With the paring of a peare,
> And drynke them without feare
> If you will have remedy."
>
> "Three syppes for the hycocke,
> And six more for the chycocke:
> Thus will my pretty pycocke
> Recover bye and bye."

Various superstitions have attached themselves in England to the Elder bush. The Tree-Mother has been thought to inhabit it; and it has been long believed that refuge may be safely taken under an Elder tree in a thunderstorm, because the cross was made therefrom, and so the lightning never strikes it. Elder was formerly buried with a corpse to protect it from witches, and even now at a funeral the driver of the hearse commonly has his whip handle made of Elder wood. Lord Bacon commended the rubbing of warts with a green Elder stick, and then burying the stick to rot in the mud. Brand says it is thought in some parts that beating with an Elder rod will check the growth of boys. A cross made of the wood if affixed to cow-houses and stables was supposed to protect cattle from all possible harm.

Belonging to the order of *Caprifoliaceous* (with leaves eaten by goats) plants, the Elder bush grows to the size of a small tree, bearing many white flowers in large flat umbels at the ends of the branches. It gives off an unpleasant soporific smell, which is said to prove harmful to those that sleep under its shade. Our summer is not here until the Elder is fully in flower, and it ends when the berries are ripe. When taken together with the berries of Herb Paris (four-leaved Paris) they have been found very useful in epilepsy. "Mark by the way," says *Anatomie of the Elder* (1760), "the berries of Herb Paris, called by some Bear, or Wolfe Grapes, is held by certain matrons as a great secret against epilepsie; and they give them ever in an unequal number, as three, five, seven, or nine, in the water of Linden tree flowers. Others also do hang a cross made of the Elder and Sallow, mutually inwrapping one another, about the children's neck as anti-epileptick." "I learned the certainty of this experiment (Dr. Blochwich) from a friend in Leipsick, who no sooner erred in diet but he was seized on by this disease; yet after he used the Elder wood as an amulet cut into little pieces, and sewn in a knot against him, he was free." Sheep suffering from the foot-rot, if able to get at the bark and young shoots of an Elder tree, will thereby cure themselves of this affection. The great Boerhaave always took off his hat when passing an Elder bush. Douglas Jerrold once, at a well-known tavern, ordered a bottle of port wine, which should be "old, but not *Elder*."

The *Dwarf Elder* (*Sambucus ebulus*) is quite a different shrub, which grows not infrequently in hedges and bushy places, with a herbaceous stem from two to three feet high. It possesses a smell which is less aromatic than that of the true Elder, and it seldom brings its fruit to ripeness. A rob made therefrom is actively purgative; one tablespoonful for a dose. The root, which has a nauseous bitter taste, was formerly used in dropsies. A decoction made from it, as well as from the inner bark, purges, and promotes free urination.

The leaves made into a poultice will resolve swellings. and relieve contusions. The odour of the green leaves will drive away mice from granaries. To the Dwarf Elder have been given the names Danewort, Danesweed, and Danesblood, probably because it brings about a loss of blood called the "Danes," or perhaps as a corruption of its stated use *contra quotidianam.* The plant is also known as Walewort, from *wal*—slaughter. It grows in great plenty about Slaughterford, Wilts, where there was a noted fight with the Danes; and a patch of it thrives on ground in Worcestershire, where the first blood was drawn in the civil war between the Parliament and the Royalists. Rumour says it will only prosper where blood has been shed either in battle, or in murder.

ELECAMPANE.

"ELECAMPANE," writes William Coles, "is one of the plants whereof England may boast as much as any, for there grows none better in the world than in England, let apothecaries and druggists say what they will." It is a tall, stout, downy plant, from three to five feet high, of the Composite order, with broad leaves, and bright, yellow flowers. Campania is the original source of the plant (*Enula campana*), which is called also Elf-wort, and Elf-dock. Its botanical title is *Helenium inula*, to commemorate Helen of Troy, from whose tears the herb was thought to have sprung, or whose hands were full of the leaves when Paris carried her off from Menelaus. This title has become corrupted in some districts to Horse-heal, or Horse hele, or Horse-heel, through a double blunder, the word *inula* being misunderstood for *hinnula*, a colt; and the term *Hellenium* being thought to have something to do with healing, or heels; and solely on this account the Elecampane has been employed by farriers to cure horses of scabs and sore heels. Though found wild only seldom, and as a local production in our copses and meadows, it is cultivated in our gardens as a medicinal and culinary herb. The name *inula* is only a corruption of the Greek *elenium*; and the herb is of ancient repute, having been described by Dioscorides. An old Latin distich thus celebrates its virtues: *Enula campana reddit præcordia sana*—"Elecampane will the spirits sustain." "Julia Augusta," said Pliny, "let no day pass without eating some of the roots of *Enula* condired, to help digestion, and cause mirth."

The *inula* was noticed by Horace, *Satire* viii., 51:—

> "Erucos virides inulas ego primus amaras
> Monstravi incoquere."

Also the *Enula campana* has been identified with the herb Moly (of Homer), *apo tou moleuein*, from its mitigating pain."

Prior to the Norman Conquest, and during the Middle Ages, the root of Elecampane was much employed in Great Britain as a medicine; and likewise it was candied and eaten as a sweetmeat. Some fifty years ago the candy was sold commonly in London, as flat, round cakes, being composed largely of sugar, and coloured with cochineal. A piece was eaten each night and morning for asthmatical complaints, whilst it was customary when travelling by a river to suck a bit of the root against poisonous exhalations and bad air. The candy may be still had from our confectioners, but now containing no more of the plant Elecampane than there is of barley in barley sugar.

Gerard says: "The flowers of this herb are in all

their bravery during June and July; the roots should be gathered in the autumn. The plant is good for an old cough, and for such as cannot breathe freely unless they hold their necks upright; also it is of great value when given in a loch, which is a medicine to be licked on. It voids out thick clammy humors, which stick in the chest and lungs." Galen says further: "It is good for passions of the huckle-bones, called sciatica.' The root is thick and substantial, having, when sliced, a fragrant aromatic odour.

Chemically, it contains a crystalline principle, resembling camphor, and called "helenin"; also a starch, named "inulin," which is peculiar as not being soluble in water, alcohol, or ether; and conjointly a volatile oil, a resin, albumen, and acetic acid. Inulin is allied to starch, and its crystallized camphor is separable into true helenin, and alantin camphor. The former is a powerful antiseptic to arrest putrefaction. In Spain it is much used as a surgical dressing, and is said to be more destructive than any other agent to the bacillus of cholera. Helenin is very useful in ulceration within the nose (ozœna), and in chronic bronchitis to lessen the expectoration. The dose is from a third of a grain to two grains.

Furthermore, Elecampane counteracts the acidity of gouty indigestion, and regulates the monthly illnesses of women. The French use it in the distillation of absinthe, and term it *l'aulnee, d'un lieu planté d'aulnes ou elle se plait.* To make a decoction, half-an-ounce of the root should be gently boiled for ten minutes in a pint of water, and then allowed to cool. From one to two ounces of this may be taken three times in the day. Of the powdered root, fróm half to one teaspoonful may be given for a dose.

A medicinal tincture (H.) is prepared from the root, of which thirty or forty drops may be taken for a dose, with two tablespoonfuls of cold water; but too large a dose will induce sickness. Elecampane is specifically curative of a sharp pain affecting the right elbow joint, and recurring daily; also of a congestive headache coming on through costiveness of the lowest bowel. Moreover, at the present time, when there is so much talk about the inoculative treatment of pulmonary consumption by the cultivated virus of its special microbe, it is highly interesting to know that the helenin of Elecampane is said to be peculiarly destructive to the bacillus of tubercular disease.

In classic times the poet Horace told how Fundanius first taught the making of a delicate sauce, by boiling in it the bitter *Inula* (Elecampane); and how the Roman stomach, when surfeited with an excess of rich viands, pined for turnips, and the appetising *Enulas acidas* from frugal Campania:—

"Quum rapula plenus
Atque acidas mavult inulas."

EYEBRIGHT.

Found in abundance in summer time on our heaths, and on mountains near the sea, this delicate little plant, the *Euphrasia officinalis*, has been famous from earliest times for restoring and preserving the eyesight. The Greeks named the herb originally from the linnet, which first made use of the leaf for clearing its vision, and which passed on the knowledge to mankind. The same Greek word, *euphrosunee*, signifies joy and gladness. The elegant little herb grows from two to six inches high, with deeply-cut leaves, and numerous white or purplish tiny flowers variegated with yellow; being partially a parasite, and preying on the roots of other plants. It belongs to the order of scrofula-curing plants; and, as proved by positive experiment (H.), the Eye-bright has been recently found to possess a distinct sphere of curative operation, within which it manifests virtues which are as unvarying as they are truly potential. It acts specifically on the mucous lining of the eyes and nose, and the uppermost throat to the top of the windpipe, causing, when given so largely as to be injurious, a profuse secretion from these parts; and, if given of reduced strength, it cures the same troublesome symptoms when due to catarrh.

An attack of cold in the head, with copious running from the eyes and nose, may be aborted straightway by giving a dose of the infusion (made with an ounce of the herb to a pint of boiling water) every two hours; as, likewise, for hay fever. A medicinal tincture (H.) is prepared from the whole plant with spirit of wine, of which an admirably useful lotion may be made together with rose water for simple inflammation of the eyes, with a bloodshot condition of their outer coats. Thirty drops of the tincture should be mixed with a wineglass-ful of rosewater for making this lotion, which may be used several times in the day.

What precise chemical constituents occur in the Eye-bright beyond tannin, mannite, and glucose, are not yet recorded. In Iceland its expressed juice is put into requisition for most ailments of the eyes. Likewise, in Scotland, the Highlanders infuse the herb in milk, and employ this for bathing weak, or inflamed eyes. In France, the plant is named *Casse lunettes*; and in Germany, *Augen trost*, or, consolation of the eye.

Surely the same little herb must have been growing freely in the hedge made famous by ancient nursery tradition:—

"Thessalus acer erat sapiens prœ civibus unus
Qui medium insiluit spineta per horrida sepem.
Effoditque oculos sibi crudelissimus ambos.
Cum vero effosos orbes sine lumine vidit
Viribus enisum totis illum altera sepes
Accipit, et raptos oculos cito reddit egenti."

"There was a man of Thessuly, and he was wondrous wise;
He jumped into a quick set hedge, and scratched out both his eyes;
Then, when he found his eyes were out, with all his might and main
He jumped into the quick set hedge, and scratched them in again."

Old herbals pronounced it "cephalic, ophthalmic, and good for a weak memory." Hildamus relates that it restored the sight of many persons at the age of seventy or eighty years. "Eyebright made into a powder, and then into an electuary with sugar, hath," says Culpeper, "powerful effect to help and to restore the sight decayed through years; and if the herb were but as much used as it is neglected, it would have spoilt the trade of the spectacle maker."

On the whole it is probable that the Eyebright will succeed best for eyes weakened by long-continued straining, and for those which are dim and watery from old age. Shenstone declared, "Famed Euphrasy may not be left unsung, which grants dim eyes to wander leagues around"; and Milton has told us in *Paradise Lost*, Book XI:—

"To nobler sights
Michael from Adam's eyes the film removed,
Then purged with *Euphrasy* and rue
The visual nerve, for he had much to see."

The Arabians knew the herb Eyebright under the name *Adhil.* It now makes an ingredient in British herbal tobacco, which is smoked most usefully for chronic bronchial colds.

Some sceptics do not hesitate to say that the Eyebright owes its reputation solely to the fact that the tiny flower bears in its centre a yellow spot, which is darker towards the middle, and gives a close resemblance to the human eye; wherefore, on the doctrine of signatures, it was pronounced curative of ocular derangements. The present Poet Laureate speaks of the herb as:—

> "The Eyebright this,
> Whereof when steeped in wine I now must eat
> Because it strengthens mindfulness."

Grandmother Cooper, a gipsy of note for skill in healing, practised the cure of inflamed and scrofulous eyes, by anointing them with clay, rubbed up with her spittle, which proved highly successful. Outside was applied a piece of rag kept wet with water in which a cabbage had been boiled. As confirmatory of this cure, we read reverently in the *Gospel of St. John* about the man "which was blind from his birth," and for whose restoration to sight our Saviour "spat on the ground, and made clay of the spittle, and anointed the eyes of the blind man with the clay." More than one eminent oculist has similarly advised that weak, ailing eyes should be daily wetted on waking with the fasting saliva. And it is well known that "mothers' marks" of a superficial character, but even of a considerable size, become dissipated by a daily licking with the mother's tongue. Old Mizaldus taught that "the fasting spittle of a whole and sound person both quite taketh away all scurviness, or redness of the face, ringworms, tetters, and all kinds of pustules, by smearing or rubbing the infected place therewith; and likewise it clean puts away thereby all painful swelling by the means of any venomous thing as hornets, spiders, toads, and such like." Healthy saliva is slightly alkaline, and contains sulphocyanate of potassium.

FENNEL.

We all know the pleasant taste of Fennel sauce when eaten with boiled mackerel. This culinary condiment is made with Sweet Fennel, cultivated in our kitchen gardens, and which is a variety of the wild Fennel growing commonly in England as the Finkel, especially in Cornwall and Devon, on chalky cliffs near the sea. It is then an aromatic plant of the umbelliferous order, but differing from the rest of its tribe in producing bright yellow flowers.

Botanically, it is the *Anethum fœniculum*, or "small fragrant hay" of the Romans, and the *Marathron* of the Greeks. The whole plant has a warm carminative taste, and the old Greeks esteemed it highly for promoting the secretion of milk in nursing mothers. Macer alleged that the use of Fennel was first taught to man by serpents. His classical lines on the subject when translated run thus:—

> "By eating herb of Fennel, for the eyes
> A cure for blindness had the serpent wise;
> Man tried the plant; and, trusting that his sight
> Might thus be healed, rejoiced to find him right."

> "Hac mansâ serpens oculos caligine purgat;
> Indeque compertum est humanis posse mederi
> Illum hominibus: atque experiendo probatum est."

Pliny also asserts that the ophidia, when they cast their skins, have recourse to this plant for restoring their sight. Others have averred that serpents wax young again by eating of the herb; "Wherefore the use of it is very meet for aged folk."

Fennel powder may be employed for making an eye-wash: half-a-teaspoonful infused in a wineglassful of cold water, and decanted when clear. A former physician to the Emperor of Germany saw a monk cured by his tutor in nine days of a cataract by only applying the roots of Fennel with the decoction to his eyes.

In the Elizabethan age the herb was quoted as an emblem of flattery; and Lily wrote, "Little things catch light minds; and fancie is a worm that feedeth first upon Fennel." Again, Milton says, in *Paradise Lost*, Book XI:—

> "The savoury odour blown,
> Grateful to appetite, more pleased my sense
> Than smell of sweetest Fennel."

Shakespeare makes the sister of Laertes say to the King, in *Hamlet*, when wishing to prick the royal conscience, "There's Fennel for you." And Falstaff commends Poins thus, in *Henry the Fourth*, "He plays at quoits well, and eats conger, and Fennel."

The Italians take blanched stalks of the cultivated Fennel (which they call *Cartucci*) as a salad; and in Germany its seeds are added to bread as a condiment, much as we put caraways in some of our cakes. The leaves are eaten raw with pickled fish to correct its oily indigestibility. Evelyn says the peeled stalks, soft and white, when "dressed like salery," exercise a pleasant action conducive to sleep. Roman bakers put the herb under their loaves in the oven to make the bread taste agreeably.

Chemically, the cultivated Fennel plant furnishes a volatile aromatic oil, a fixed fatty principle, sugar, and some starch in the root; also a bitter resinous extract. It is an admirable corrective of flatulence; and yields an essential oil, of which from two to four drops taken on a lump of sugar will promptly relieve griping of the bowels with distension. Likewise a hot infusion, made by pouring half-a-pint of boiling water on a teaspoonful of the bruised seeds will comfort belly ache in the infant, if given in teaspoonful doses sweetened with sugar, and will prove an active remedy in promoting female monthly regularity, if taken at the periodical times, in doses of a wineglassful three times in the day. Gerard says, "The green leaves of the Fennel eaten, or the seed made into a ptisan, and drunk, do fill women's brestes with milk; also the seed if drunk asswageath the wambling of the stomacke, and breaketh the winde." The essential oil corresponds in composition to that of anise, but contains a special camphoraceous body of its own; whilst its vapour will cause the tears and the saliva to flow. A syrup prepared from the expressed juice was formerly given for chronic coughs.

W. Coles teaches in *Nature's Paradise*, that "both the leaves, seeds, and roots, are much used in drinks and broths for those that are grown fat, to abate their unwieldinesse, and make them more gaunt and lank." The ancient Greek name of the herb, *Marathron*, from *maraino*, to grow thin, probably embodied the same notion. "In warm climates," said Matthiolus, "the stems are cut, and there exudes a resinous liquid, which is collected under the name of fennel gum."

The Edinburgh *Pharmacopœia* orders "Sweet Fennel seeds, combined with juniper berries and caraway seeds, for making with spirit of wine, the 'compound spirit of juniper,' which is noted for promoting a copious flow of urine in dropsy." The bruised plant, if applied externally, will speedily relieve toothache or earache. This likewise proves of service as a poultice to resolve chronic swellings. Powdered Fennel is an ingredient in the modern laxative "compound liquorice powder" with senna. The flower, surrounded by its four leaves, is called in the South of England, "Devil in a bush." An old proverb of ours, which is still believed in New England, says, that "Sowing Fennel is sowing sorrow."

A modern distilled water is now obtained from the cultivated plant, and dispensed by the druggist. The whole herb has been supposed to confer longevity, strength and courage. Longfellow wrote a poem about it to this effect.

The fine-leaved Hemlock Water Dropwort (*Œnanthe Phellandrium*), is the Water Fennel.

FERNS.

ONLY some few of our native Ferns are known to possess medicinal virtues, though they may all be happily pronounced devoid of poisonous or deleterious properties. As curative simples, a brief consideration will be given here to the common male and female Ferns, the Royal Fern, the Hart's Tongue, the Maidenhair, the common Polypody, the Spleenwort, and the Wall Rue. Generically, the term "fern" has been referred to the word "feather," because of the pinnate leaves, or to *farr*, a bullock, from the use of the plants as litter for cattle. Ferns are termed *Filices*, from the Latin word *filum*, a thread, because of their filamentary fronds. Each of those now particularized owes its respective usefulness chiefly to its tannin; while the few more specially endowed with healing powers yield also a peculiar chemical acid "filicic," which is fatal to worms. In an old charter, A.D. 855, the right of pasturage on the common Ferns was called "fearnleswe," or *Pascua porcorum*, the pasturage of swine (from *fearrh*, a pig). Matthiolus when writing of the ferns, male and female, says, *Utriusque radice sues pinguescunt.* In some parts of England Ferns at large are known as "Devil's brushes"; and to bite off close to the ground the first Fern which appears in the Spring, is said, in Cornwall, to cure toothache, and to prevent its return during the remainder of the year.

The common Male Fern (*Filix mas*) or Shield Fern, grows abundantly in all parts of Great Britain, and has been known from the times of Theophrastus and Dioscorides, as a specific remedy for intestinal worms, particularly the tape worm. For medicinal purposes, the green part of the rhizome is kept and dried; this is then powdered, and its oleo-resin is extracted by ether. The green fixed oil thus obtained, which is poisonous to worms, consists of the glycerides of filocylic and filosmylic acids, with tannin, starch, gum, and sugar. The English oil of Male Fern is more reliable than that which is imported from the Continent. Twenty drops made into an emulsion with mucilage should be given every half-hour on an empty stomach, until sixty or eighty drops have been taken. It is imprudent to administer the full quantity in a single dose. The treatment should be thus pursued when the vigour of the parasite has been first reduced by a low diet for a couple of days, and is lying within the intestines free from alimentary matter; a purgative being said to assist the action of the plant, though it is, independently, quite efficacious. The knowledge of this remedy had become lost, until it was repurchased for fifteen thousand francs, in 1775, by the French king, under the advice of his principal physicians, from Madame Nouffer, a surgeon's widow in Switzerland, who employed it as a secret mode of cure with infallible success. Her method consisted in giving from one to three drams of the powdered root, after using a clyster, and following the dose up with a purge of scammony and calomel. The rhizome should not be used medicinally if more than a year old. A medicinal tincture (H.) is now prepared from the root-stock with proof spirit, in the autumn when the fronds are dying.

The young shoots and curled leaves of the Male Fern, which is distinguished by having one main rib, are sometimes eaten like asparagus; whilst the fronds make an excellent litter for horses and cattle. The seed of this and some other species of Fern is so minute (one frond producing more than a million) as not to be visible to the naked eye. Hence, on the doctrine of signatures, the plant—like the ring of Gyges, found in a brazen horse—has been thought to confer invisibility. Thus Shakespeare says, *Henry IV.*, Act II., Scene 1, "We have the receipt of Fern seed; we walk invisible."

Bracken or Brakes, which grows more freely than any other of the Fern tribe throughout England, is the *Filix fœmina*, or common Female Fern. The fronds of this are branched, whilst the male plant having only one main rib, is more powerful as an astringent, and antiseptic; "the powder thereof freely beaten healeth the galled necks of oxen and other cattell." Bracken is also named botanically, *Pteris aquilina*, because the figure which appears in its succulent stem when cut obliquely across at the base, has been thought to resemble a spread eagle; and, therefore, Linnæus termed the Fern *Aquilina*. Some call it, for the same reason, "King Charles in the oak tree"; and in Scotland the symbol is said to be an impression of the Devil's foot.

Again, witches are reputed to detest this Fern, since it bears on its cut root the Greek letter X, which is the initial of *Christos*.

In Ireland it is called the Fern of God, because of the belief that if the stem be cut into three sections, on the first of these will be seen the letter G; on the second O; and on the third D.

An old popular proverb says about this Bracken :—

> "When the Fern is as high as a spoon
> You may sleep an hour at noon,
> When the Fern is as high as a ladle
> You may sleep as long as you're able,
> When the Fern is looking red
> Milk is good with faire brown bread."

The Bracken grows almost exclusively on waste places and uncultivated ground; or, as Horace testified in Roman days, *Neglectis urenda filix innascitur agris*. It contains much potash; and its ashes were formerly employed in the manufacture of soap. The young tops of the plant are boiled in Hampshire for hogs' food, and the peculiar flavour of Hampshire bacon has been attributed to this custom. The root affords much starch, and is used medicinally. "For thigh aches" [sciatica], says an old writer, "smoke the legs thoroughly with Fern braken."

During the Seventeenth Century it was customary to set growing Brakes on fire with the belief that this would produce rain. A like custom of "firing the Bracken" still prevails to-day on the Devonshire moors. By an official letter the Earl of Pembroke admonished the High Sheriff of Stafford to forbear the burning of Ferns during a visit of Charles I., as "His Majesty desired that the country and himself may enjoy fair weather as long as he should remain in those parts."

In northern climates a coarse kind of bread is made

from the roots of the Brake Fern; whilst in the south the young shoots are often sold in bundles as a salad. (Some writers give the name of Lady Fern, not to the Bracken, but to the *Asplenium filix fœmina*, because of its delicate and graceful foliage.) The Bracken has branched riblets, and is more viscid, mucilaginous, and diuretic, than the Male Fern.

Its ashes when burnt contain much vegetable alkali which has been used freely in making glass.

It was customary to "watch the Fern" on Midsummer eve, when the plant put forth at dusk a blue flower, and a wonderful seed at midnight, which was carefully collected, and known as "wish seed." This gave the power to discover hidden treasures, whilst to drink the sap conferred perpetual youth.

The Royal Fern (*Osmunda regalis*), grows abundantly in many parts of Great Britain, and is the stateliest of Ferns in its favourite watery haunts. It needs a soil of bog earth, and is incorrectly styled "the flowering Fern," from its handsome spikes of fructification. One of its old English names is "Osmund, the Waterman"; and the white centre of its root has been called the heart of Osmund. This middle part boiled in some kind of liquor was supposed good for persons wounded, dry-beaten, and bruised, or that have fallen from some high place. The name "Osmund" is thought to be derived from *os*, the mouth, or *os*, bone, and *mundare*, to cleanse, or from *gross mond kraut*, the Greater Moonwort; but others refer it to Saint Osmund wading a river, whilst bearing the Christ on his shoulders. The root or rhizome has a mucilaginous slightly bitter taste. The tender sprigs of the plant at their first coming are "good to be put into balmes, oyles, and healing plasters." Dodonœus says, "the harte of the root of

Osmonde is good against squattes, and bruises, heavie and grievous falles, and whatever hurte or dislocation soever it be." "A conserve of these buds," said Dr. Short of Sheffield, 1746, "is a specific in the rickets; and the roots stamped in water or gin till the liquor becometh a stiff mucilage, has cured many most deplorable pains of the back, that have confined the distracted sufferers close to bed for several weeks." This mucilage was to be rubbed over the vertebræ of the back each night and morning for five or six days together. Also for rickets, "take of the powdered roots with the whitest sugar, and sprinkle some thereof on the child's pap, and on all his liquid foods." "It maketh a noble remedy," said Dr. Bowles, "without any other medicine." The actual curative virtues of this Fern are most probably due to the salts of lime, potash, and other earths, which it derives in solution from the bog soil, and from the water in which it grows. On July 25th it is specially dedicated to St. Christopher, its patron saint.

The Hart's Tongue or Hind's Tongue, is a Fern of common English growth in shady copses on moist banks, it being the *Lingua cervina* of the apothecaries, and its name expressing the shape of its fronds. This, the *Scolopendrium vulgare*, is also named "Button-hole," "Horse tongue," and in the Channel Islands "Godshair." The older physicians esteemed it as a very valuable medicine; and Galen gave it for diarrhœa or dysentery. By reason of its tannin it will restrain bleedings, "being commended," says Gerard, "against the bloody flux." People in rural districts make an ointment from its leaves for burns and scalds. It was formerly, in company with the common Maidenhair Fern, one of the five great capillary herbs. Dr. Tuthill Massy advises the drinking, in Bright's disease, of as much as three half-pints daily of an infusion of this Fern, whilst always taking care to gather the young shoots. Also, in combination (H.) with the American Golden Seal (*Hydrastis canadensis*), the Hart's Tongue has served in not a few authenticated cases to arrest the progress of that formidable disease, diabetes mellitus. Its distilled water will quiet any palpitations of the heart, and will stay the hiccough ; it will likewise help the falling of the palate (relaxed throat), or stop bleeding of the gums if the mouth be gargled therewith.

From the *Ophioglossum vulgatum*, "Adder's tongue," or "Christ's Spear," when boiled in olive oil is produced a most excellent greene oyle, or rather a balsam for greene wounds, comparable to oyle of St. John's Wort, if it doth not far surpasse it." A preparation from this plant known as the "green oil of charity," is still in request as a vulnerary, and remedy for wounds.

The true Maidenhair Fern (*Adiantum capillus veneris*), of exquisite foliage, and of a dark crimson colour, is a stranger in England, except in the West country. But we have in greater abundance the common Maidenhair (*Asplenium trichomanes*), which grows on old walls, and which will act as a laxative medicine; whilst idiots are said to have taken it remedially, so as to recover their senses. The true Maidenhair is named *Adiantum*, from the Greek: *Quod denso imbre cadente destillans foliis tenuis non insidet humor*, "Because the leaves are not wetted even by a heavily falling shower of rain." "In vain," saith Pliny, "do you plunge the Adiantum into water, it always remains dry." This veracious plant doth "strengthen and embellish the hair." It occurs but rarely with us, on damp rocks, and walls near the sea. The Maidenhair is called *Polytrichon* because it brings forth a multitude of hairs;

Calitrichon because it produces black and faire hair; *Capillus veneris* because it fosters grace and love.

From its fine hairlike stems, and perhaps from its attributed virtues in toilet use, this Fern has acquired the name of "Our Lady's Hair" and "Maria's Fern." "The true Maidenhair," says Gerard, "maketh the hair of the head and beard to grow that is fallen and pulled off." From this graceful Fern a famous elegant syrup is made in Franco called *Capillaire*, which is given as a favourite medicine in pulmonary catarrh. It is flavoured with orange flowers, and acts as a demulcent with slightly stimulating effects. One part of the plant is gently boiled with ten parts of water, and with nineteen parts of white sugar. Dr. Johnson says Boswell used to put *Capillaire* into his port wine. Sir John Hill instructed us that (as we cannot get the true Maidenhair fresh in England) the fine syrup made in France from their Fern in perfection, concocted with pure Narbonne honey, is not by any means to be thought a trifle, because barley water, sweetened with this, is one of the very best remedies for a violent cold. But a tea brewed from our more common Maidenhair will answer the same purpose for tedious coughs. Its leaves are sweet, mucilaginous, and expectorant, being, therefore, highly useful in many pulmonary disorders.

The common Polypody Fern, or "rheum-purging Polypody" grows plentifully in this country on old walls and stumps of trees, in shady places. In Hampshire it is called "Adder's Tongue," as derived from the word *attor*, poison; also Wall-fern, and formerly in Anglo-Saxon Ever-fern, or Boar-fern. In Germany it is said to have sprung from the Virgin's milk, and is named *Marie bregue.* The fresh root has been used successfully in decoction, or powdered, for melancholia;

also of late for general rheumatic swelling of the joints. By the ancients it was employed as a purgative. Six drachms by weight of the root should be infused for two hours in a pint of boiling water, and given in two doses. This is the Oak Fern of the herbalists, not that of modern botanists *(Polypodium dryopteris)*, it being held that such Fern plants as grew upon the roots of an oak tree were of special medicinal powers, *Quod nascit super radices quercûs est efficacius.* The true Oak Fern (*Dryopteris*) grows chiefly in mountainous districts among the mossy roots of old oak trees, and sometimes in marshy places. If its root is bruised and applied to the skin of any hairy part, whilst the person is sweating, this will cause the hair to come away. Dioscorides said, "The root of Polypody is very good for chaps between the fingers." "It serveth," writes Gerard, "to make the belly soluble, being boiled in the broth of an old cock, with beets or mallows, or other like things, that move to the stool by their slipperiness." Parkinson says: "A dram or two, if need be, of the powdered dry roots taken fasting, in a cupful of honeyed water, worketh gently as a purge, being a safe medicine, fit for all persons and seasons, which daily experience confirmeth." "Applied also to the nose it cureth the disease called polypus, which by time and sufferance stoppeth the nostrils." The leaves of the Polypody when burnt furnish a large proportion of carbonate of Potash.

The Spleenwort (*Asplenium ceterach*—an Arabian term), or Scaly Fern, or Finger Fern, grows on old walls, and in the clefts of moist rocks. It is also called "Miltwaste," because supposed to cure disorders of the milt, or spleen :—

> "The Finger Fern, which being given to swine,
> It makes their milt to melt away in fine."

Very probably this reputed virtue has mainly become attributed to the plant, because the lobular milt-like shape of its leaf resembles the form of the spleen. "No herbe maie be compared therewith," says one of the oldest Herbals, "for his singular virtue to help the sicknesse or grief of the splene." Pliny ordered: "It should not be given to women, because it bringeth barrenness." Vitruvius alleged that in Crete the flocks and herds were found to be without spleens, because they browsed on this fern. The plant was supposed when given medicinally to diminish the size of the enlarged spleen or "ague-cake."

The Wall Rue *(Ruta muraria)* is a white Maidenhair Fern, and is named by some *Salvia vitæ.* It is a small herb, somewhat nearly of the colour of Garden Rue, and is likewise good for them that have a cough, or are shortwinded, or be troubled with stitches in the sides. It stayeth the falling or shedding of the hair, and causeth them to grow thick, fair, and well coloured. This plant is held by those of judgment and experience, to be as effectual a capillary herb as any whatever. Also, it helpeth ruptures in children. Matthiolus "hath known of divers holpen therein by taking the powder of the herb in drink for forty days together." Its leaves are like those of Rue, and the Fern has been called Tentwort from its use as a specific or sovereign remedy for the cure of rickets, a disease once known as "the taint."

The generic appellations of the several species of Ferns are derived thus: *Aspidium,* from *aspis,* a shield, because the spores are enclosed in bosses; *Pteris,* from *pteerux,* a wing, having doubly pinnate fronds; or from *pteron,* a feather, having feathery fronds; *Scolopendrium,* because the fructification is supposed to resemble the feet of *Scolopendra,* a genus of mydrapods; and *Polypody,* many footed, by reason of the pectinate fronds.

There grows in Tartary a singular polypody Fern, of which the hairy root is easily made to simulate in form a small sheep. It rises above the ground with excrescences resembling a head and tail, whilst having four leg-like fronds. Fabulous stories are told about this remarkable Fern root; and in China its hairy down is so highly valued as a styptic for fresh bleeding cuts and wounds, that few families will be without it. Dr. Darwin, in his *Loves of the Plants*, says about this curious natural production, the *Polypodium Barometz*:—

"Cradled in snow, and fanned by Arctic air
Shines, gentle Barometz, thy golden hair;
Rooted in earth each cloven hoof descends,
And round and round her flexile neck she bends:
Crops the green coral moss, and hoary thyme,
Or laps with rosy tongue the melting rime;
Eyes with mute tenderness her distant dam,
Or seems to bleat—a vegetable Lamb."

FEVERFEW.

THE Feverfew is one of the wild Chamomiles *(Pyrethrum Parthenium)*, or *Matricaria*, so called because especially useful for motherhood. Its botanical names come from the Latin *febrifugus*, putting fever to flight, and *parthenos*, a virgin. The herb is a Composite plant, and grows in every hedgerow, with numerous small heads of yellow flowers, having outermost white rays, but with an upright stem; whereas that of the true garden Chamomile is procumbent. The whole plant has a pungent odour, and is particularly disliked by bees. A double variety is cultivated in gardens for ornamental purposes.

The herb Feverfew is strengthening to the stomach, preventing hysteria and promoting the monthly functions of women. It is much used by country mediciners, though insufficiently esteemed by the doctors of to-day.

In Devonshire the plant is known as "Bachelor's buttons," and at Torquay as "Flirtwort," being also sometimes spoken of as "Feathyfew," or "Featherfull."

Gerard says it may be used both in drinks, and bound on the wrists, as of singular virtue against the ague.

As "Feverfue," it was ordered, by the Magi of old, "to be pulled from the ground with the left hand, and the fevered patient's name must be spoken forth, and the herbarist must not look behind him." Country persons have long been accustomed to make curative uses of this herb very commonly, which grows abundantly throughout England. Its leaves are feathery and of a delicate green colour, being conspicuous even in mid-winter. Chemically, the Feverfew furnishes a blue volatile oil, containing a camphoraceous stearopten, and a liquid hydrocarbon, together with some tannin, and a bitter mucilage.

The essential oil is medicinally useful for correcting female irregularities, as well as for obviating cold indigestion. The herb is also known as "Maydeweed," because useful against hysterical distempers, to which young women are subject. Taken generally it is a positive tonic to the digestive and nervous systems. Our chemists make a medicinal tincture of Feverfew, the dose of which is from ten to twenty drops, with a spoonful of water, three times a day. This tincture, if dabbed on the parts with a small sponge, will immediately relieve the pain and swelling caused by bites of insects or vermin. In the official guide to Switzerland directions are given to take "a little powder of the plant called *Pyrethrum roseum*, and make it into a paste with a few drops of spirit, then apply this to the hands and face, or any exposed part of the body, and let it dry: no mosquito or fly will then touch you." Or if two teaspoonfuls of the tincture are mixed with half a pint of cold water, and if all parts of the body likely to be exposed to the bites of insects are freely sponged therewith they will remain unassailed. Feverfew is manifestly the progenitor of the true Chamomilla *(Anthemis nobilis)*, from which the highly useful Camomile "blows," so commonly employed in domestic medicine, are obtained, and its flowers, when dried, may be applied to the same purposes. An infusion of them made with boiling water and allowed to become cold, will allay any distressing sensitiveness to pain in a highly nervous subject, and will afford relief to the faceache or earache of a dyspeptic or rheumatic person. This Feverfew (*Chrysanthemum parthenium*), is best calculated to pacify those who are liable to sudden, spiteful, rude irascibility, of which they are conscious, but say they cannot help it, and to soothe fretful children. "Better is a dinner of such herbs, where love is, than a stalled ox, and hatred therewith."

FIGS.

"IN the name of the Prophet 'Figs'" was the pompous utterance ascribed to Dr. Johnson, whose solemn magniloquent style was simulated as Eastern cant applied to common business in *Rejected Addresses*, by the clever humorists, Horace and James Smith, 1812. The tree which produces this fruit belongs to the history of mankind. In Paradise Adam partook of figs, and covered his nakedness with the leaves.

Though indigenous to Western Asia, Figs have been cultivated in most countries from a remote period, and will ripen in England during a warm summer if screened from north-east winds. The figtree flourishes best with us on our sea coasts, bathed by the English Channel, by reason of the salt-laden atmosphere. Near Gosport, and at Fig Valleys, in the neighbourhood of Worthing, there are orchards of figtrees; but they remain barren in this country as far as affording seed to be raised anew from the ripened fruit. The first figtrees introduced into England are still alive and productive in the gardens of the Archbishop of Canterbury, at Lambeth, having been planted there by Cardinal Pole in the time of Henry the Eighth. We call the Sunday before Easter "Fig Sunday," probably because of our Saviour's quest of the fruit when going from Bethany the next day.

By the Jews a want of blossom on the Fig tree was considered a grievous calamity. On the Saturday preceding Palm Sunday (says Miss Baker), the market at Northampton is abundantly supplied with figs, and more of the fruit is purchased at this time than throughout the rest of the year. Even charity children are regaled in some parts with figs on the said Sunday; whilst in Lancashire fig pies made of dried figs with sugar and treacle are eaten beforehand in Lent.

In order to become fertilised, figs (of which the sexual apparatus lies within the fruit) must have their outer skin perforated by certain gnats of the Cynips tribe, which then penetrate to the interior whilst carrying with them the fertilising pollen; but these gnats are not found in this country. Producers of the fruit abroad bearing the said fact in view tie some of the wild fruit when tenanted by the Culex fly to the young cultivated figs.

Foreign figs are dried in the oven so as to destroy the larvæ of the Cynips insect, and are then compressed into small boxes. They consist in this state almost exclusively of mucilage and sugar.

Only one kind of Fig comes to ripeness with us in England, the great blue Fig, as large as a Catherine pear. "It should be grown," says Gerard, "under a hot wall, and eaten when newly gathered, with bread, pepper, and salt; or it is excellent in tarts." This fruit is soft, easily digested, and corrective of strumous disease. Dried Turkey Figs, as imported, contain glucose (sugar), starch, fat, pectose, gum, albumen, mineral matter, cellulose, and water. They are used by our druggists as an ingredient in confection of senna for a gentle laxative effect. When split open, and applied as hot as they can be borne against gumboils, and similar suppurative gatherings, they afford ease, and promote maturation of the abscess; and likewise they will help raw, unhealthy sores to heal. The first poultice of Figs on record is that employed by King Hezekiah 260 years before Christ, at the instance of the prophet Isaiah, who ordered to "take a lump of Figs; and they took it, and laid it on the boil, and the King recovered" (2 Kings xx. 7).

The Fig is said to have been the first fruit eaten as food by man. Among the Greeks it formed part of the ordinary Spartan fare, and the Athenians forbade exportation of the best Figs, which were highly valued at table. Informers against those who offended in this respect were called *Suko phantai*, or Fig discoverers—our *Sycophants.*

Bacchus was thought to have acquired his vigour and corpulency from eating Figs, such as the Romans gave to professed wrestlers and champions for strength and good sustenance.

Dodonœus said concerning Figs, *Alimentum amplius quam cœteri prœbent*; and Pliny spoke of them as the best restorative for those brought low by languishing disease, with loss of their colour. It was under the Perpul tree (*Ficus religiosa*) Buddha attained Nirvada.

The botanical name *ficus* has been derived from the Greek verb *phuo* to generate, and the husbandry of Figs was called by the Latins "caprification." The little fig-bird of the Roman Campagna pays a yearly visit in September to the fig orchards on our Sussex coast.

When eaten raw, dried Figs prove somewhat aperient, and they are apt to make the mouth sore whilst masticating them. Their seeds operate mechanically against constipation, though sometimes irritating the lining membrane of the stomach and bowels. Grocers prepare from the pulp of these foreign dried figs, when mixed with honey, a jam called "figuine," which is wholesome, and will prevent costiveness if eaten at breakfast with bread.

The pulp of Turkey Figs is mucilaginous, and has been long esteemed as a pectoral emollient for coughs: also when stewed and, added to ptisans, for catarrhal troubles of the air passages, and of other mucous canals.

In its fresh green state the fruit secretes a milky acrid juice, which will destroy warts; this afterwards becomes saccharine and oily. The dried Figs of the shops give no idea of the fresh fruit as enjoyed in Italy at breakfast, which then seem indeed a fruit of paradise, and which contain a considerable quantity of grape sugar. In the *Regimen of the School of Salerne* (eleventh century) we read :—

> "Scrofa, tumor, glandes, ficus cataplasma sedet,
> Swines' evil, swellings, kernels, a plaster of figs will heal."

Barley water boiled with dried Figs (split open), liquorice root, and raisins, forms the compound decoction of barley prescribed by doctors as a capital demulcent;

and an admirable gargle for inflamed sore throat may be made by boiling two ounces of the Figs in half-a-pint of water, which is to be strained when cool. Figs cooked in milk make an excellent drink for costive persons.

In the French codex a favourite pectoral medicine is composed of Figs, stoned dates, raisins, and jujubes.

Formerly the poisoned Fig was used in Spain as a secret means for getting rid of an enemy. The fruit was so common there that to say "a fig for you!" and "I give you the fig" became proverbial expressions of contempt. *In fiocchi* (in gala costome), is an Italian phrase which we now render as "in full fig."

The *Water Figwort*, a common English plant which grows by the sides of ditches, and belongs to the scrofula-curing order, has acquired its name because supposed to heal sores in the fundament when applied like figs as a poultice. It further bears the name of *Water Betony (page* 50), under which title its curative excellence against piles, and for scrofulous glands in the neck has been already described. The whole plant, yielding its juice, may be blended with lard to be used as an ointment; and an infusion of the roots, made with boiling water, an ounce to a pint, may be taken as a medicine—a wineglassful three times in the day.

In Ireland it is known as "Rose noble," also as Kernelwort, because the kernels, or tubers attached to the roots have been thought to resemble scrofulous glands in the neck. "Divers do rashly teach that if it be hanged about the necke, or else carried about one it keepeth a man in health." In France the sobriquet *herbe du seige*, given to this plant, is said to have been derived from its famous use in healing all sorts of wounds during the long siege of Rochelle under Louis XIII.

The Water Figwort may be readily known by the winged corners of its stems, which, though hollow and succulent, are rigid when dead, and prove very troublesome to anglers. The flowers are much frequented by wasps: and the leaves are employed to correct the taste of senna.

FLAG (Common).

OUR English water Flags are true whigs of the old school, and get their generic name because hanging out their banners respectively of dark blue and yellow.

Each is also called *Iris*, as resembling the rainbow in beauty of colour. The land Flag (*Iris versicolor*) is well known as growing in swamps and moist meadows, with sword-shaped leaves, and large purple heads of flowers, bearing petals chiefly dark blue, and veined with green, yellow, or white. The water Flag (*Iris pseudacorus*) is similar of growth, and equally well known by its brilliant heads of yellow flowers, with blade-like leaves, being found in wet places and water courses. The root of the Blue Flag, "Dragon Flower," or "Dagger Flower," contains chemically an "oleo-resin," which is purgative to the liver in material doses, and specially alleviative against bilious sickness when taken of much reduced strength by reason of its acting as a similar. The official dose of this "iridin" is from one to three grains. A liability to the formation of gall stones may be remedied by giving one grain of the oleo-resin (iridin) every night for twelve nights.

A medicinal tincture (H.) is made which holds this Iris in solution; and if three or four drops are taken immediately, with a spoonful of water, and the same dose is repeated in half-an-hour if still necessary, an attack of bilious vomiting, with sick headache, and a film before the eyes, will be prevented, or cut short. The remedy is, under such circumstances, a trustworthy substitute for calomel, or blue pill. Orris powder, which is so popular in the nursery, and for the toilet table with ladies, on account of its fresh "violet" scent, is made from the root of this Iris, being named from the genitive *ireos*.

Louis VII. of France chose this Blue Flag as his heraldic emblem, and hence its name, *fleur de lys*, has been subsequently borne on the arms of France. The flower was said to have been figured on a shield sent down from heaven to King Louis at Clovis, when fighting against the Saracens. *Fleur de Louis* has become corrupted to *fleur de lys*, or *fleur de lis*.

The Purple Flag was formerly dedicated to the Virgin Mary. A certain knight more devout than learned could never remember more than two words of the Latin prayer addressed to the Holy Mother; these were *Ave Maria*, which the good old man repeated day and night until he died. Then a plant of the blue Iris sprang up over his grave, displaying on every flower in golden letters these words, *Ave Maria*. When the monks opened the tomb they found the root of the plant resting on the lips of the holy knight whose body lay buried below.

The Yellow Flag, or Water Flag, is called in the north, "Seggs." Its flowers afford a beautiful yellow dye; and its seeds, when roasted, can be used instead of coffee. The juice of the root is very acrid when sniffed up the nostrils, and causes a copious flow of water therefrom, thus giving marked relief for obstinate congestive headache of a dull, passive sort. The root is very astringent, and will check diarrhœa by its infusion; also it is of service for making ink. In the south of England the plant is named "Levers." It contains much tannin.

The "Stinking Flag," or "Gladdon," or "Roast Beef," because having the odour of this viand, is another British species of Flag, abundant in southern England, where it grows in woods and shady places. Its leaves, when bruised, emit a strong smell like that of carrion, which is very loathsome. The plant bears the appellations, *Iris fœtidissima*, *Spatula fœtida*, and "Spurgewort," having long, narrow leaves, which stink when rubbed. Country folk in Somersetshire purge themselves to good purpose with a decoction made from the root. The term "glad," or "smooth," refers to the surface of the leaves, or to their sword-like shape, from *gladiolus* (a small sword), and the plant bears flowers of a dull, livid purple, smaller than those of the other flags.

Lastly, there is the Sweet Flag (*Acorus calamus*), though this is not an Iris, but belongs botanically to the family of *Arums*. It grows on the edges of lakes and streams all over Europe, as a highly aromatic, reedy plant, with an erect flowering stem of yellowish green colour. Its name comes from the Greek, *koree*, or "pupil of the eye," because of its being used in ailments of that organ.

Calamus was the Roman term for a reed; and formerly this sweet Flag, by reason of its pleasant odour like that of violets, was freely strewn on the floor of a cathedral at times of church festivals, and in many private houses instead of rushes. The root is a powerful cordial against flatulence, and passive indigestion, with headache. It contains a volatile oil, and a bitter principle, "acorin;" so that a fluid extract is made by the chemists, of which from thirty to forty drops may be given as a dose, with a tablespoonful of water, every half-hour for several consecutive times. The candied root is much employed for like uses in Turkey and India. It is sold as a favourite medicine in every Indian Bazaar; and Ainslie says it is reckoned so valuable in the bowel complaints of children, that there is a penalty incurred by every druggist who will not open his door in the middle of the night to sell it if demanded.

The root stocks are brought to this country from Germany, being used by mastication to clear the urine when it is thick and loaded with dyspeptic products; also for flavouring beer, and scenting snuff.

Their ash contains potash, soda, zinc, phosphoric acid, silica, and peroxide of iron. In the *Times* April 24th, 1856, Dr. Graves wrote commending for the soldiers when landing at Galipoli, and not able to obtain costly quinine, the Sweet Flag—*acorus calamus*—as their sheet anchor against ague and allied maladies arising from *marsh miasmata*. The infusion of the root should be given, or the powdered root in doses of from ten to sixty grains. (*See* RUSHES.)

FLAX (LINSEED).

THE common Flax plant, from which we get our Linseed, is of great antiquity, dating from the twenty-third century before Christ, and having been cultivated in all countries down to the present time. But it is exhausting to the soil in England, and therefore not favoured in home growth for commercial uses. The seeds come to us chiefly from the Baltic. Nevertheless, the plant (*Linum usitatissimum*) is by no means uncommon in our cornfields, flowering in June, and ripening its seed in September. Provincially it is called "Lint" and "Lyne." A rustic proverb says "if put in the shoes it preserves from poverty"; wherever found it is probably an escape from cultivation.

The word "flax" is derived from *filare*, to spin, or, *filum*, a thread; and the botanical title, *linum*, is got from the Celtic *lin* also signifying thread. The fibres of the bark are separated from the woody matter by soaking it in water, and they then form tow, which is afterwards spun into yarn, and woven into cloth. This water becomes poisonous, so that Henry the Eighth prohibited the washing of flax in any running stream.

The seeds are very rich in linseed oil, after expressing which, the refuse is oil-cake, a well-known fattening food for cattle. The oil exists chiefly in the outer skins of the seeds, and is easily extracted by boiling water, as in the making a linseed poultice. These seeds contain gum, acetic acid, acetate and muriate of potash, and other salts, with twenty-two parts per cent. of the oil. They were taken as food by the ancient Greeks and Romans, whilst Hippocrates knew the demulcent properties of linseed. An infusion of the seeds has long been given as Linseed tea for soothing a sore chest or throat in severe catarrh, or pulmonary complaints; also the crushed seed is used for making poultices. Linseed oil has laxative properties, and forms, when mixed with lime water, or with spirit of turpentine, a capital external application to recent burns or scalds.

Tumours of a simple nature, and sprains, may be usefully rubbed with Linseed oil; and another principal service to which the oil is put is for mixing the paints of artists. To make Linseed tea, wash two ounces of Linseed by putting them into a small strainer, and pouring cold water through it; then pare off as thinly as possible the yellow rind of half a lemon; to the Linseed and lemon rind add a quart of cold water, and allow them to simmer over the fire for an hour-and-a-half; strain away the seeds, and to each half-pint of the tea add a teaspoonful of sugar, or sugar candy, with some lemon juice, in the proportion of the juice of one lemon to each pint of tea.

The seeds afford but little actual nourishment, and are difficult of digestion; they provoke troublesome flatulence, though sometimes used fraudulently for adulterating pepper. Flax seed has been mixed with corn for making bread, but it proved indigestible and hurtful to the stomach. In the sixteenth century during a scarcity of wheat, the inhabitants of Middleburgh had recourse to Linseed for making cakes, but the death of many citizens was caused thereby, it bringing about in those who partook of the cakes dreadful swellings on the body and face. There is an Act of Parliament still in force which forbids the steeping of Flax in rivers, or any waters which cattle are accustomed to drink, as it is found to communicate a poison destructive to cattle, and to the fish inhabiting such waters. In Dundee a hank of yarn is worn round the loins as a cure for lumbago, and girls may be seen with a single thread of yarn round the head as an infallible specific for tic douloureux.

The Purging Flax (*Linum catharticum*), or Mill Mountain (*Kamailinon*), or Ground Flax, is a variety of the Flax common on our heaths and pastures, being called also Fairy Flax from its delicacy, and Dwarf Flax. It contains a resinous, purgative principle, and is known to country folk as a safe, active purge. They infuse the herb in water, which they afterwards take medicinally Also a tincture is made (H.) from the entire fresh plant, which may be given curatively for frequent, watery, painless diarrhœa, two or three drops for a dose with water every hour or two until the flux is stayed.

FOXGLOVE.

THE purple Foxglove (*Digitalis purpurea*) which every one knows and admires for its long graceful spikes of elegant bell-shaped brilliant blossoms seen in our woods and hedges, is also called the Thimble Flower, or the Finger Flower, from the resemblance of these blossoms to a thimble or to the fingers of a glove. The word *digitalis* refers likewise to the digits, or fingers of a gauntlet. In France the title is *Gants de Notre Dame*, the gloves of our Lady the Virgin. Some writers give Folks' Glove, or Fairies' Glove as the proper English orthography, but this is wrong. Our name of the plant comes really from the Anglo-Saxon, Foxesglew or Fox music, in allusion to an ancient musical instrument composed of bells which were hanging from an arched support, *a tintinnabulum*, which this plant with its pendent bell-shaped flowers so exactly represents.

In Ireland the Foxglove is known as the Great Herb, and Lusmore, also the Fairy Cap ; and in Wales it is the Goblin's Gloves ; whilst in the North of Scotland it is the Dead men's Bells. We read in the *Lady of the Lake* there grew by Loch Katrine :--

> "Night shade and Foxglove side by side,
> Emblems of punishment and pride."

In Devonshire the plant is termed Poppy, because when one of the bell-shaped flowers is inflated by the breath whilst the top edges are held firmly together, the wind bag thus formed, if struck smartly against the other hand, goes off with a sounding pop. The peasantry also call it "Flop a dock." Strangely enough, the Foxglove, so handsome and striking in a landscape, is not mentioned by Shakespeare, or by either of the old English poets. The "long purples" of Shakespeare refers to the *orchis mascula.*

Chemically, the Foxglove contains a dangerous, active, medicinal principle *digitalin*, which acts powerfully on the heart, and on the kidneys, but this should never be given in any preparation of the plant except under medical guidance, and then only with much caution. Parkinson speaks highly of the bruised herb, or of its expressed juice, for scrofulous swellings when applied outwardly in the form of an ointment. An officinal tincture is made from the plants collected in the spring, when two years old; also, in some villages the infusion is employed as a homely remedy to cure a cold, the herb being known as "Throttle Wort;" but this is not a safe thing to do, for medical experience shows that the watery infusion of Foxglove acts much more powerfully than the spirituous tincture, which is eight times stronger, and from this fact it may fairly be inferred that the presence of alcohol, as in the tincture, directly opposes the specific action of the plant. This herb bears further in some districts the names "Flop Top," "Cow Flop," and "Flabby Dock." It was stated in the *Times Telescope*, 1822, "the women of the poorer class in Derbyshire used to indulge in copious draughts of Foxglove tea, as a cheap means of obtaining the pleasures of intoxication. This was found to produce a great exhilaration of the spirits, with other singular effects on the system. So true is the maxim, *ubi virus, ibi virtus.*

No animal will touch the plant, which is biennial, and will only develop its active principle *digitalin*, when getting some sunshine, but remains inert when grown altogether in the shade. Therefore its source of production for medicinal purposes is very important.

FUMITORY.

THE common Fumitory (*Fumaria officinalis*) is a small grey-green plant, bearing well known little flowers, rose coloured, and tipped with purple, whilst standing erect in every cornfield, vineyard, or such-like manured place throughout Great Britain. It is so named from the Latin *fumus terræ*, earth smoke, which refers either to the appearance of its pretty glaucous foliage on a dewy summer morning, or to the belief that it was produced not from seed but from vapours rising out of the earth. The plant continues to flower throughout the year, and was formerly much favoured for making cosmetic washes to purify the skin of rustic maidens in the spring time:—

> "Whose red and purpled mottled flowers
> Are cropped by maids in weeding hours
> To boil in water, milk, or whey,
> For washes on a holiday;
> To make their beauty fair and sleek,
> And scare the tan from summer's cheek."

In many parts of Kent the Fumitory bears the name of "Wax Dolls," because its rose coloured flowers, with their little, dark, purple heads, are by no means unlike the small waxen toys given as nurslings to children.

Dioscorides affirmed: "The juice of Fumitory, of that which groweth among barley, with gum arabic, doth take away unprofitable hairs that prick, being first plucked away, for it will not suffer others to grow in their places." "It helpeth," says Gerard, "in the summer time those that are troubled with scabs."

Pliny said it is named because causing the eyes to water as smoke does. In Shakespeare the name is written Fumiter. It continues to flower throughout the year, and its presence is thought to indicate good deep rich land. There is also a "ramping" Fumitory (*capreolata*) which climbs; being found likewise in fields and waste places, but its infusion produces purgative effects.

The whole plant has a saline, bitter, and somewhat acrid taste. It contains "fumaric acid," and the alkaloid "fumarina," which are specially useful for scrofulous diseases of the skin. A decoction of the herb makes a curative lotion for the milk-crust which disfigures the scalp of an infant, and for grown up persons troubled with chronic eruptions on the face, or freckles.

The fresh juice may be given as a medicine; or an infusion made with an ounce of the plant to a pint of boiling water, one wineglassful for a dose twice or three times in the day.

By the ancients Fumitory was named *Capnos*, smoke: Pliny wrote "*Claritatem facit inunctis oculis delachrymationemque, ceu fumus, unde nomen.*" They esteemed the herb specially useful for dispelling dimness of the sight, and for curing other infirmities of the eyes.

The leaves, which have no particular odour, throw up crystals of nitre on their surface when cool. The juice may be mixed with whey, and taken as a common drink, or as a medicinal beverage for curing obstinate skin eruptions, and for overcoming obstructions of the liver and digestive organs. Dr. Cullen found it most useful in leprous skin disease. The juice from the fresh herb may be given two ounces in the day, but the virtues remain equally in the dried plant. Its smoke was said by the ancient exorcists to have the power of expelling evil spirits. The famous physician, John of Milan, extolled Fumitory as a sovereign remedy against malarious fever.

It is a remarkable fact, that the colour of the hair and the complexion seem to determine the liability, or otherwise, of a European to West Coast fever in Africa. A man with harsh, bright-coloured red hair, such as is common in Scotland, has a complete immunity, though running the same risks as another man, dark and with a dry skin, who seems absolutely doomed. A red-haired European will, as a rule, keep his health where even the natives are attacked. Old negresses have secret methods of cure which can, undoubtedly, save life even in cases which have become hopeless to European medical science.

GARLIC, LEEK, and ONION.

SEEMING at first sight out of place among the lilies of the field, yet Garlic, the Leek, and the Onion are true members of that noble order, and may be correctly classified together with the favoured tribe, "Clothed more grandly than Solomon in all his glory." They possess alike the same properties and characteristics, though in varying degrees, and they severally belong to the genus *Allium*, each containing "allyl," which is a radical rich in sulphur.

The homely Onion may be taken first as the best illustration of the family. This is named technically *Allium cepa*, from *cep*, a head (of bunched florets which it bears). Lucilius called it *Flebile cæpe*, because the pungency of its odour will provoke a flow of tears from the eyes. As Shakespeare says, in *Taming of the Shrew*:—

> "Mine eyes smell onions;
> I shall weep anon."

The Egyptians were devoted to Onions, which they ate more than two thousand years before the time of Christ. They were given to swear by the Onion and

Garlic in their gardens. Herodotus tells us that during the building of the pyramids nine tons of gold were spent in buying onions for the workmen. But it is to be noted that in Egypt the Onion is sweet and soft; whereas, in other countries it grows hard, and nauseous, and strong.

By the Greeks this bulb was called Krommuon, "*apo tou Meuein tas koras*," because of shutting the eyes when eating it. In Latin its name *unio*, signified a single root without offsets.

Raw Onions contain an acrid volatile oil, sulphur, phosphorus, alkaline earthy salts, phosphoric and acetic acids, with phosphate and citrate of lime, starch, free uncrystallized sugar, and lignine. The fresh juice is colourless, but by exposure to the air becomes red. A syrup made from the juice with honey is an excellent medicine for old phlegmatic persons in cold weather, when their lungs are stuffed, and the breathing is hindered.

Raw Onions increase the flow of urine, and promote perspiration, insomuch, that a diet of them, with bread, has many a time cured dropsy coming on through a chill at first, or from exposure to cold. They contain the volatile principle, "sulphide of allyl," which is acrid and stimulating. If taken in small quantities, Onions quicken the circulation, and assist digestion; but when eaten more prodigally they disagree.

In making curative Simples, the Onion (and Garlic) should not be boiled, else the volatile essential oil, on which its virtues chiefly depend, will escape during the process.

The principal internal effects of the Onion, the Leek, and Garlic, are stimulation and warmth, so that they are of more salutary use when the subject is of a cold temperament, and when the vital powers are feeble, than when the body is feverish, and the constitution ardently excitable. "They be naught," says Gerard, "for those that be cholericke; but good for such as are replete with raw and phlegmatick humors." *Vous tous qui etes gros, et gras, et lymphatiques, avec l'estomac paresseux, mangez l'oignon cru; c'est pour vous que le bon Dieu l'a fait.*

Onions, when eaten at night by those who are not feverish, will promote sleep, and induce perspiration. The late Frank Buckland confirmed this statement. He said, "I am sure the essential oil of Onions has soporific powers. In my own case it never fails. If I am much pressed with work, and feel that I am not disposed to sleep, I eat two or three small Onions, and the effect is magical." The Onion has a very sensitive organism, and absorbs all morbid matter that comes in its way. During our last epidemic of cholera it puzzled the sanitary inspectors of a northern town why the tenants of one cottage in an infected row were not touched by the plague. At last some one noticed a net of onions hanging in the fortunate house, and on examination all these proved to have become diseased. But whilst welcoming this protective quality, the danger must be remembered of eating an onion which shows signs of decay, for it cannot be told what may have caused this distemper.

When sliced, and applied externally, the raw Onion serves by its pungent and essential oil to quicken the circulation, and to redden the skin of the particular surface treated in this way; very usefully so in the case of an unbroken chilblain, or to counteract neuralgic pain; but in its crude state the bulb is not emollient or demulcent. If employed as a poultice for ear-ache, or broken chilblains, the Onion should be roasted, so as to modify its acrid oil. When there is a constant and painful discharge of fetid matter from the ear, or where an abscess is threatened, with pain, heat, and swelling, a hot poultice of roasted Onions will be found very useful, and will mitigate the pain. The juice of a sliced raw Onion is alkaline, and will quickly relieve the acid venom of a sting from a wasp, or bee, if applied immediately to the part.

A tincture is made (H.) from large, red, strong Onions for medicinal purposes. As a warming expectorant in chronic bronchitis, or asthma, or for a cold which is not of a feverish character, from half to one teaspoonful of this tincture may be given with benefit three or four times in the day in a wineglassful of hot water, or hot milk. Likewise, a jorum (*i.e.*, an earthen bowl) of hot Onion broth taken at bed time, serves admirably to soothe the air passages, and to promote perspiration, after the first feverish stage of catarrh or influenza has passed by. To make this, peel a large Spanish Onion, and divide it into four parts; then put them into a saucepan, with half a saltspoonful of salt, and two ounces of butter, and a pint of cold water; let them simmer gently until quite tender; next pour all into a bowl which has been made hot, dredging a little pepper over; and let the porridge be eaten as hot as it can be taken.

The allyl and sulphur in the bulbs, together with their mucilaginous parts, relieve the sore mucous membranes, and quicken perspiration, whilst other medicinal virtues are exercised at the same time on the animal economy.

By eating a few raw parsley sprigs immediately afterwards, the strong smell which onions communicates to the breath may be removed and dispelled. Lord

Bacon averred "the rose will be sweeter if planted in a bed of onions." So nutritious does the Highlander find this vegetable, that, if having a few raw bulbs in his pocket, with oat-cake, or a crust of bread, he can travel for two or three days together without any other food. Dean Swift said :—

> "This is every cook's opinion,
> No savoury dish without an onion,
> But lest your kissing should be spoiled,
> Your onions must be fully boiled."

Provings have been made by medical experts of the ordinary red Onion in order to ascertain what its toxical effects are when pushed to an excessive degree, and it has been found that Onions, Leeks, or Garlic, when taken immoderately, induce melancholy and depression, with severe catarrh. They dispose to sopor, lethargy, and even insanity. The immediate symptoms are extreme watering of the eyes after frequent sneezing, confusion of the head, and heavy defluxion from the nose, with pains in the throat extending to the ears; in a word, all the accompaniments of a bad cold, sneezings, lacrymation, pains in the forehead, and a hoarse, hacking cough. These being the effects of taking Onions in a harmful quantity, it is easy to understand that when the like morbid symptoms have arisen spontaneously from other causes, as from a sharp catarrh of the head and chest, then modified forms of the Onion are calculated to counteract them on the law of similars, so that a cure is promptly produced. On which principle the Onion porridge is a scientific remedy, as food, and as physic, during the first progress of a catarrhal attack; and *pari passu* the medicinal tincture of the red Onion may be likewise curatively given.

Spanish Onions, which are imported into this country in the winter, are sweet and mucilaginous. A peasant in Spain will munch an onion just as an English labourer eats an apple.

At the present day Egyptians take onions, roasted, and each cut into four pieces, with small bits of baked meat, and slices of an acid apple, which the Turks call *kebobs*. With this sweet and savoury dish they are so delighted, that they trust to enjoy it in paradise. The Israelites were willing to return to slavery and brick-making for their love of the Onion; and we read that Hecamedes presented some of the bulbs to Patrochus, in *Homer*, as a regala. These are supplied liberally to the antelopes and giraffes in our Zoological Gardens, which animals dote on the Onion.

A clever paraphrase of the word Onion may be read in the lines :—

> "Charge! Stanley, charge! On! Stanley, on!
> Were the last words of Marmion.
> If *I* had been in Stanley's place
> When Marmion urged him to the chase,
> In me you quickly would descry
> What draws a tear from many an eye."

For chilblains apply onions with salt pounded together, and for inflamed or protruding piles, raw Onion pulp, made by bruising the bulb, if kept bound to the parts by a compress, and renewed as needed, will afford certain relief.

The Garlic (*Allium sativum*), Skorodon of the Greeks, which was first cultivated in English gardens in 1540, takes its name from *gar*, a spear; and *leac*, a plant, either because of its sharp tapering leaves, or perhaps as "the war plant," by reason of its nutritive and stimulating qualities for those who do battle. It is known also to many as "Poor-man's Treacle," or "Churls Treacle," from being regarded by rustics as a treacle, or antidote to the bite of any venomous reptile.

The bulb, consisting of several combined cloves, is stimulating, antispasmodic, expectorant, and diuretic. Its active properties depend on an essential oil which may be readily obtained by distillation. A medicinal tincture is made (H.) with spirit of wine, of which from ten to twenty drops may be taken in water several times a day. Garlic proves useful in asthma, whooping-cough, and other spasmodic affections of the chest. For an adult, one or more cloves may be eaten at a time. The odour of the bulb is very diffusible, even when it is applied to the soles of the feet its odour is exhaled by the lungs.

When bruised and mixed with lard, it makes a most useful opodeldoc to be rubbed in for irritable spines or indolent scrofulous tumours or gout, until the skin surface becomes red and glowing. If employed thus over the chest (back and front) of a child with whooping-cough, it proves eminently helpful.

Raw Garlic, when applied to the skin, reddens it, and the odour sniffed into the nostrils will revive an hysterical sufferer. It formed the principal ingredient in the "Four thieves' vinegar," which was adopted so successfully at Marseilles for protection against the plague, when prevailing there. This originated with four thieves, who confessed that, whilst protected by the liberal use of aromatic vinegar during the plague, they plundered the dead bodies of its victims with complete security. Or, according to another explanation of the name, an old tract, printed in 1749, testifies that one, Richard Forthave, who lived in Bishopsgate Street, invented and sold a vinegar which had such a run that he soon grew famous, and that his surname became thus corrupted in the course of time.

But long before the plague at Marseilles (1722) vinegar was employed as a disinfectant. With Cardinal Wolsey it was a constant custom to carry in his hand an orange emptied of its pulp, and containing a sponge soaked in vinegar made aromatic with spices, so as to protect himself from infection when passing through the crowds which his splendour and his office attracted.

It is related that during a former outbreak of infectious fever in Somer's Town and St. Giles's, the French priests, who constantly used Garlic in all their dishes, visited the worst cases in the dirtiest hovels with impunity, while the English clergy, who were similarly engaged, but who did not eat onions in like fashion, caught the infection in many instances, and fell victims to the disease.

For toothache and earache, a clove of Garlic stripped of its skin, and cut in the form of a suppository, if thrust in the ear of the aching side, will soon assuage the pain. If introduced into the lower bowel, it will help to destroy thread worms, and when swallowed it abolishes round worms.

As a condiment, Garlic undoubtedly aids digestion by stimulating the circulation, with a consequent increase of saliva and gastric juice. The juice from the bulbs can be employed for cementing broken glass or china, by means of its mucilage.

Dr. Bowles, a noted English physician of former times, made use of Garlic with much success as a secret remedy for asthma. He concocted a preserve from the boiled cloves with vinegar and sugar, to be kept in an earthen jar. The dose was a bulb or two with some of the syrup, each morning when fasting.

The pain of rheumatic parts may be much relieved by simply rubbing them with cut Garlic.

Garlic emits the most acrimonious smell of all the onion tribe. When leprosy prevailed in this country, Garlic was a prime specific for its relief, and as the victims had to "pil," or peel their own garlic, they were nicknamed "Pil Garlics," and hence it came about that anyone shunned like a leper had this epithet applied to him. Stow says, concerning a man growing old: "He will soon be a peeled garlic like myself."

The strong penetrating odour and taste of this plant, though offensive to most English palates, are much relished by Russians, Poles, and Spaniards, and especially by the Jews. But the Greeks detested Garlic. It is true the Attic husbandmen ate it from remote times, probably in part to drive away by its odour venomous creatures from assailing them; but persons who partook of it were not allowed to enter the temples of Cybele, says Athenæus; and so hated was garlic, that to have to eat it was a punishment for those that had committed the most horrid crimes. Horace, among the Romans, was made ill by eating garlic at the table of Mæcenas; and afterwards (in his third *Epode*) he reviled the plant as, *Cicutis allium nocentius*, "Garlic more poisonous than hemlock." Sir Theodore Martin has thus spiritedly translated the passage:—

"If his old father's throat any impious sinner,
Has cut with unnatural hand to the bone,
Give him garlick—more noxious than hemlock—at dinner;
Ye gods! what strong stomachs the reapers must own!"

The singular property is attributed to Garlic, that if a morsel of the bulb is chewed by a man running a race, it will prevent his competitors from getting ahead of him. Hungarian jockeys sometimes fasten a clove of garlic to the bits of their racers; and it is said that the horses which run against those thus baited, fall back the moment they smell the offensive odour. If a leg of mutton, before being roasted, has a small clove of Garlic inserted into the knuckle, and the joint is afterwards served with haricot beans (soaked for twenty-four hours before being boiled), it is rendered doubly delicious. In Greece snails dressed with Garlic are now a favourite dish.

A well known *chef* is said to have chewed a small clove of Garlic when he wished to impart its delicate flavour to a choice *plât*, over which he then breathed lightly. Dumas relates that the whole atmosphere of Provence is impregnated with the perfume of Garlic, and is exceedingly wholesome to inhale.

As an instance of lunar influences (which undoubtedly affect our bodily welfare), it is remarkable that if Garlic is planted when the moon is in the full, the bulb will be round like an onion, instead of being composed, as it usually is, of several distinct cloves.

Homer says it was to the virtues of the Yellow Garlic (Moly ?) Ulysses owed his escape from being changed by Circe into a pig, like each of his companions.

The Crow Garlic, *vineale*, and the purple striped, *oleraceum*, grow wild in this country. When the former of these is eaten by birds it so stupefies them that they may be taken with the hand.

Concerning the cure of nervous headache by Garlic (and its kindred medicinal herb *Asafœtida*), an old charm reads thus:—

"Give onyons to Saynt Cutlake,
And Garlycke to Saynt Cyryake;
If ye will shun the headake,
Ye shall have them at Queenhyth."

The Asafœtida (*Ferula Asafœtida*) grows in Western Thibet, and exudes a gum which is used medicinally, coming as a milky juice from the incised root and soon coagulating; it is then exported, having a very powerful odour of garlic which may be perceived a long distance away. Phosphorus and sulphur are among its constituent elements, and, because of the latter, says Dr. Garrod after much observation, he regards Asafœtida as one of the most valuable remedies known to the physician. From three to five grains of the gum in a pill, or half-a-teaspoonful of the tincture, with a small wineglassful of warm milk, may be given for a dose.

Some of the older writers esteemed it highly as an aromatic flavouring spice, and termed it *cibus deorum*, food of the gods. John Evelyn says (in his *Acetaria*) "the ancient Silphium thought by many to be none other than the fetid asa, was so highly prized for its taste and virtues, that it was dedicated to Apollo at Delphi, and stamped upon African coins as a sacred plant."

Aristophanes extolled its juice as a restorer of masculine vigour, and the Indians at this day sauce their viands with it. Nor are some of our skilful cooks ignorant how to condite it, with the applause of those who are unaware of the secret. The Silphium, or *laserpitium* of the Romans, yielded what was a famous restorative, the "Cyrenaic juice." Pareira tells us he was assured by a noted gourmet that the finest relish which a beef steak can possess, may be communicated to it by rubbing the gridiron on which the steak is to be cooked, with Asafœtida.

The gum when given in moderate doses, acts on all parts of the body as a wholesome stimulant, leading among other good results, to improvement of the vision, and enlivening the spirits. But its use is apt to produce eructations smacking of garlic, which may persist for several hours; and, if it be given in over doses, the effects are headache and giddiness. When suitably administered, it quickens the appetite and improves the digestion, chiefly with those of a cold temperament, and languid habit. Smollet says the Romans stuffed their fowls for the table with Asafœtida. In Germany, Sweden, and Italy, it is known as "Devil's Dung."

The Leek (*Allium porrium*) bears an Anglo-Saxon name corrupted from Porleac, and it is also called the Porret, having been the Prason of the Greeks. It was first made use of in England during 1562. This was a food of the poor in ancient Egypt, as is shown by an inscription on one of the Pyramids, whence was derived the phrase, "to eat the Leek"; and its loss was bewailed by the Israelites in their journey through the Desert. It was said by the Romans to be prolific of virtue, because Latona, the mother of Apollo, longed after leeks. The Welsh, who take them much, are observed to be very fruitful. They dedicate these plants to St. David, on whose day, March 1st, in 640, the Britons (who were known to each other by displaying in their caps, at the inspiration of St. David, some leeks, "the fairest emblym that is worne," plucked in a garden near the field of action) gained a complete victory over the Saxons.

The bulb contains some sulphur, and is, in its raw state, a stimulating expectorant. Its juice acts energetically on the kidneys, and dissolves the calculous formations of earthy phosphates which frequently form in the bladder.

For chilblains, chapped hands, and sore eyes, the juice of a leek squeezed out, and mixed with cream, has been found curative. Old Tusser tells us, in his *Husbandry for March*:—

> "Now leeks are in season, for pottage full good,
> That spareth the milch cow, and purgeth the blood."

and a trite proverb of former times bids us :—

> "Eat leeks in Lide [March] and ramsons in May,
> Then all the year after physicians can play."

Ramsons, or the Wild Garlic (*Allium ursinum*), is broad leaved, and grows abundantly on our moist meadow banks, with a strong smell of onions when crushed or bruised. It is perennial, having egg-shaped or lance-like leaves, whilst bearing large, pearly-white blossoms with acute petals. The name is the plural of "Ramse," or "Ram," which signifies strong-smelling, or rank. And the plant is also called "Buck Rams," or "Buck Rampe," in allusion to its spadix or spathe. "The leaves of Ramsons," says Gerard, "are stamped and eaten with fish, even as we do eat greene sauce made with sorrell." This is "Bear's Garlic," and the Star Flower of florists.

Leeks were so highly esteemed by the Emperor Nero, that his subjects gave him the sobriquet of "Porrophagus." He took them with oil for several days in each month to clear his voice, eating no bread on those days. *Un remede d'Empereur (Neron) pour se debarrasser d'un rhume,—et de commère pour attendre le meme but—fut envelopper un oignon dans une feuille de chou et le faire cuire sous la cendre ; puis l'ecrasser, le reduire en pulpe, le mettre dans une tasse de lait, ou une decoction chaude de redisse ; se coucher ; et se tenir chaudement, au besoin recidiver matin et soir.*

The Scotch leek is more hardy and pungent than that

grown in England. It was formerly a favourite ingredient in the Cock-a-Leekie soup of Caledonia, which is so graphically described by Sir Walter Scott, in the *Fortunes of Nigel.*

A "Herby" pie, peculiar to Cornwall, is made of leeks and pilchards, or of nettles, pepper cress, parsley, mustard, and spinach, with thin slices of pork. At the bottom of the Squab pie mentioned before was a Squab, or young Cormorant, "which diffused," says Charles Kingsley, "through the pie, and through the ambient air, a delicate odour of mingled guano and polecat." That "lovers live by love, as larks by leeks," is an old saying; and in the classic story of Pyramus and Thisbe, reference is made to the beautiful emerald green which the leaves of the leek exhibit. "His eyes were as green as leeks." Among the Welsh farmers, it is a neighbourly custom to attend on a certain day and plough the land of a poor proprietor whose means are limited—each bringing with him one or more leeks for making the soup or broth.

The *Schalot,* or *Eschalotte,* is another variety of the onion tribe, which was introduced into England by the Crusaders, who found it growing at Ascalon. And Chives (*Allium schœnoprasum*) are an ever green perennial herb of the onion tribe, having only a mild, alliaceous flavour. Epicures consider the Schalot to be the best seasoning for beef steaks, either by taking the actual bulb, or by rubbing the plates therewith.

Again, as a most common plant in all our hedgerows, is found the Poor Man's Garlic, or Sauce-alone (*Erisymum alliaria*), from *eruo,* to cure, a somewhat coarse and most ordinary member of the onion tribe, which goes also by the names of "Jack by the hedge" and "Garlick-wort," and belongs to the cruciferous order of plants. When bruised, it gives out a strong smell of garlic, and when eaten by cows it makes their milk taste powerfully of onions. The Ancients, says John Evelyn, used "Jack by the hedge" as a succedaneum to their Scordium, or cultivated Garlic.

This herb grows luxuriantly, bearing green, shining, heart-shaped leaves, and headpieces of small, white-flowering bunches. It was named "Saucealone," from being eaten in the Springtime with meat, whilst having so strong a flavour of onions, that it served alone of itself for sauce. Perhaps (says Dr. Prior) the title "Jack by the hedge" is derived from "jack," or "jakes," an old English word denoting a privy, or house of office, and this in allusion to the fetid smell of the plant, and the usual place of its growth.

When gathered and eaten with boiled mutton, after having been first separately boiled, it makes an excellent vegetable, if picked as it approaches the flowering state. Formerly this herb was highly valued as an antiscorbutic, and was thought a most desirable pot herb.

(The *Erysimum officinale* (Hedge Mustard) and the *Vervain* (Verbena) make Count Mattæi's empirical nostrum *Febrifugo:* but this *Erysimum* is not the same plant as the Jack by the hedge.)

GOOSEBERRY.

THE Gooseberry (*Ribes grossularia*) gets its name from *krüsbar*, which signifies a cross, in allusion to the triple spine of the fruit or berry, which is commonly cruciform. This is a relic of its first floral days, preserved like the apron of the blacksmith at Persia, when he came to the throne. The term *grossularia* implies a resemblance of the fruit to *grossuli*, small unripe figs.

Frequently the shrub, which belongs to the same natural order as the Currant (*Ribes*), grows wild in the hedges and thickets of our Eastern counties, bearing then only a small, poor berry, and not supposed to be of native origin.

In East Anglia it is named Fabe, Feap, Thape, or Theab berry, probably by reason of a mistake which arose through an incorrect picture. The Melon, in a well-known book of Tabernæmontanus, was figured to look like a large gooseberry, and was headed, *Pfebe.* And this name was supposed by some wiseacre to be that of the gooseberry, and thus became attached to the said fruit. Loudon thinks it signifies Feverberry, because of the cooling properties possessed by the gooseberry, which is scarcely probable.

In Norfolk, the green, unripe fruit is called Thape, and the schoolboys in that county well know Thape pie, made from green Gooseberries. The French call the fruit *Groseille*, and the Scotch, Grosert. It contains, chemically, citric acid, pectose, gum, sugar, cellulose, albumen, mineral matter, and water. The quantity of flesh-forming constituents is insignificant. Its pectose, under heat, makes a capital jelly.

In this country, the Gooseberry was first cultivated at the time of the Reformation, and it grows better in Great Britain than elsewhere, because of the moist climate. The original fruit occurred of the hairy sort, like Esau, as the *Uva crispa* of Fuschius, in Henry the Eighth's reign; and there are now red, white, and yellow cultivated varieties of the berry.

When green and unripe, Gooseberries are employed in a sauce, together with bechamel, and aromatic spices, this being taken with mackerel and other rich fish, as an acid corrective condiment. Also, from the juice of the green fruit, "which cureth all inflammations," may be concocted an excellent vinegar.

Gooseberry-fool, which comes to our tables so acceptably in early summer, consists of the unripe fruit *foulé* (that is, crushed or beaten up) with cream and milk. Similarly the French have a *foulé des pommes*, and a *foulé des raisins*. To "play old Gooseberry" with another man's property is conjectured to mean smashing it up, and reducing it, as it were, to Gooseberry-fool.

The young and tender leaves of the shrub, if eaten raw in a salad, drive forth the gravel. And from the red Gooseberry may be prepared an excellent light jelly, which is beneficial for sedentary, plethoric, and bilious subjects. This variety of the fruit, whether hairy or smooth, is grown largely in Scotland, but in France it is little cared for.

The yellow Gooseberry is richer and more vinous of taste, suiting admirably, when of the smooth sort, for making Gooseberry wine; which is choice, sparkling, and wholesome, such as that wherewith Goldsmith's popular *Vicar of Wakefield* used to regale Farmer Flamborough and the blind piper, having "lost neither the recipe nor the reputation." They were soothed in return by the touching ballads of *Johnny Armstrong's Last Good Night*, and *Cruel Barbara Allen*.

Gooseberry Shows are held annually in Lancashire, and excite keen competition; but after exhibition, the successful berries are "topped and tailed," so as to disqualify them from being shown elsewhere. Southey, in *The Doctor*, speaks about an obituary notice in a former Manchester newspaper, of a man who "bore a severe illness with Christian fortitude, and was much esteemed among Gooseberry growers." Prizes are given for the biggest and heaviest berries, which are produced with immense pains as to manuring, and the growth of cool chickweed around the roots of the bushes. At the same time each promising berry is kept submerged in a shallow vessel of water placed beneath it so as to compel absorption of moisture, and thus to enlarge its size. Whimsical names, such as "Golden Lion," "The Jolly Angler," and "Crown Bob," etc., are bestowed on the prize fruit. Cuttings from the parent plant of a prize Gooseberry become in great request; and thus the pedigree scions of a single bush have been known to yield as much as thirty-two pounds sterling to their possessor. The *Gooseberry Book* is a regular Manchester annual.

A berry weighing as heavy as thirty-seven pennyweight has been exhibited; and a story is told of a Middleton weaver, who, when a thunder-storm was gathering, lay awake as if for his life, and at the first patter of rain against the window panes, rushed to the rescue of his Gooseberry bushes with his bed quilt. Green Gooseberries will help to abate the strange longings which sometimes beset pregnant women.

In Devon the rustics call Gooseberries "Deberries," and in Sussex they are familiarly known to village lads as Goosegogs.

An Irish cure for warts is to prick them with a Gooseberry thorn passed through a wedding ring.

By some subtle bodily action wrought through a suggestion made to the mind, warts undoubtedly disappear as the result of this and many another equally trivial proceeding; which being so, why not the more serious skin affections, and larger morbid growths?

The poet Southey wrote a *Pindaric Ode upon a Gooseberry*

Pie, beginning "Gooseberry Pie is best," with the refrain:—

> "And didst thou scratch thy tender arms,
> Oh, Jane! that I should dine"?

GOOSEFOOT.

AMONG Curative Simples, the Goosefoot, or *Chenopod* order of British plants, contributes two useful herbs, the *Chenopodium bonus Henricus* (Good King Henry), and the *Chenopodium vulvaria* (Stinking Goosefoot).

This tribe derives its distinctive title from the Greek words, *cheen*, a goose, and *pous*, a foot, in allusion to the resemblance borne by its leaves to the webbed members of that waddling bird which raw recruits are wont to bless for their irksome drill of the goose-step. Incidentally, it may be said that goosegrease, got from the roasted bird, is highly emollient, and very useful in clysters; it also proves easily emetic.

The Goosefoot herbs are common weeds in most temperate climates, and grow chiefly in salt marshes, or on the sea-shore. Other plants of this tribe are esculent vegetables, as the Spinach, Beet, and Orach. They all afford "soda" in abundance.

The *Good King Henry* (Goosefoot) grows abundantly in waste places near villages, being a dark green, succulent plant, about a foot high, with thickish arrow-shaped leaves, which are cooked as spinach, especially in Lincolnshire. It is sometimes called Blite, from the Greek *bliton*, insipid; and, as Evelyn says, in his *Acetaria*, "it is well named, being insipid enough."

Why the said Goosefoot has been named "Good King Henry," or, "Good King Harry," is a disputed point. A French writer declares "this humble plant which grows on our plains without culture will confer a more lasting duration on the memory of *Henri Quatre* than the statue of bronze placed on the Pont Neuf, though fenced with iron, and guarded by soldiers." Dodœus says the appellation was given to distinguish the plant from another, a poisonous one, called *Malus Henricus*, "Bad Henry." Other authors have referred it to our Harry the Eighth, and his sore legs, for which the leaves were applied as a remedy; but this idea does not seem of probable correctness. Frowde tells us "the constant irritation of his festering legs made his terrible temper still more dreadful. Warned of his approaching dis-solution, and consumed with the death-thirst, he called for a cup of white wine, and, turning to one of his attendants, cried, 'All is lost!'—and these were his last words." The substantive title, *Henricus*, is more likely derived from "heinrich," an elf or goblin, as indicating certain magical virtues in the herb.

It is further known as English Marquery, or Mercury, and *Tota bona*, or, Allgood, the latter from a conceit of the rustics that it will cure all hurts; "wherefore the leaves are now a constant plaster among them for every green wound." It bears small flowers of sepals only, and is grown by cottagers as a pot herb. The young shoots peeled and boiled may be eaten as asparagus, and are gently laxative. The leaves are often made into broth, being applied also externally by country folk to heal old ulcers; and the roots are given to sheep having a cough.

Both here and in Germany this Goosefoot is used for feeding poultry, and it has hence acquired the sobriquet of Fat-hen.

The term, English Mercury, has been given because of its excellent remedial qualities against indigestion, and bears out the proverb: "Be thou sick or whole, put

Mercury in thy koole." Poultices made from the herb are applied to cleanse and heal chronic sores, which, as Gerard teaches, "they do scour and mundify." Certain writers associate it with our *good* King Henry the Sixth.

There is made in America, from an allied plant, the oak-leaved Goosefoot (*Chenopodium glaucum*), or from the aphis which infests it, a medicinal tincture used for expelling round worms.

The *Stinking Goosefoot*, called therefore, *Vulvaria*, and *Garosmus*, grows often on roadsides in England, and is known as Dog's Orach. It is of a dull, glaucous, or greyish-green aspect, and invested with a greasy mealiness which when touched exhales a very odious and enduring smell like that of stale salt fish, this being particularly attractive to dogs, though swine refuse the plant. It has been found very useful in hysteria, the leaves being made into a conserve with sugar; or Dr. Fuller's famous *Electuarium hystericum* may be compounded by adding forty-eight drops of oil of amber (*Oleum succini*) to four ounces of the conserve. Then a piece of the size of a chestnut should be taken when needed, and repeated more or less often as required. It further promotes the monthly flow of women. But the herb is possessed *odoris virosi intolerabilis*, of a stink which remains long on the hands after touching it. The whole plant is sprinkled over with the white, pellucid meal, and contains much "trimethylamine," together with osmazome, and nitrate of potash; also it gives off free ammonia. The title, Orach, given to the Stinking Goosefoot, a simple of a "most ancient, fish-like smell," and to others of the same tribe, is a corruption of *aurum*, gold, because their seeds were supposed to cure the ailment known popularly as the "yellow jaundice." These plants afford no nutriment, and, therefore, each bears the name, *atriplex*—*a*, not, *trephein*, to nourish:—

"Atriplicem tritum cum nitro, melle, et aceto
Dicunt appositum calidum sedare podagram
Ictericis dicitque Galenus tollere morbum
Illius semen cum vino sæpius haustum."

"With vinegar, honey, and salt, the Orach
Made hot, and applied, cures a gouty attack;
Whilst its seeds for the jaundice, if mingled with wine,
—As Galen has said—are a remedy fine."

"Orach is cooling," writes Evelyn, "and allays the pituit humors." "Being set over the fire, neither this nor the lettuce needs any other water than their own moisture to boil them in." The Orach hails from Tartary, and is much esteemed in France. It was introduced about 1548.

GOOSEGRASS.

"GOOSEY, goosey, gander, whither do ye wander?" says an old nursery rhyme by way of warning to the silly waddling birds not to venture into hedgerows, else will they become helplessly fettered by the tough, straggling coils of the Clivers, Goosegrass, or, Hedgehcriff, growing so freely there, and a sad despoiler of feathers.

The medicinal Goosegrass (*Galium aparine*), which is a highly useful curative Simple, springs up luxuriantly about fields and waste places in most English districts. It belongs to the Rubiaceous order of plants, all of which have a root like madder, affording a red dye. This hardy Goosegrass climbs courageously by its slender, hairy stems through the dense vegetation of our hedges into open daylight, having sharp, serrated leaves, and producing small white flowers, "pearking on the tops of the sprigs." It is one of the Bedstraw tribe, and bears a number of popular titles, such as Cleavers, Clithers, Robin run in the grass, Burweed, Loveman, Gooseherriff, Mutton chops, Clite, Clide, Clitheren, and Goosebill, from the sharp, serrated leaves, like the rough-edged mandibles of a goose.

Its stalks and leaves are covered with little hooked bristles, which attach themselves to passing objects, and by which it fastens itself in a ladder-like manner to adjacent shrubs, so as to push its way upwards in the hedgerows.

Goosegrass has obtained the sobriquet of Beggar's lice, from clinging closely to the garments of passers by, as well as because the small burs resemble these disgusting vermin; again it is known to some as Harriff, or, Erriff, from the Anglo-Saxon "hedge rife," a taxgather, or robber, because it plucks the wool from the sheep as they pass through a hedge; also Grip-grass, Catchweed, and Scratchweed. Furthermore, this Bedstraw has been called Goose-grease, from a mistaken belief that obstructive ailments of geese can be cured therewith. It is really a fact that goslings are extremely fond of the herb.

The botanical name, *Aparine*, bears the same meaning, being derived from the Greek verb, *apairo*, to lay hold of. The generic term, *Galium*, comes from the Greek word *gala*, milk, which the herb was formerly employed to curdle, instead of rennet.

The flowers of this Bedstraw bloom towards August, about the time of the Feast of the Annunciation, and a legend says they first burst into blossom at the birth of our Saviour. Bedstraw is, according to some, a corruption of Beadstraw. It is certain that Irish peasant girls often repeat their "aves" from the round seeds of the Bedstraw, using them for beads in the absence of a rosary;

and hence, perhaps, has been derived the name our Lady's Be(a)dstraw. But straw (so called from the Latin *sterno*, to strew, or, scatter about) was formerly employed as bedding, even by ladies of rank: whence came the expression of a woman recently confined being "in the straw." Children style the *Galium Aparine* Whip tongue, and Tongue-bleed, making use of it in play to draw blood from their tongues.

This herb has a special curative reputation with reference to cancerous growths and allied tumours. For open cancers an ointment is made from the leaves and stems wherewith to dress the ulcerated parts, and at the same time the expressed juice of the plant is given internally. Dr. Tuthill Massy avers that it often produces a cure in from six to twelve months, and advises that the decoction shall be drank regularly afterwards in the Springtime.

Dr. Quinlan, at St. Vincent's Hospital, Dublin, successfully employed poultices made with the fresh juice, and applied three times in the day, to heal chronic ulcers on the legs. Its effects, he says, in the most unlikely cases, were decisive and plain to all.

He gave directions that whilst a bundle of ten or twelve stalks is grasped with the left hand, this bundle should be cut into pieces of about half-an-inch long, by a pair of scissors held in the right hand. The segments are then to be bruised thoroughly in a mortar, and applied in the mass as a poultice beneath a bandage.

Dr. Thornton, in his excellent *Herbal* (1810), says: "After some eminent surgeons had failed, he ordered the juice of Cleavers, mixed with linseed, to be applied to the breast, in cases of supposed cancer of that part, with a teaspoonful of the juice to be taken every night and morning whilst fasting; by which plan, after a short time, he dispersed very frightful tumours in the breast."

The herb is found, on analysis, to contain three distinct acids—the tannic acid (of galls), the citric acid (of lemons), and the special rubichloric acid of the plant.

"In cancer," says Dr. Boyce, "five fluid ounces of the fresh juice of the plant are to be taken twice a day, whilst constantly applying the bruised leaves, or their ointment, to the sore."

Some of our leading druggists now furnish curative preparations made from the fresh herb. These include the *succus*, or juice, to be swallowed; the decoction, to be applied as a lotion; and the ointment, for curative external use. Both in England and elsewhere the juice of this Goosegrass constitutes one of the Spring juices taken by country people for scorbutic complaints. And not only for cancerous disease, but for many other foul, illconditioned ulcers, whether scrofulous or of the scurvy nature, this Goosegrass has proved itself of the utmost service, its external application being at all times greatly assisted by the internal use of the juice, or of a decoction made from the whole herb.

By reason of its acid nature, this Galium is astringent, and therefore of service in some bleedings, as well as in diarrhœa, and for obesity.

Gerard writes: "The herb, stamped with swine's grease, wasteth away the kernels by the throat; and women do usually make pottage of Cleavers with a little mutton and oatmeal, to cause leanness, and to keep them from fatness." Dioscorides reported that: "Shepherds do use the herb to take hairs out of the milk, if any remain therein."

Considered generally, the *Galium aparine* exercises acid, astringent, and diuretic effects, whilst it is of special value against epilepsy, and cancerous sores, as already declared; being curative likewise of psoriasis, eczema, lepra, and other cutaneous diseases. The dose of the authorised officinal juice is from one to two tea-spoonfuls, and from five to twenty grains of the prepared extract.

The title *Galium* borne by Bedstraws has been derived from the Greek *gala*, milk, because they all possess to some extent the power of curdling milk when added to it. Similarly the appellation "Cheese rennet," or, Cheese running (from *gerinnen*, to coagulate), is given to these plants. Highlanders make special use of the common Yellow Bedstraw for this purpose, and to colour their cheese.

From the Yellow Bedstraw (*Galium verum*), which is abundant on dry banks chiefly near the sea, and which may be known by its diminutive, puffy stems, and its small golden flowers, closely clustered together in dense panicles, "an ointment," says Gerard, "is prepared, which is good for anointing the weary traveller."

Because of its bright yellow blossoms, this herb is also named "Maid's hair," resembling the loose, unsnooded, golden hair of maidens. In Henry VIII's reign "maydens did wear silken callis to keep in order their hayre made yellow with dye." For a like reason the Yellow Bedstraw has become known as "Petty mugget," from the French *petit muguet*, a little dandy, as applied in ridicule to effeminate young men, the *Jemmy Jessamies*, or "mashers" of the period. Old herbalists affirmed that the root of this same Bedstraw, if drunk in wine, stimulates amorous desires, and that the flowers, if long smelt at, will produce a similar effect.

This is, *par excellence*, the Bedstraw of *our Lady*, who

gave birth to her son, says the legend, in a stable, with nothing but wild flowers for the bedding.

Thus, in the old Latin hymn, she sings right sweetly:—

"Lectum stravi tibi soli: dormi, nate bellule!
Stravi lectum fœno molli: dormi, mi animule!
Ne quid desit sternam rosis: sternam fœnum violis,
Pavimentum hyacinthis; et præsepe liliis."

"Sleep, sweet little babe, on the bed I have spread thee;
Sleep, fond little life, on the straw scattered o'er!
'Mid the petals of roses, and pansies I've laid thee,
In crib of white lilies; blue bells on the floor."

GOUTWEED.

A PASSING word should certainly be given to the Goutweed, or, Goatweed, among Herbal Simples. It is, though but little regarded, nevertheless, a common and troublesome garden weed, of the Umbelliferous tribe, and thought to possess certain curative virtues. Botanically it is the *Œgopodium podagraria*, signifying, by the first of these names, Goatsfoot, and by the second, a specific power against gout. The plant is also known as Herb Gerard, because dedicated to St. Gerard, who was formerly invoked to cure gout, against which this herb was employed. Also it has been named Ashweed, wild Master-wort, and Gout-wort. The herb grows about a foot high, with white flowers in umbels, having large, thrice-ternate, aromatic leaves, and a creeping root. These leaves are sometimes boiled, and eaten, but they possess a strong, disagreeable flavour. Culpeper says: "It is not to be supposed that Goutweed hath its name for nothing; but upon experiment to heal the gout, and sciatica; as also joint aches, and other cold griefs; *the very bearing it about one easeth the pains of the gout, and defends him that bears it from disease.*" Hill recommends the root and fresh buds of the leaves as excellent in fomentations and poultices for pains; and the leaves, when boiled soft, together with the roots, for application about the hip in sciatica.

No chemical analysis of the Goutweed is yet on record.

"Herbe Gerard groweth of itself in gardens without setting, or sowing; and is so fruitful in his increase that where once it hath taken root, it will hardly be gotten out again, spoiling and getting every yeere more ground —to the annoying of better herbes."

GRAPES (see also VINE).

GRAPES, the luscious and refreshing fruit of the Vine, possess certain medicinal properties and virtues which give them a proper place among Herbal Simples. The name Vine comes from *viere*, to twist, being applied with reference to the twining habits of the parent stock; as likewise to "with," and "withy."

The fruit consists of pulp, stones, and skin. Within the pulp is contained the grape sugar, which differs in some respects chemically from cane sugar, and which is taken up straightway into our circulation when eaten, without having to be changed slowly by the saliva, as is the case with cane sugar. Therefore it happens that the grape sugar warms and fattens speedily, with a quick repair of waste, when the strength and the structures are consumed by fever, Grapes then being most grateful to the sufferer. But they do not suit inflammatory subjects at other times, or gouty persons at any time, as well as cane sugar, which has to undergo slower chemical conversion before it furnishes heat and sustenance. And in this respect, grape sugar closely resembles the glucose, or sweet principle of honey.

The fruit also contains a certain quantity of "fruit sugar," which is chemically identical with cane sugar; and, because of the special syrupy juice of its pulp, the Grape adapts itself to quick alcoholic fermentation.

The important ingredients of Grapes are sugar (grape and fruit), gum, tannin, bitartrate of potash, sulphate of potash, tartrate of lime, magnesia, alum, iron, chlorides of potassium and sodium, tartaric, citric, racemic, and malic acids, some albumen, and azotized matters, with water.

But the wine grower is glad to see his *must* deposit the greater part of these chemical ingredients in the "tartar," a product much disliked, and therefore named *Sal Tartari*, or Hell Salt; and *Cremor Tartari*, Hell Scum (Cream of Tartar).

In Italy, the vine furnishes oil as well as wine, this being extracted from the grape stones, and reckoned superior to any other sort, whether for the table or for purposes of lighting. It has no odour, and burns without smoke. The stones also yield volatile essences, which are developed by crushing, and which give bouquet to the several wines, whilst the skin affords colouring matter and tannin, of more or less astringency.

Grapes supply but little actual nutritious matter for building up the solid structures of the body; they act as gentle laxatives; though their stones, and the leaves of the vine, are astringent. These latter were formerly employed to stop bleedings, and when dried and powdered, for arresting dysentery in cattle.

In Egypt the leaves are used, when young and tender, for enveloping balls of hashed meat, at good tables. The sap of the vine, named *lacryma*, "a tear," is an excellent application to weak eyes, and for specs of the cornea. The juice of the unripe fruit, which is verjuice (as well as that of the wild crabapple), was much esteemed by the ancients, and is still in good repute for applying to bruises and sprains.

When taken in any quantity, Grapes act freely on the kidneys, and promote a flow of urine. The vegetable acids of the fruit become used up as such, and are neutralised in the system by combining with the earthy salts found therein, and they pass off in the urine as alkaline carbonates. With full-blooded, excitable persons, grapes in any quantity are apt to produce palpitation, and to quicken the circulation for a time. Also with persons of slow and feeble energies, having a languid digestion (and especially if predisposed to acid fermentation in the stomach), Grapes are apt to disagree. They send their glucose straightway into the circulation combined with acids found in the stomach, and create considerable distress of heartburn and dyspepsia. "Thus," says Dr. King Chambers, "is generated acidity of the stomach, parent of gout, and of all its hideous crew." Likewise wine, especially if sweet, new, or full-bodied, when taken by such persons at a meal, is absorbed but slowly by the stomach, and much of the sugar, with some alcohol, becomes converted by fermentation into acetic acid, which further causes the oily ingredients in the food which has been swallowed to turn rancid. "Things sweet to taste prove to digestion sour." But otherwise, with a person in good health, and not given to gout or rheumatism, Grapes are an excellent food for supplying warmth as combustion material, by their ready-made sugar; whilst the essential flavours of the fruit are cordial, and whilst a surplus of the glucose serves to form fat for storage.

What is known as the *Grape-cure*, is pursued in the Tyrol, in Bavaria, on the banks of the Rhine, and elsewhere—the sick person being ordered to eat from three to six pounds of grapes a day. But the relative proportions of the sugar and acids in the various kinds of grapes have important practical bearings on the results obtained, determining whether wholesome purgation shall follow, or whether tonic and fattening effects shall be produced. In the former case, sufferers from sluggish liver and torpid biliary functions, with passive local congestions, will benefit most by taking the grapes not fully ripe, and not completely sweet; whilst in the latter instance, those invalids will gain special help from ripe and sweet grapes, who require quick supplies of animal heat and support to resist rapid waste of tissue, as in chronic catarrh of the lungs, or mucous catarrh of the bowels.

The most important constituent to be determined is the quantity of grape sugar, which varies according to the greater or less warmth of the climate. Tokay Grapes are the sweetest; next are those of southern France; then of Moselle, Bohemia, and Heidelberg; whilst the fruit of the Vine in Spain, Italy, and Madeira, is not commended for curative purposes. The Grapes are eaten three, four, or five times a day, during the promenade; those which are not sweet produce a diuretic and laxative effect; seeing, moreover, that their reaction is alkaline, the "cure" thereby is particularly suitable for persons troubled with gravel and acid gout.

After losses of blood, and in allied states of exhaustion, the restorative powers of the grape-cure are often strikingly exhibited. Formerly, the German doctors kept their patients, when under this mode of treatment, almost entirely without other food. But it is now found that light, wholesome nourishment, properly chosen, and taken at regular times, even with some moderate allowance of Bordeaux wine, may be permitted in useful conjunction with the grapes. Children do not, as a rule, bear the grape-cure well. One sort of grape, the Bourdelas, or Verjus, being intensely sour when green, is never allowed to ripen, but its large berries are made to yield their acid liquor for use instead of vinegar or lemon juice, in sauces, drinks, and medicinal preparations.

A vinegar poultice, applied cold, is an effectual remedy for sprains and bruises, and will arrest the progress of scrofulous enlargements of bones. It may be made with vinegar and oatmeal, or with the addition of bread crumb."—*Pharmacopœia Chirurgica*, 1794.

"Other fruits may please the palate equally well, but it is the proud prerogative of the kingly grape to minister also to the mind." This served to provide one of the earliest offerings to the Deity, seeing that "Bread and wine were brought forth to Abraham by Melchisedec, the Priest of the Most High God."

The Vine (*Vitis vinifera*) was almost always to the front in the designs drawn by the ancients. Thus, miniatures and dainty little pictures were originally encircled with representations of its foliage, and we still name such small exquisite illustrations, "vignettes," from the French word, *vigne*.

The large family of Muscat grapes get their distinctive title not because of any flavour of musk attached to them, but because the sweet berries are particularly attractive to flies (*muscæ*), a reason which induced the Romans to name this variety, *Vitis apiaria.* "*On attrape plus de mouches avec le miel qu' avec le vinaigre*"—say the French.

In Portugal, grape juice is boiled down with quinces into a sort of jam—the progenitor of all marmalades.

The original grape vine is supposed to have been indigenous to the shores of the Caspian Sea.

If eaten to excess, especially by young persons, grapes will make the tongue and the lining membrane of the mouth sore, just as honey often acts. For this reason, both grapes and honey do good to the affection known as thrush, with sore raw mouth, and tongue in ulcerative white patches, coming on as a derangement of the health.

GRASSES.

OUR abundant English grasses furnish nutritious herbage and farinaceous seeds, whilst their stems and leaves prove useful for textile purposes. Furthermore, some few of them possess distinctive medicinal virtues, with mucilaginous roots, and may be properly classed among Herbal Simples.

The Sweet-scented Vernal Grass (Anthoxanthum, with Yellow Anthers) gives its delightfully characteristic odour to newly mown meadow hay, and has a pleasant aroma of Woodruff. But it is specially provocative of hay fever and hay asthma with persons liable to suffer from these distressing ailments. Accordingly, a medicinal tincture is made (H.) from this grass with spirit of wine, and if some of the same is poured into the open hand-palms for the volatile aroma to be sniffed well into the nose and throat, immediate relief is afforded during an attack. At the same time three or four drops of the tincture should be taken as a dose with water, and repeated at intervals of twenty or thirty minutes, as needed.

The flowers contain "coumarin," and their volatile pollen impregnates the atmosphere in early summer. The sweet perfume is due chiefly to benzoic acid, such as is used for making scented pastilles, or Ribbon of Bruges for fumigation.

Again, the Couch Grass, Dog Grass, or Quilch (*Triticum repens*) found freely in road-sides, fields, and waste places, has been employed from remote times as a vulnerary, and to relieve difficulties of urination. Our English wheat has been evolved therefrom.

In modern days its infusion—of the root—is generally regarded as a soothing diuretic, helpful to the bladder and kidneys. Formerly, this was a popular drink to purify the blood in the Spring. But no special constituents have been discovered in the root besides a peculiar sugar, a gum-like principle, *triticin*, and some lactic acid. The decoction may be made from the whole fresh plant, or from the dried root sliced, two to four ounces being put in a quart of water, reduced to a pint by boiling. A wineglassful of this may be given for a dose. It certainly palliates irritation of the urinary passages, and helps to relieve against gravel. A liquid extract is also dispensed by the druggists, of which from one to two teaspoonfuls are given in water.

The French specially value this grass for its stimulating fragrancy of vanilla and rose perfumes in the decoction. They use the Cocksfoot Grass (*Dactylis*), or *pied de poule*, in a similar way, and for the same purposes.

Also the "bearded Darnel," *Lolium temulentum* ("intoxicated"), a common grass-weed in English cornfields, will produce medicinally all the symptoms of drunkenness. The French call it *Ivraie* for this reason, and with us it is known as Ray Grass, or in some provincial districts as "Cheat." The old Sages supposed it to cause blindness, hence with the Romans, *lolio victitare,* to live on Darnel, was a phrase applied to a dim-sighted person. Gerard says, "the new bread wherein Darnell is eaten hot, causeth drunkenness."

From *lolium* the term Lollard given in reproach to the Waldenses, and the followers of Wickliffe, indicated that they were pernicious weeds choking and destroying the pure wheat of the gospel. Milne says the expression in Matthew xiii. *v.* 25, would have been better translated "darnel" than "tares."

A general trembling, followed by inability to walk, hindered speech, and presently profound sleep, with subsequent headache and vomiting, are the symptoms produced by Darnel when taken in a harmful quantity. So that medicinally a tincture of the plant may be expected, if given in small diluted doses, to quickly dispel intoxication from alcoholic drinks; also to prove useful for analogous congestion of the brain coming on as an illness, and for dimness of vision. Chemically, it contains an acrid fixed oil, and a yellow glucoside.

There is some reason to suspect that the old custom of using Darnel to adulterate malt and distilled liquors has not been wholly abandoned. Farmers in Devonshire are fond of the Ray Grass, which they call "Eaver" or "Iver"; and "Devon-ever" is noted likewise in Somersetshire.

GROUNDSEL.

COMMON Groundsel is so well known throughout Great Britain, that it needs scarcely any description. It is very prolific, and found in every sort of cultivated ground, being a small plant of the Daisy tribe, but without any outer white rays to its yellow flower-heads. These are compact little bundles, at first of a dull yellow colour, until presently the florets fall off and leave the white woolly pappus of the seeds collected together, somewhat resembling the hoary hairs of age. They have suggested the name of the genus "senecio," from the Latin *senex*, an old man :—

> "Quod canis simili videatur flore capillis;
> Cura facit canos quamvis vir non habet annos."

> "With venerable locks the Groundsel grows;
> Hard care more quick than years white head-gear shows."

In the fifteenth century this herb went by the name of Grondeswyle, from *grund*, ground, and *swelgun*, to swallow, and to this day it is called in Scotland Grundy Swallow, or Ground Glutton.

Not being attractive to insects or visited by them the Groundsel is fertilized by the wind. It flowers throughout the whole year, and is the favourite food of many small birds, being thus given to canaries, and to other domesticated songsters.

The weed, named at first "Ascension," is called in the Eastern counties by corruption "Senshon" and "Simson." Its leaves are fleshy, with a bitter saline taste, whilst the juice is slightly acrid, but emollient. In this country farriers give it to horses for bot-worms, and in Germany it is employed as a vermifuge for children. A weak infusion of the whole plant with boiling water makes a simple and easy purgative dose, but a strong infusion will act as an emetic. For the former purpose two drachms by weight of the fresh plant should be boiled in four fluid ounces of water, and the same decoction serves as a useful gargle for a sore throat from catarrh. Chemically it contains senecin and seniocine.

In the hands of Simplers the Groundsel formerly held high rank as a herb of power. An old herbal prescribes against toothache to "dig up Groundsel with a tool that hath no iron in it, and touch the tooth five times with the plant, then spit thrice after each touch, and the cure will be complete." Hill says "the fresh roots if smelled when first taken out of the ground, are an immediate cure for many forms of headache." To apply the bruised leaves will serve for preventing boils, and the plant, if taken as a sallet with vinegar, is good for sadness of the heart. Gerard says "Women troubled with the mother (womb) are much eased by baths made of the leaves, and flowers of this, and the kindred Ragworts."

A decoction of Groundsel serves as a famous application for healing chapped hands. In Cornwall if the herb is to be used as an emetic they strip it upwards, if for a purgative downwards. "Lay by your learned receipts," writes Culpeper, "this herb alone shall do the deed for you in all hot diseases, first safely, second speedily."

HAWTHORN (Whitethorn).

THE Hawthorn, or Whitethorn, is so welcome year by year as a harbinger of Summer, by showing its wealth of sweet-scented, milk-white blossoms, in our English hedgerows, that every one rejoices when the Mayflower comes into bloom. Its brilliant haws, or fruit, later on are a botanical advance on the blackberry and wild raspberry, which belong to the same natural order. It has promoted itself to the possession of a single carpel or seed-vessel to each blossom, producing a separate fruit, this being a stony apple in miniature.

But the word "haw" is misapplied, because it really means a "hedge," and not a fruit; whilst "hips," which are popularly connected with "haws," are the fruit-capsules of the wild Dog-rose. Haws, when dried, make an infusion which will act on the kidneys; they are astringent, and serve, as well as the flowers, in decoction, to cure a sore throat.

The Hawthorn bush was chosen by Henry the Seventh for his device, because a small crown from the helmet of Richard the Third was discovered hanging thereon. Hence arose the legend "Cleve to thy crown though it hangs on a bush." In some districts it is called Hazels, Gazels, and Halves; and in many country places the villagers believe that the blossom of the Hawthorn still bears the smell of the great plague of London. It was formerly thought to be scathless—a tree too sacred to be touched.

Botanically, the Hawthorn is called *Cratægus oxyacantha*, these names signifying *kratos*, strength or hardness (of the wood); and *oxus*, sharp—*akantha*, a thorn. It is the German *Hage-dorn* or Hedge thorn, showing that from a very early period in the history of the Germanic races, their land was divided into plots by means of hedges.

The Hawthorn is also named Whitethorn, from the whiteness of its rind; and Quickset from its growing in a hedge as a "quick" or living shrub, when contrasted with a paling of dead wood. An old English name for the buds of the Hawthorn when just expanding, was Ladies' Meat; and in Sussex it is called the Bread and Cheese tree.

In many parts of England charms or incantations are

employed to prevent a thorn from festering in the flesh, as :—

> "Happy the man that Christ was born,
> He was crownéd with a thorn,
> He was piercéd through the skin
> For to let the poison in;
> But His five wounds, so they say,
> Closed before He passed away;
> In with healing, out with thorn!
> Happy man that Christ was born."

The flowers are fertilised for the most part by carrion insects, and a certain undertone of decomposition may be detected (says Grant Allen) by keen nostrils in the scent of the Mayflower. It is this curious element, in what seems otherwise a pure and delicious perfume, which attracts the meat-eating insects, or rather those insects which lay their eggs and hatch out their larvæ in decaying animal matter. The meat-fly comes first abroad just at the time when the Mayblossom breaks into bloom.

A Greek bride was sometimes decked with a sprig of Hawthorn, as emblematic of a flowery future, with thorns intermingled. It is supposed that "the Jewes maden," for our Saviour, "a croune of the branches of Albespyne, that is, Whitethorn, that grew in the same garden, and therefore hath the Whitethorn many vertues" being called in France *l'epine noble.*

The shadows in the moon are popularly thought to represent a man laden with a bundle of thorns in punishment of theft :—

> "Rusticus in lunâ quem sarcina deprimit una,
> Monstrat per spinas nulli prodesse rapinas."

> "A thievish clown by cruel thorns opprest
> Shows in the moon that honesty pays best."

HEMLOCK and HENBANE.

THE Spotted Hemlock (*Conium maculatum*), and the Sickly-smelling Henbane (*Hyoscyamus niger*), are plants of common wild growth throughout England, especially the former, and are well known to everyone familiar with our Herbal Simples. But each is so highly narcotic as a medicine, and yet withal so safely useful externally to allay pain, as well as to promote healing, that their outward remedial forms of application must not be overlooked among our serviceable herbs. Nevertheless, for internal administration, these herbs lie altogether beyond the pale of domestic uses, except in the hands of a doctor.

The Hemlock is an umbelliferous plant of frequent growth in our hedges and roadsides, with tall, hollow stalks, powdered blue at the bottom, whilst smooth and splashed about with spotty streaks of a reddish purple. It possesses foliage resembling that of the garden carrot, but feathery and more delicately divided.

The name has been got from *healm*, or *haulm*, straw, and *leac*, a plant, because of the dry hollow stalks which remain after flowering is done. In Kent and Essex, the Hemlock is called Kecksies, and the stalks are spoken of as Hollow Kecksies.

Keckis, or Kickes, of Humblelockis are mentioned by our oldest herbalists. In a book about herbs, of the fourteenth century, two sorts of Hemlock are specified—one being the Grete Homeloc, which is called "Kex," or "Wode Whistle," being of no use except for poor men's fuel, and children's play.

Botanically, it bears the name of *Conium maculatum* (spotted), the first of these words coming from the Greek, *konos*, a top, and having reference to the giddiness which the juice of hemlock causes toxically in the human brain. The unripe fruit of this plant possesses its peculiar medicinal properties in a greater degree than any other part, and the juice expressed therefrom is more reliably medicinal than the tincture made with spirit of wine, from the whole plant.

Soil, situation, and the time of year, materially affect the potency of Hemlock. Being a biennial plant, it is not poisonous in this country to cattle during the first year, if they eat its leaves.

The herb is always uncertain of action unless gathered of the true "maculatum" sort, when beginning to flower. Its juice should be thickened in a water bath, or the leaves carefully dried, and kept in a well-stoppered bottle, not exposed to the light. Cole says, "if asses chance to feed on Hemlock, they will fall so fast asleep that they seem to be dead, insomuch that some, thinking them to be dead indeed, have flayed off their skins; yet after the Hemlock had done operating they had stirred and wakened out of their sleep."

The dried leaves of the plant, if put into a small bag, and steeped in boiling water for a few minutes, and then applied hot to a gouty part, will quickly relieve the pain; also, they will help to soften the hard concretions which form about gouty joints. If the fresh juice of the Hemlock is evaporated to a thick syrup, and mixed with lanoline (the fat of sheep's wool), to make an ointment, it will afford wonderful relief to severe itching within and around the fundament; but it must be thoroughly applied. For a poultice some of this thickened juice may be added to linseed meal and boiling water, previously mixed well together.

Conium plasters were formerly employed to dry up the breast milk, and are now found of service to subdue palpitations of the heart.

An extract of Hemlock, blended with potash, is kept by the chemists, to be mixed with boiling water, for inhalation to ease a troublesome spasmodic cough, or an asthmatic attack. In Russia and the Crimea, this plant is so inert as to be edible; whereas in the South of Europe it is highly poisonous.

Chemically, the toxic action of Hemlock depends on its alkaloids, "coniine," and "methyl-coniine."

Vinegar has proved useful in neutralising the poisonous effects of Hemlock, and it is said if the plant is macerated or boiled in vinegar it becomes altogether inert.

For inhalation to subdue whooping-cough, three or four grains of the extract should be mixed with a pint of boiling water in a suitable inhaler, so that the medicated vapour may be inspired through the mouth and nostrils.

To make a Hemlock poultice, when the fresh plant cannot be procured, mix an ounce of powdered hemlock leaves (from the druggist) with three ounces of linseed meal; then gradually add half a pint of boiling water whilst constantly stirring.

Herb. gatherers sometimes mistake the wild Cicely (*Myrrhis odorata*) for the Hemlock; but this Cicely has a furrowed stem without spots, and is hairy, with a highly aromatic flavour. The bracts of Hemlock, at the base of the umbels, go only half way round the stem. The rough Chervil is also spotted, but hairy, and its stem is swollen below each joint. Under proper medical advice, the extract and the juice of Hemlock may be most beneficially given internally in cancer, and as a nervine sedative.

The Hemlock was esteemed of old as Herba Benedicta, a blessed herb, because "where the root is in the house the devil can do no harm, and if anyone should carry the plant about on his person no venomous beast can harm him." The Eleusinian priests who were required to remain chaste all their lives, had the wisdom to rub themselves with Hemlock.

Poultices may be made exclusively with the fresh leaves (which should be gathered in June) or with the dried leaflets when powdered, for easing and healing cancerous sores. Baron Stoerck first brought the plant into repute (1760) as a medicine of extraordinary efficacy for curing inveterate scirrhus, cancer, and ulcers, such as were hitherto deemed irremediable.

Likewise the *Cicuta virosa*, or Water Hemlock, has proved curative to many similar glandular swellings. This is also an umbelliferous plant, which grows commonly on the margins of ditches and rivers in many parts of England. It gets its name from *cicuta* (a shepherd's pipe made from a reed), because of its hollow stems. Being hurtful to cows it has acquired the title of Cowbane.

The root when incised secretes from its wounded bark a yellow juice of a narcotic odour and acrid taste. This has been applied externally with benefit for scirrhous cancer, and to ease the pain of nervous gout. But when taken internally it is dangerous, being likely to provoke convulsions, or to produce serious narcotic effects. Nevertheless, goats eat the herb with impunity :—

> "Nam videre licet pinguescere sœpe cicutam,
> Barbigeras pecudes; hominique est acre venenum."

The leaves smell like celery or parsley, these being most toxical in summer, and the root in spring. The potency of the plant depends on its cicutoxin, a principle derived from the resinous constituents, and which powerfully affects the organic functions through the spinal cord. It was either this or the Spotted Hemlock, which was used as the State poison of the Greeks for causing the death of Socrates.

For a fomentation with the Water Hemlock half-a-pound of the fresh leaves, or three ounces of the dried leaves should be boiled in three pints of water down to a quart; and this will be found very helpful for soothing and healing painful cancerous, or scrofulous sores. Also the juice of the herb mixed with hot lard, and strained, will serve a like useful purpose.

For pills of the herb take of its inspissated juice half-an-ounce, and of the finely powdered plant enough when mixed together to make from forty to sixty pills. Then for curing cancer, severe scrofula, or syphilitic sores, give from one to twenty of these pills in twenty-four hours (*Pharmacopeia Chirurgica*, 1794).

An infusion of the plant will serve when carefully used, to relieve nervous and sick headache. If the fresh, young, tender leaves are worn under the soles of the feet, next the skin, and are renewed once during the day, they will similarly assuage the discomfort of a nervous headache. The oil with which the herb abounds is not poisonous.

The *Black Henbane* grew almost everywhere about England, in Gerard's day, by highways, in the borders of fields, on dunghills, and in untoiled places. But now it has become much less common as a rustic herb in this country. We find it occasionally in railway cuttings, and in rubbish on waste places, chiefly on chalky ground, and particularly near the sea. The plant is biennial, rather large, and dull of aspect, with woolly sea-green leaves, and bearing bell-shaped flowers of a lurid, creamy colour, streaked and spotted with purple. It is one of the Night-shade tribe, having a heavy, oppressive, sub-fetid odour, and being rather clammy to the touch. This herb is also called Hogsbean, and its botanical name, *Hyoscyamus*, signifies "the bean of the hog," which animal eats it with impunity, though to mankind it is a poisonous plant. It has been noticed in Sherwood Forest, that directly the turf is pared Henbane springs up.

"To wash the feet," said Gerard, "in a decoction of Henbane, as also the often smelling to the flowers, causeth sleep." Similarly famous anodyne necklaces were made from the root, and were hung about the necks of children to prevent fits, and to cause an easy breeding of the teeth. From the leaves again was prepared a famous sorcerer's ointment. "These, the seeds, and the juice," says Gerard, "when taken internally, cause an unquiet sleep, like unto the sleep of drunkenness, which continueth long, and is deadly to the patient."

The herb was known to the ancients, being described by Dioscorides and Celsus. Internally, it should only be prescribed by a physician, and is then of special service for relieving irritation of the bladder, and to allay maniacal excitement, as well as to subdue spasm.

The fresh leaves crushed, and applied as a poultice, will quickly relieve local pains, as of gout or neuralgia. In France the plant is called *Jusquiame*, and in Germany it is nicknamed Devil's-eye.

The chemical constituents of Henbane are "hyoscyamine," a volatile alkaloid, with a bitter principle, "hyoscypricin" (especially just before flowering), also nitrate of potash, which causes the leaves, when burnt, to sparkle with a deflagration, and other inorganic salts. The seeds contain a whitish, oily albumen.

The leaves and viscid stem are produced only in

each second year. The juice when dropped into the eye will dilate the pupil.

Druggists prepare this juice of the herb, and an extract; also, they dispense a compound liniment of Henbane, which, when applied to the skin-surface on piline, is of great service for relieving obstinate rheumatic pains.

In some rural districts the cottony leaves of Henbane are smoked for toothache, like tobacco, but this practice is not free from risk of provoking convulsions, and even of causing insanity.

Gerard writes, with regard to the use of the seed of Henbane by mountebanks, for obstinate toothache: "Drawers of teeth who run about the country and pretend they cause worms to come forth from the teeth by burning the seed in a chafing dish of coals, the party holding his mouth over the fume thereof, do have some crafty companions who convey small lute strings into the water, persuading the patient that those little creepers came out of his mouth, or other parts which it was intended to ease." Forestus says: "These pretended worms are no more than an appearance of worms which is always seen in the smoak of Henbane seed."

> "Sic dentes serva; porrorum collige grana:
> No careas thure; cum *hyoscyamo* ure:
> Sic que per embotum fumun cape dente remotum."
>
> *Regimen sanitatis salernitanum* (Translated 1607).

> "If in your teeth you happen to be tormented,
> By means some little worms therein do brede,
> Which pain (if need be tane) may be prevented
> By keeping cleane your teeth when as ye fead.
> Burn Frankonsence (a gum not evil scented),
> Put Henbane into this, and onyon seed,
> And with a tunnel to the tooth that's hollow,
> Convey the smoke thereof, and ease shall follow."

By older writers, the Henbane was called Henbell and Symphonica, as implying its resemblance to a ring of bells (*Symphonia*), which is struck with a hammer. It has also been named *Faba Jovis* (Jupiter's bean). Only within recent times has the suffix "bell" given place to "bane," because the seeds are fatal to poultry and fish. In some districts horsedealers mix the seed of Henbane with their oats, in order to fatten the animals.

An instance is narrated where the roots of Henbane were cooked by mistake at a monastery for the supper of its inmates, and produced most strange results. One monk would insist on ringing the large bell at midnight, to the alarm of the neighbourhood; whilst of those who came to prayers at the summons, several could not read at all, and others read anything but what was contained in their breviaries.

Some authors suppose that this is the noxious herb intended by Shakespeare, in the play of *Hamlet*, when the ghost of the murdered king makes plaint, that:

> "Sleeping within mine orchard,
> My custom always of the afternoon,
> Upon my sécure hour thy uncle stole,
> With juice of cursed *hebenon* in a vial,
> And in the porches of mine ear did pour
> The leprous distilment."

But others argue more correctly that the name used here is a varied form of that by which the yew is known in at least five of the Gothic languages, and which appears in Marlow and other Elizabethan writers, as "hebon." "This tree," says Lyte, "is altogether venomous and against man's nature; such as do but only sleepe under the shadow thereof, become sicke, and sometimes they die."

HONEY.

BEING essentially of floral origin, and a vegetable product endowed with curative properties, Honey may be fairly ranked among Herbal Simples. Indeed, it is the nectar of flowers, partaking closely of their flavours and odours, whilst varying in taste, colour, scent, and medicinal attributes, according to the species of the plant from which it is produced.

The name Honey has been derived from a Hebrew word *ghoneg*, which means literally "delight." Historically, this substance dates from the oldest times of the known world. We read in the book of Genesis, that the land of Canaan where Abraham dwelt, was flowing with milk and honey; and in the Mosaic law were statutes regulating the ownership of bees.

Among the ancients Honey was used for embalming the dead, and it is still found contained in their preserved coffins.

Aristœus, a pupil of Chiron, first gathered Honey from the comb, and it was the basis of the seasoning of Apicius: whilst Pythagoras, who lived to be ninety, took latterly only bread and Honey. "Whoever wishes," said an old classic maxim, "to preserve his health, should eat every morning before breakfast young onions with honey."

Tacitus informs us that our German ancestors gave credit for their great strength and their long lives to the Mead, or Honey-beer, on which they regaled themselves. Pliny tells of Rumilius Pollio, who enjoyed marvellous health and vitality, when over a hundred years old. On being presented to the Emperor Augustus, who enquired what was the secret of his wondrous longevity, Pollio answered *Interus melle, exterus oleo*, "the eating of Honey, and anointing with oil."

At the feasts of the gods, described by Ovid, the delicious Honey-cakes were never wanting, these being made of meal, Honey, and oil, whilst corresponding in number to the years of the devout offerer.

Pure Honey contains chemically about seventy per cent. of glucose (analogous to grape sugar) or the crystallizable part which sinks to the bottom of the jar, whilst the other portion above, which is non-crystallizable, is levulose, or fruit sugar, almost identical with the brown syrup of the sugar cane, but less easy of digestion. Hence, the proverb has arisen "of oil the top, of wine the middle, of Honey the bottom."

The odour of Honey is due to a volatile oil associated with a yellow colouring matter *melichroin*, which is separated by the floral nectaries, and becomes bleached on exposure to the sunlight. A minute quantity of an animal acid lends additional curative value for sore throat, and some other ailments.

Honey has certain claims as a food which cane sugar does not possess. It is a heat former, and a producer of vital energy, both in the human subject, and in the industrious little insect which collects the luscious fodder. Moreover, it is all ready for absorption straightway into the blood after being eaten, whereas cane sugar must be first masticated with the saliva, or spittle, and converted somewhat slowly into honey sugar before it can be utilised for the wants of the body. In this way the superiority of Honey over cane sugar is manifested, and it may be readily understood why grapes, the equivalent of Honey in the matter of their sugar, have an immediate effect in relieving fatigue by straightway contributing power and caloric.

Aged persons who are toothless may be supported almost exclusively on sugar. The great Duke of

Beaufort, whose teeth were white and sound at seventy, whilst his general health was likewise excellent, had for forty years before his death a pound of sugar daily in his wine, chocolate, and sweetmeats. A relish for sugar lessens the inclination for alcohol, and seldom accompanies the love of strong drink.

With young children, cane sugar is apt to form acids in the stomach, chiefly acetic, by a process of fermentation which causes pain, and flatulence, so that milk sugar should be given instead to those of tender years who are delicate, as this produces only lactic acid, which is the main constituent of digestive gastric juice.

When examined under a microscope Honey exhibits in addition to its crystals (representing glucose, or grape sugar), pollen-granules of various forms, often so perfect that they may be referred to the particular plants from which the nectar has been gathered.

As good Honey contains sugar in a form suitable for such quick assimilation, it should be taken generally in some combination less easily absorbed, otherwise the digestion may be upset by too speedy a glut of heat production, and of energy. Therefore the bread and Honey of time-honoured memory is a sound form of sustenance, as likewise, the proverbial milk and Honey of the Old Testament. This may be prepared by taking a bowl of new milk, and breaking into it some light wheaten bread, together with some fresh white Honeycomb. The mixture will be found both pleasant and easy of digestion.

Our forefathers concocted from Honey boiled with water and exposed to the sun (after adding chopped raisins, lemon peel, and other matters) a famous fermented drink, called mead, and this was termed metheglin (*methu*, wine, and *aglaion*, splendid) when the finer

Honey was used, and certain herbs were added so as to confer special flavours.

> "Who drank very hard the whole night through
> Cups of strong mead, made from honey when new,
> Metheglin they called it, a mighty strong brew,
> Their whistles to wet for the morrow."

Likewise, the old Teutons prepared a Honey wine, (hydromel), and made it the practice to drink this for the first thirty days after marriage; from which custom has been derived the familiar Honeymoon, or the month after a wedding.

Queen Elizabeth was particularly fond of mead, and had it made every year according to a special recipe of her own, which included the leaves of sweet briar, with rosemary, cloves, and mace.

Honey derived from cruciferous plants, such as rape, ladies' smock, and the wallflower, crystallizes quickly, often, indeed, within the comb before it is removed from the hive; whilst Honey from labiate plants, and from fruit trees in general, remains unchanged for several months after being extracted from the comb.

As a heat producer, if taken by way of food, one pound of Honey is equal to two pounds of butter; and when cod liver oil is indicated, but cannot be tolerated by the patient, Honey may sometimes be most beneficially substituted.

In former times it was employed largely as a medicine, and applied externally for the healing of wounds. When mixed with flour, and spread on linen, or leather, it has long been a simple remedy for bringing boils to maturity. In coughs and colds it makes a serviceable adjunct to expectorant medicines, whilst acting at the same time as sufficiently laxative. For sore throats it may be used in gargles with remarkable benefit; and when mixed with vinegar it forms the old-fashioned oxymel, always popular against colds of the chest and throat.

"Honeywater" distilled from Honey, incorporated with sand, is an excellent wash for promoting the growth of the hair, either by itself, or when mixed with spirit of rosemary. Rose Honey (rhodomel) made from the expressed juice of rose petals with Honey, was formerly held in high esteem for the sick.

Bee propolis, or the glutinous resin manufactured by bees for fixing the foundations of their combs, will afford relief to the asthmatic by its fumes when burnt. It consists largely of resin, and yields benzoic acid.

Basilicon, kingly ointment, or resin ointment, is composed of bees wax, olive oil, resin, Burgundy pitch, and turpentine. This is said to be identical with the famous "Holloway's Ointment," and is highly useful when the stimulation of indolent sores is desired.

A medicinal tincture of superlative worth is prepared by Homœopathic practitioners from the sting of the Honey bee. This makes a most valuable and approved medicine for obviating erysipelas, especially of the head and face; likewise, for a puffy sore throat with much swelling about the tonsils; also for dropsy of the limbs which has followed a chill, or is connected with passive inactivity of the kidneys. Ten drops of the diluted tincture, first decimal strength, should be given three or four times in the day, with a tablespoonful of cold water. This remedy is known as the tincture of *Apis mellifica.* For making it the bees are seized when emerging from the hive, and they thus become irritated, being ready to sting. They are put to death with a few drops of chloroform, and then have their Honey-bags severed. These are bruised in a mortar with glycerine, and bottled in spirit of wine, shaking them for several days, and lastly filtering the tincture.

Boiling water poured on bees (workers) when newly killed makes bee-tea, which may be taken to relieve strangury, and a difficult passage of urine, as likewise for dropsy of the heart and kidneys. Also of such bees when dried and powdered, thirty grains will act as a dose to promote a free flow of the urine.

Honey, especially if old, will cause indigestion when eaten by some persons, through an excessive production of lactic acid in the stomach; and a superficial ulceration of the mouth and tongue, resembling thrush, will ensue; it being at the same time a known popular fact, that Honey by itself, or when mixed with powdered borax (which is alkaline) will speedily cure a similar sore state within the mouth arising through deranged health.

As long ago as when Soranus lived, the contemporary of Galen (160 A.D.) Honey was declared to be "an easy remedy for the thrush of children," but he gravely attributed its virtues in this respect to the circumstance that bees collected the Honey from flowers growing over the tomb of Hippocrates, in the vale of Tempe.

The sting venom of bees has been found helpful for relieving rheumatic gout in the hands, and elsewhere through toxicating the tender and swollen limbs by means of lively bees placed over the parts in an inverted tumbler, and then irritating the insects so as to make them sting. A custom prevails in Malta of inoculation by frequent bee stinging, so as to impart at length a protective immunity against rheumatism, this being confirmatory of the fact known to bee keepers elsewhere, that after exposure to attacks from bees, often repeated throughout a length of time, most persons will acquire a convenient freedom from all future disagreeable effects. An Austrian physician has based on these methods an infallible cure for acute rheumatism.

In Shakespeare's *Twelfth Night*, Sir Toby Belch asks to have a "song for sixpence," the third verse of which has been thought to run thus :—

"The King was in his counting house
Counting out his money,
The Queen was in the parlour
Eating bread and Honey."

"Mel mandit, panemque, morans regina culinâ,
Dulcia plebeiâ non comedenda nuru."

A plain cake, currant or seed, made with Honey in place of sugar is a pleasant addition to the tea-table and a capital preventive of constipation.

"All kinds of precious stones cast into Honey become more brilliant thereby," says St. Francis de Sales in *The Devout Life*, 1708, "and all persons become more acceptable when they join devotion to their graces."

HOP.

THE Hop (*Humulus lupulus*) belongs to the Nettle tribe (*Cannabineæ*) of plants, and grows wild in our English hedges and copses ; but then it bears only male flowers. When cultivated it produces the female catkins, or strobiles which are so well known as Hops, and are so largely used for brewing purposes.

The plant gets its first name *Humulus* from *humus*, the rich moist ground in which it chooses to grow, and its affix *lupulus* from the Latin *lupus* a wolf, because (as Pliny explained), when produced among osiers, it strangles them by its light climbing embraces as the wolf does a sheep.

The word Hop comes from the Anglo-saxon *hoppan* to climb. The leaves and the flowers afford a fine brown dye, and paper has been made from the bine, or stalk, which sprouts in May, and soon grows luxuriantly; as said old Tusser (1557):—

> "Get into thy Hop-yard, for now it is time
> To teach Robin Hop on his pole how to climb."

The Hop, says Cockayne, was known to the Saxons, and they called it the *Hymele,* a name enquired-for in vain among Hop growers in Worcestershire and Kent.

Hops were first brought to this country from Flanders, in 1524:—

> "Turkeys, Carp, Hops, Pickerel, and Beer,
> Came into England all in one year."

So writes old Izaak Walton! Before Hops were used for improving and preserving beer our Saxon ancestors drank a beverage made from malt, but clarified in a measure with Ground Ivy which is hence named Alehoof. This was a thick liquor about which it was said:—

> "Nil spissius est dum bibitur; nil clarius dum mingitur,
> Unde constat multas fæces in ventre relinqui."

The Picts made beer from heather, but the secret of its manufacture was lost when they became exterminated, since it had never been divulged to strangers. Kenneth offered to spare the life of a father, whose son had been just slain, if he would reveal the method; but, though pardoned, he refused persistently. The inhabitants of Tola, Jura, and other outlying districts, now brew a potable beer by mixing two-thirds of heath tops with one of malt. Highlanders think it very lucky to find the white heather, which is the badge of the Captain of Clan Ronald.

At first Hops were unpopular, and were supposed to engender melancholy. Therefore Henry the Eighth issued an injunction to brewers not to use them. "Hops," says John Evelyn in his *Pomona*, 1670, "transmuted our wholesome ale into beer, which doubtless much altered our constitutions. This one ingredient, by some suspected not unworthily, preserves the drink indeed, but repays the pleasure with tormenting diseases, and a shorter life."

Hops, such as come into the market, are the chaffy capsules of the seeds, and turn brown early in the autumn. They possess a heavy fragrant aromatic odour, and a very bitter pungent taste. The yellow glands at the base of the scales afford a volatile strong-smelling oil, and an abundant yellow powder which possesses most of the virtues of the plant. Our druggists prepare a tincture from the strobiles with spirit of wine, and likewise a thickened extract.

Again, a decoction of the root is esteemed by some as of equal benefit with Sarsaparilla.

The lassitude felt in hot weather at its first access, or in early spring, may be well met by an infusion of the leaves, strobiles and stalks as Hop tea, taken by the wineglassful two or three times in the day, whilst sluggish derangements of the liver and spleen may be benefited thereby.

Lupulin, the golden dust from the scales (but not the pollen of the anthers, as some erroneously suppose), is given in powder, and acts as a gentle sedative if taken at bedtime. This is specific against sexual irritability and its attendant train of morbid symptoms, with mental depression and vital exhaustion. It contains "lupulite," a volatile oil, and a peculiar resin, which is somewhat acrid, and penetrating of taste.

Each of the Simples got from the Hop will allay pain and conduce to sleep; they increase the firmness of the pulse, and reduce its frequency.

Also if applied externally, Hops as a poultice, or when steeped in a bag, in very hot water as a stupe, will relieve muscular rheumatism, spasm, and bruises.

Hop tea, when made from the flowers only, is to be brewed by pouring a pint of boiling water on an ounce of the Hops, and letting it stand until cool. This is an excellent drink in delirium tremens, and will give prompt ease to an irritable bladder. Sherry in which some Hops have been steeped makes a capital stomachic cordial. A pillow, *Pulvinar Humuli*, stuffed with newly dried Hops was successfully prescribed by Dr. Willis for George the Third, when sedative medicines had failed to give him sleep; and again for our Prince of Wales at the time of his severe typhoid fever, 1871, in conjunction then with a most grateful draught of ale which had been heretofore withheld. The crackling of dry Hop flowers when put into a pillow may be prevented by first sprinkling them with a little alcohol.

Persons have fallen into a deep slumber after remaining for some time in a storehouse full of hops; and in certain northern districts a watery extract from the flowers is given instead of opium. It is useful to know that for sound reasons a moderate supper of bread and butter, with crisp fresh lettuces, and light home-brewed ale which contains Hops, is admirably calculated to promote sleep, except in a full-blooded plethoric person. *Lupulin*, the glandular powder from the dried strobiles, will induce sleep without causing constipation, or headache. The dose is from two to four grains at bedtime on a small piece of bread and butter, or mixed with a spoonful of milk.

The year 1855 produced a larger crop of cultivated Hops than has been known before or since. When Hop poles are shaken by the wind there is a distant electrical murmur like thunder.

Hop tea in the leaf is now sold by grocers, made from a mixture of the Kentish and Indian plants, so as to combine in its infusion, the refreshment of the one herb with the sleep-inducing virtues of the other. The hops are brought direct from the farmers, just as they are picked. They are then laid for a few hours to wither, after which they are put under a rolling apparatus, which in half-an-hour makes them look like tea leaves, both in shape and colour. They are finally mixed with Indian and Ceylon teas.

The young tops of the Hop plant if gathered in the spring and boiled, may be eaten as asparagus, and make a good pot-herb: they were formerly brought to market tied up in small bundles for table use.

A popular notion has, in some places, associated the Hop and the Nightingale together as frequenting the same districts.

Medicinally the Hop is tonic, stomachic, and diuretic, with antiseptic effects; it prevents worms, and allays the disquietude of nervous indigestion. The popular nostrum "Hop Bitters" is thus made: Buchu leaves, two ounces; Hops, half-a-pound; boil in five quarts of water, in an iron vessel, for an hour; when lukewarm add essence of Winter-green (*Pyrola*), two ounces, and one pint of alcohol. Take one tablespoonful three times in the day, before eating. White Bryony root is likewise used in making the Bitters.

HOREHOUND (White and Black).

THE herb Horehound occurs of two sorts, white and black, in our hedge-rows, and on the sides of banks, each getting its generic name, which was originally Harehune, from *hara*, hoary, and *hune*, honey; or, possibly, the name Horehound may be a corruption of the Latin *Urinaria*, since the herb has been found efficacious in cases of strangury, or difficult making of water.

The White Horehound (*Marrubium*) is a common square-stemmed herb of the Labiate order, growing in waste places, and of popular use for coughs and colds, whether in a medicinal form, or as a candied sweetmeat. Its botanical title is of Hebrew derivation, from *marrob*, a bitter juice. The plant is distinguished by the white woolly down on its stems, by its wrinkled leaves, and small white flowers.

It has a musky odour, and a bitter taste, being a much esteemed Herbal Simple, but very often spuriously imitated. It affords chemically a fragrant volatile oil, a bitter extractive "marrubin," and gallic acid.

As a homely remedy it is especially given for coughs accompanied with abundant thick expectoration, and for chronic asthma. In Norfolk scarcely a cottage garden can be found without its Horehound corner; and Horehound beer is much drunk there by the natives. Horehound tea may be made by pouring boiling water on the fresh leaves, an ounce to a pint, and sweetening this with honey: then a wineglassful should be taken three or four times in the day. Or from two to three teaspoonfuls of the expressed juice of the herb may be given for a dose.

Candied Horehound is best made from the fresh plant by boiling it down until the juice is extracted, and then adding sugar before boiling this again until it has become thick enough of consistence to pour into a paper case, and to be cut into squares when cool. Gerard said: "Syrup made from the greene fresh leaves and sugar is a most singular remedy against the cough and wheezing of the lungs. It doth wonderfully, and above credit, ease such as have been long sicke of any consumption of the lungs; as hath been often proved by the learned physicians of our London College."

When given in full doses, an infusion of the herb is laxative. If the plant be put in new milk and set in a place pestered with flies, it will speedily kill them all. And according to Columella, the Horehound is a serviceable remedy against the Cankerworm in trees: *Profuit et plantis latices infundere amaros marrubii.*

The Marrubium was called by the Egyptian Priests the "Seed of Horus," or "the Bull's Blood," and "the Eye of the Star." It was a principal remedy in the Negro Cœsar's Antidote for vegetable poisons.

The Black Horehound (*Ballota nigra*), so called from its dark purple-coloured flowers, is likewise of common growth about our roadsides and waste places. Its botanical title comes from the Greek *ballo*, to reject, because of its disagreeable odour, particularly when burnt. The herb is sometimes known as Madwort, being supposed to act as an antidote to the bite of a mad dog. In Beaumont and Fletcher's *Faithful Shepherdess*, we read of:—

> "Black Horehound, good
> For Sheep, or Shepherd bitten by a wood-
> dog's venomed tooth."

If its leaves are applied externally as a poultice, they will relieve the pain of gout, and will mollify angry boils. In Gotha the plant is valued for curing chronic skin diseases, particularly of a fungoid character, such as ringworm; also for diseases of cattle. "This," says Meyrick "is one of those neglected English herbs which are possessed of great virtues, though they are but little known, and still less regarded. It is superior to most things as a remedy in hysteria, and for low spirits." Drayton said (*Polybion*, 1613):—

> "For comforting the spleen and liver—get for juice,
> Pale Horehound."

The Water Horehound (*Lycopus*), or Gipsy wort, which grows frequently in our damp meadows and on the sides of streams, yields a black dye used for wool, or silk, and with which gipsies stain their skins, as well as with Walnut juice. "This is called Gipsy Wort," says Lyte, "because the rogues and runagates, which name themselves Egyptians, do colour themselves black with this herbe." Each of the Horehounds is a labiate plant; and this, the water variety, bears flesh coloured flowers, whilst containing a volatile oil, a resin, a bitter principle, and tannin. Its medicinal action is astringent, with a reduced frequency of the pulse, and some gentle sedative effects, so that any tendency to coughing, etc., will be allayed. Half-an-ounce of the plant to a pint of boiling water will make the infusion.

HORSE RADISH (*Radix*, a Root).

THE Horse Radish of our gardens is a cultivated cruciferous plant of which the fresh root is eaten, when scraped, as a condiment to correct the richness of our national roast beef. This plant grows wild in many parts of the country, particularly about rubbish, and the sides of ditches; yet it is probably an introduction, and not a native. Its botanical name, *Cochlearia armoracia*, implies a resemblance between its leaves and an old-fashioned spoon, *cochleare*; also that the most common place of its growth is *ar*, near, *mor*, the sea.

Our English vernacular styles the plant "a coarse root," or a "Horse radish," as distinguished from the eatable radish (root), the *Raphanus sativus*. Formerly it was named Mountain Radish, and Great Raifort. This is said to be one of the five bitter herbs ordered to be eaten by the Jews during the Feast of the Passover, the other four being Coriander, Horehound, Lettuce, and Nettle.

Not a few fatal cases have occurred of persons being poisoned by taking Aconite root in mistake for a stick of Horse radish, and eating it when scraped. But the two roots differ materially in shape, colour, and taste, so as to be easily discriminated : furthermore the leaves of the Aconite—supposing them to be attached to the root—are not to be mistaken for those of any other plant, being completely divided to their base into five wedge-shaped lobes, which are again sub-divided into three. Squire says it seems incredible that the Aconite Root should be mistaken for Horse Radish unless we remember that country folk are in the habit of putting back again into the ground Horse Radish which has been scraped, until there remain only the crown and a remnant of the root vanishing to a point, these bearing resemblance to the tap root of Aconite.

The fresh root of the Horse radish is a powerful stimulant by reason of its ardent and pungent volatile principle, whether it be taken as a medicament, or be applied externally to any part of the body. When scraped it exhales a nose-provoking odour, and possesses a hot biting taste, combined with a certain sweetness: but on exposure to the air it quickly turns colour, and loses its volatile strength; likewise, it becomes vapid, and inert by being boiled. The root is expectorant, antiscorbutic, and, if taken at all freely, emetic. It contains a somewhat large proportion of sulphur, as shown by the black colour assumed by metals with which it comes into touch. Hence it promises to be of signal use for relieving chronic rheumatism, and for remedying scurvy.

Taken in sauce with oily fish or rich fatty viands, scraped Horse radish acts as a corrective spur to complete digestion, and at the same time it will benefit a relaxed sore throat, by contact during the swallowing. In facial neuralgia scraped Horse radish applied as a poultice, proves usefully beneficial: and for the same purpose some of the fresh scrapings may be profitably held in the hand of the affected side, which hand will become in a short time bloodlessly benumbed, and white.

When sliced across with a knife the root of the Horse radish will exude some drops of a sweet juice which may be rubbed with advantage on rheumatic, or palsied limbs. Also an infusion of the sliced root in milk, almost boiling, and allowed to cool, makes an excellent and safe cosmetic; or the root may be infused for a longer time in cold milk, if preferred, for use with a like purpose in view. Towards the end of the last century Horse radish was known in England as Red cole, and in the previous century it was eaten habitually at table, sliced, with vinegar.

Infused in wine the root stimulates the whole nervous system, and promotes perspiration, whilst acting likewise as a diuretic. For rheumatic neuralgia it is almost a specific, and for palsy it has often proved of service. Our druggists prepare a "compound spirit of Horse radish," made with the sliced fresh root, orange peel, nutmeg, and spirit of wine. This proves of effective use in strengthless, languid indigestion, as well as for chronic rheumatism; it stimulates the stomach, and promotes the digestive secretions. From one to two teaspoonfuls may be taken two or three times in the day, with half a wineglassful of water, at the end of a principal meal, or a few minutes after the meal. An infusion of the root made with boiling water and taken hot readily proves a stimulating emetic. Until cut or bruised the root is inodorous; but fermentation then begins, and develops from the essential oil an ammoniacal odour and a pungent hot bitter taste which were not pre-existing.

Chemically the Horse radish contains a volatile oil, identical with that of mustard, being highly diffusible and pungent by reason of its "myrosin." One drop of this volatile oil will suffice to odorise the atmosphere of a whole room, and, if swallowed with any freedom, it excites vomiting. Other constituents of the root are a bitter resin, sugar, starch, gum, albumen, and acetates.

A mixture of the fresh juice, with vinegar, if applied externally, will prove generally of service for removing freckles.

Bergius alleges that by cutting the root into very small pieces without bruising it, and then swallowing a tablespoonful of these fragments every morning without chewing them, for a month, a cure has been effected in chronic rheumatism, which had seemed otherwise intractable.

For loss of the voice and relaxed sore throat the

infusion of Horse radish makes an excellent gargle; or it may be concentrated in the form of a syrup, and mixed for the same use—a teaspoonful, with a wineglassful of cold water.

Gerard said of the root: "If bruised and laid to the part grieved with the sciatica, gout, joyntache, or the hard swellings of the spleen and liver, it doth wonderfully help them all." If the scraped root be macerated in vinegar, it will form a mixture (which may be sweetened with glycerine to the taste) very effective against whooping cough. In pimply acne of the skin, to touch each papula with some of the Compound Spirit of Horse Radish now and again will soon effect a general cure of the ailment.

HOUSE LEEK (Crassulaceæ).

THE House Leek (*Sempervivum tectorum*), or "never dying" flower of our cottage roofs, which is commonly known also as Stone-crop, grows plentifully on walls and the tops of small buildings throughout Great Britain, in all country districts. It is distinguished by its compact rose-shaped arrangement of seagreen succulent leaves lying sessile in a somewhat flattened manner, and by its popularity among country folk on account of these bland juicy leaves, and its reputed protective virtues. It possesses a remarkable tenacity of life, *quem sempervivam dicunt quoniam omni tempore viret*, this being in allusion to its prolonged vitality; for which reason it is likewise called Ayegreen, and Sengreen (*semper*, green).

History relates that a botanist tried hard for eighteen months to dry a plant of the House Leek for his herbarium, but failed in this object. He afterwards restored it to its first site when it grew again as if nothing had interfered with its ordinary life.

The plant was dedicated of old to Thor, or Jupiter, and sometimes to the Devil. It bore the titles of Thor's beard, Jupiter's eye, Joubarb, and Jupiter's beard, from its massive inflorescence which resembles the sculptured beard of Jove; though a more recent designation is St. George's beard.

> "Quem sempervivam dicunt quoniam viret omni
> Tempore—'Barba Jovis' vulgari more vocatur,
> Esse refert similem predictœ Plinius istam."
>
> *Macer.*

The Romans took great pleasure in the House Leek, and grew it in vases set before the windows of their houses. They termed it *Buphthalmon*, *Zoophthalmon*, and *Stergethron*, as one of the love medicines; it being further called *Hypogeson*, from growing under the eaves; likewise *Ambrosia* and *Ameramnos*. The plant is indigenous to the Greek Islands, being sometimes spoken of as "Imbreke" and "Home Wort."

It has been largely planted about the roofs of small houses throughout the country, particularly in Scotland, because supposed to guard against lightning and thunderstorms; likewise as protective against the enchantments of sorcerers; and, in a more utilitarian spirit, as preservative against decay. Hence the House Leek is known as Thunderbeard, and in Germany *Donnersbart* or *Donderbloem*, from "Jupiter the thunderer."

The English name House Leek denotes *leac* (Anglo-Saxon) a plant growing on the house; and another appellation of its genus, *sedum*, comes from the Latin *sedare*, to soothe, and subdue inflammations, etc.

The thick leaves contain an abundant acidulous astringent juice, which is mucilaginous, and affords malic acid, identical with that of the Apple. This juice, in a dose of from one to three drams, has proved useful in dysentery, and in some convulsive diseases. Galen extolled it as a capital application for erysipelas and shingles. Dioscorides praised it for weak and inflamed eyes, but in large doses it is emetic and purgative.

In rural districts the bruised leaves of the fresh plant or its juice are often applied to burns, scalds, contusions, and sore legs, or to scrofulous ulcers; as likewise for chronic skin diseases, and enlarged or cancerous lymphatic glands. By the Dutch the leaves are cultivated with a dietetic purpose for mixing in their salads.

With honey the juice assuages the soreness and ulcerated condition within the mouth in thrush. Gerard says: "The juice being gently rubbed on any place stung by nettles, or bees, or bitten by any venomous creature, doth presently take away the pain. Being applied to the temples and forehead it easeth also the headache and distempered heat of the brain through want of sleep."

The juice, moreover, is excellently helpful for curing corns and warts, if applied from day to day after they have been scraped. As Parkinson teaches, "the juice takes away cornes from the toes and feet if they be bathed therewith every day, and at night emplastered as it were with the skin of the same House Leek."

The plant may be readily made to cover all the roof of a building by sticking on the offsets with a little moist earth, or cowdung. It bears purple flowers, and its leaves are fringed at their edges, being succulent and pulpy. Thus the erect gay-looking blossoms, in contrast to the light green foliage arranged in the form of full blown double roses, lend a picturesque appearance to the roof of even a cow-byre, or a hovel.

The House Leek (*Sedum majus*), and the Persicaria Water-pepper (Arsmart), if their juices be boiled together, will cure a diarrhœa, however obstinate, or inveterate. The famous empirical *anti-Canceroso nostrum* of Count Mattæi is authoritatively said to consist of the *Sedum acre* (Betony stone-crop), the *Sempervivum tectorum* (House Leek), *Sedum telephium* (Livelong), the *Matricaria* (Feverfew), and the *Nasturtium Sisymbrium* (Water-cress).

The *Sedum Telephium* (Livelong, or Orpine), called also Roseroot and Midsummer Men, is the largest British species of Stone-crop. Being a plant of augury its leaves are laid out in pairs on St. John's Eve, these being named after courting couples. When the leaves are freshly assorted those which keep together promise well for their namesakes, and those which fall apart, the reverse.

The special virtues of this *Sedum* are supposed to have been discovered by Telephus, the son of Hercules. Napoleon, at St. Helena, was aware of its anti-cancerous reputation, which was firmly believed in Corsica. The plant contains lime, sulphur, ammonia, and (perhaps) mercury. It remains long alive when hung up in a room. The designation Orpine has become perversely applied to this plant which bears pink blossoms, the word having been derived from *Orpin*, gold pigment, a yellow sulphuret of the metal arsenic, and it should appertain exclusively to yellow flowers. The Livelong *Sedum* was formerly named Life Everlasting. It serves to keep away moths.

Doctors have found that the expulsive vomiting provoked by doses of the *Sedum acre* (Betony stone-crop), will serve in diphtheria to remove such false membrane clinging in patches to the throat and tonsils, as threatens suffocation: and after this release afforded by copious vomiting, the diphtheritic foci are prevented from forming again.

The *Sedum Acre* (or Biting Stone-crop) is also named Pepper crop, being a cyme, or head of flowers, which furnishes a pungent taste like that of pepper. This further bears the names of Ginger (in Norfolk), Jack of the Buttery, Gold Dust, Creeping Tom, Wall Pepper, Pricket or Prick Madam, Gold Chain, and Biting Mouse Tail. It was formerly said "the savages of Caledonia use this plant for removing the sloughs of cancer."

The herb serves admirably to make a gargle for scurvy of the gums, and a lotion for scrofulous, or syphilitic ulcers. The leaves are thick and very acrid, being crowded together. This and the *Sedums album* and *reflexum* were ingredients in a famous worm-expelling medicine, or *theriac* (treacle), which conferred the title "Jack of the Buttery," as a corruption of "*Bot. theriaque.*"

The several Stone-crops are so named from *crop*, a top, or bunch of flowers, these plants being found chiefly in tufts upon walls or roofs. From their close growth originally on their native rocks they have acquired the generic title of *Sedum*, from *sedere* (to sit).

HYSSOP.

THE cultivated Hyssop, now of frequent occurrence in the herb-bed, and a favourite plant there because of its fragrance, belongs to the labiate order, and possesses cordial qualities which give it rank as a Simple. It has pleasantly odorous striped leaves which vary in colour, and possess a camphoraceous odour, with a warm aromatic bitter taste. This is of comparatively recent introduction into our gardens, not having been cultivated until Gerard's time, about 1568, and not being a native English herb.

The *Ussopos* of Dioscorides, was named from *azob*, a holy herb, because used for cleansing sacred places. Hence it is alluded to in this sense scripturally: "Purge me with Hyssop, and I shall be clean: wash me, and I shall be whiter than snow" (Psalm li. 7). Solomon wrote "of all trees, from the Cedar in Lebanon to the Hyssop that springeth out of the wall." The healing virtues of the plant are due to a particular volatile oil which admirably promotes expectoration in bronchial catarrh and asthma. Hyssop tea is a grateful drink well adapted to improve the tone of a feeble stomach, being brewed with the green tops of the herb. The same parts of the plant are sometimes boiled in soup to be given for asthma. The leaves and flowers are of a warm pungent taste, and of an agreeable aromatic smell; therefore if the tops and blossoms are reduced to a powder and added to cold salad herbs they give a comforting cordial virtue.

There was formerly made a distilled water of Hyssop, which may still be had from some druggists, it being deemed a good pectoral medicine. In America an infusion of the leaves is used externally for the relief of muscular rheumatism, as also for bruises and discoloured contusions. The herb was sometimes called Rosemary in the East, and was hung up to afford protection from the evil eye, as well as to guard against witches.

To make Hyssop tea, one drachm of the herb should be infused in a pint of boiling water, and allowed to become cool. Then a wineglassful is to be given as a dose two or three times in the day.

Of the essential oil of Hyssop, from one to two drops

should be the dose. Pliny said: "Hyssop mixed with figs, purges; with honey, vomits." If the herb be steeped in boiling water and applied hot to the part, it will quickly remove the blackness consequent upon a bruise or blow, especially in the case of "black" or blood-shot eyes.

Parkinson says that in his day "the golden hyssop was of so pleasant a colour that it provoked every gentlewoman to wear them in their heads, and on their arms with as much delight as many fine flowers can give." The leaves are striped conspicuously with white or yellow; for which reason, and because of their fragrance, the herb is often chosen to be planted on graves. The green herb, bruised and applied, will heal cuts promptly. Its tea will assist in promoting the monthly courses for women. Hyssop grows wild in middle and southern Europe.

The Hedge Hyssop (*Gratiola officinalis*), or Water Hyssop, is quite a different plant from the garden pot-herb, and belongs to the scrofula-curing order, with far more active medicinal properties than the Hyssop proper. The commonly recognized Hedge Hyssop bears a pale yellow, or a pale purple flower, like that of the Foxglove; and the whole plant has a very bitter taste. A medicinal tincture (H.) is made from the entire herb, of which from eight to ten drops may be taken with a tablespoonful of cold water three times in the day. It will afford relief against nervous weakness and shakiness, such as occur after an excessive use of coffee or tobacco. The title "gratiola," is from *dei gratiâ*, "by the grace of God."

The juice of the plant purges briskly, and may be usefully employed in some forms of dropsy. Its decoction is milder of action, and proves beneficial in cases of jaundice. In France the plant is cultivated as a perfume, and it is said to be an active ingredient in the famous *Eau médicinale* for gout.

Of the dried leaves from five to twenty-five grains will act as a drastic vermifuge to expel worms. The root resembles ipecacuanha in its effects, and in moderate quantities, as a powder or decoction, helps to stay bloody fluxes and purgings. The flowers are sometimes of a blood-red hue, and the whole plant contains a special essential oil.

"Whoso taketh," says Parkinson, "but one scruple of *Gratiola* (Hedge Hyssop) bruised, shall perceive evidently his effectual operation and virtue in purging mightily, and that in great abundance, watery, gross, and slimy tumours." *Caveat qui sumpserit.* On the principle of affinities, small diluted doses of the tincture, or decoction, or of the dried leaves, prove curative in cases of fluxes from the lower bowels, where irritation within the fundament is frequent, and where there is considerable nervous exhaustion, especially in chronic cases of this sort.

IVY, Common (*Araliaceæ*).

THE clergyman of fiction in the sixth chapter of Dickens' memorable *Pickwick*, sings certain verses which he styles "indifferent" (the only verse, by the way, to be found in all that great writer's stories), and which relate to the Ivy, beginning thus :—

> "Oh! a dainty plant is the Ivy green,
> That creepeth o'er ruins old."

The well known common Ivy (*Hedera helix*), which clothes the trunks of trees and the walls of old buildings so picturesquely throughout Great Britain, gets its botanical name most probably from the Celtic word *hædra* "a cord," or from the Greek *hedra* "a seat," because sitting close, and its vernacular title from *iw* "green," which is also the parent of "yew." In Latin it is termed *abiga*, easily corrupted to "iva"; and the Danes knew it as Winter-grunt, or Winter-green, to which appellation it may still lay a rightful claim, being so conspicuously green at the coldest times of the year when trees are of themselves bare and brown.

By the ancients the Ivy was dedicated to Bacchus, whose statues were crowned with a wreath of the plant, under the name Kissos, and whose worshippers decorated themselves with its garlands. The leaves have a peculiar faintly nauseous odour, whilst they are somewhat bitter, and rough of taste. The fresh berries are rather acid, and become bitter when dried. They are much eaten by our woodland birds in the spring.

A crown of Ivy was likewise given to the classic poets of distinction, and the Greek priests presented a wreath of the same to newly married persons. The custom of decorating houses and churches with Ivy at Christmastide, was forbidden by one of the early councils on account of its Pagan associations. Prynne wrote with reference to this decree :—

"At Christmas men do always Ivy get,
And in each corner of the house it set,
But why make use then of that Bacchus weed?
Because they purpose Bacchus-like to feed."

The Ivy, though sending out innumerable small rootlets, like suckers, in every direction (which are really for support) is not a parasite. The plant is rooted in the soil and gets its sustenance therefrom.

Chemically, its medicinal principles depend on the special balsamic resin contained in the leaves and stems, as well as constituting the aromatic gum.

Ivy flowers have little or no scent, but their yield of nectar is particularly abundant.

When the bark of the main stems is wounded, a gum will exude, and may be collected : it possesses astringent and mildly aperient properties. This was at one time included as a medicine in the Edinburgh *Pharmacopœia*, but it has now fallen out of such authoritative use. Its chemical principle is "hederin." The gum is anti-spasmodic, and promotes the monthly flow of women.

An infusion of the berries will relieve rheumatism, and a decoction of the leaves applied externally will destroy vermin in the heads of children.

Fresh Ivy leaves will afford signal relief to corns when they shoot, and are painful. Good John Wesley, who dabbled in "domestic medicine," and with much sagacity of observation, taught that having bathed the feet, and cut the corns, and having mashed some fresh Ivy leaves, these are to be applied: then by repeating the remedial process for fifteen days the corns will be cured.

During the Great Plague of London, Ivy berries were given with some success as possessing antiseptic virtues, and to induce perspiration, thus effecting a remission of the symptoms. Cups made from Ivywood have been employed from which to drink for disorders of the spleen, and for whooping cough, their method of use being to be kept refilled from time to time with water (cold or hot), which the patient is to constantly sip.

Ivy gum dissolved in vinegar is a good filling for a hollow tooth which is causing neuralgic toothache: and an infusion of the leaves made with cold water, will, after standing for twenty-four hours, relieve sore and smarting eyes if used rather frequently as a lotion. A decoction of the leaves and berries will mitigate a severe headache, such as that which follows hard drinking over night. And it may have come about that from some rude acquaintance with this fact the bacchanals adopted goblets carved out of Ivywood.

This plant is especially hardy, and suffers but little from the smoke and the vitiated air of a manufacturing town. Chemically, such medicinal principles as the Ivy possesses depend on the special balsamic resin contained in its leaves and stems; as well as on its particular gum. Bibulous old Bacchus was always represented in classic sculpture with a wreath of Ivy round his laughing brows; and it has been said that if the foreheads of those whose potations run deep were bound with frontlets of Ivy the nemesis of headache would be prevented thereby. But legendary lore teaches rather that the infant Bacchus was an object of vengeance to Juno, and that the nymphs of Nisa concealed him from her wrath, with trails of Ivy as he lay in his cradle.

At one time our taverns bore over their doors the sign of an Ivybush, to indicate the excellence of the liquor supplied within. From which fact arose the saying that "good wine needs no bush," "*Vinum vendibile hederâ non est opus.*" And of this text Rosalind cleverly avails herself in *As You Like It*, "If it be true" says she, "that good wine needs no bush,"—"'tis true that a good play needs no epilogue."

IVY (Ground).

THIS common, and very familiar little herb, with its small Ivy-like aromatic leaves, and its striking whorls of dark blue blossoms conspicuous in early spring time, comes into flower pretty punctually about the third or fourth of April, however late or early the season may be. Its name is attributed to the resemblance borne by its foliage to that of the true Ivy (*Hedera helix*). The whole plant possesses a balsamic odour, and an aromatic taste, due to its particular volatile oil, and its characteristic resin, as a fragrant labiate herb. It remaineth green not only in summer, but also in winter, at all times of the year.

From the earliest days it has been thought endowed with singular curative virtues chiefly against nervous headaches, and for the relief of chronic bronchitis. Ray tells of a remarkable instance in the person of a Mr. Oldacre who was cured of an obstinate chronic headache by using the juice or the powdered leaves of the Ground Ivy as snuff: *Succus hujus plantæ naribus attractus cephalalgiam etiam vehementissimam et inveteratam non lenit tantum, sed et penitus aufert*; and he adds in further praise of the herb: *Medicamentum hoc non satis potest laudari; si res ex usu æstimarentur, auro æquiparandum.* An infusion of the fresh herb, or, if made in winter, from its dried leaves, and drank under the name of Gill tea, is a favourite remedy with the poor for coughs of long standing, accompanied with much phlegm. One ounce of the herb should be infused in a pint of boiling water, and a wineglassful of this when cool is to be taken three or four times in the day. The botanical name of the plant is *Nepeta glechoma*, from Nepet, in Tuscany, and the Greek *gleechon*, a mint.

Resembling Ivy in miniature, the leaves have been used in weaving chaplets for the dead, as well as for adorning the Alestake erected as a sign at taverns. For this reason, and because formerly in vogue for clearing the ale drank by our Saxon ancestors, the herb acquired the names of Ale hoof, and Tun hoof ("tun" signifying a garden, and "hoof" or "hufe" a coronal or chaplet), or Hove, "because," says Parkinson, "it spreadeth as a garland upon the ground." Other titles which have a like meaning are borne by the herb, such as "Gill go by the ground," and Haymaids, or Hedgemaids; the word "gill" not only relating to the fermentation of beer, but meaning also a maid. This is shown in the saying, "Every Jack should have his Gill, or Jill"; and the same notion was conveyed by the sobriquet "haymaids." Again in some districts the Ground Ivy is called "Lizzy run up the hedge," "Cat's-foot" (from the soft flower heads), "Devil's candlesticks," "Aller," and in Germany "Thundervine," also in the old English manuscripts "Hayhouse," "Halehouse," and "Horshone." The whole plant was employed by our Saxon progenitors to clarify their so-called beer, before hops had been introduced for this purpose; and the place of refreshment where the beverage was sold bore the name of a "Gill house."

In *A Thousand Notable Things*, it is stated, "The juice of Ground Ivy sniffed up into the nostrils out of a spoon, or a saucer, purgeth the head marvellously, and taketh away the greatest and oldest pain thereof that is: the medicine is worth gold, though it is very cheap."

Small hairy tumours may often be seen in the autumn on the leaves of the Ground Ivy occasioned (says Miss Pratt) by the punctures of the *cynips glechomæ* from which these galls spring. They have a strong flavour of the plant, and are sometimes eaten by the peasantry of France. The volatile oil on which the special virtues of the Ground Ivy depend exudes from small glandular dots on the under surface of the leaves. This is the active ingredient of Gill tea made by country persons, and sweetened with honey, sugar, or liquorice. Also the expressed juice of the herb is equally effectual, being diaphoretic, diuretic, and somewhat astringent against bleedings.

Gerard says that in his day "the Ground Ivy was commended against the humming sound, and ringing noises of the ears by being put into them, and for those that are hard of hearing. Also boiled in mutton broth it helpeth weak and aching backs." Dr. Thornton tells us in his *Herbal* (1810) that "Ground Ivy was at one time amongst the 'cries' of London, for making a tea to purify the blood," and Dr. Pitcairn extolled this plant before all other vegetable medicines for the cure of consumption. Perhaps the name Ground Ivy was transferred at first to the *Nepeta* from the Periwinkle, about which we read in an old distich of Stockholm:—

"Parvenke is an erbe green of colour,
In time of May he bereth blo flour,
His stalkes are so feynt and feye
That nevermore groweth he heye:
On the grounde he rynneth and growe
As doth the erbe that *hyth tunhowe*;
The lef is thicke, schinende and styf
As is the grene Ivy leef:
Uniche brod, and nerhand rownde;
Men call it the *Ivy of the grounde.*"

In the *Organic Materia Medica* of Detroit, U.S.A., 1890, it is stated, "Painters use the Ground Ivy (*Nepeta glechoma*) as a remedy for, and a preventive of lead colic." An infusion is given (the ounce to a pint of boiling water)—one wineglassful for a dose repeatedly. In the relief which it affords as a snuff made from the dried leaves to congestive headache of a passive continued sort, this benefit is most probably due partly to the special titillating aroma of the plant, and partly to the copious defluxion of mucus and tears from the nasal passages, and the eyes.

JOHN'S WORT.

THE wild Saint John's Wort (*Hypericum perforatum*) is a frequent plant in our woods and hedgebanks, having leaves studded with minute translucent vesicles, which seem to perforate their structure, and which contain a terebinthinate oil of fragrant medicinal virtues.

The name *Hypericum* is derived from the two Greek words, *huper eikon*, "over an apparition," because of its supposed power to exorcise evil spirits, or influences; whence it was also formerly called *Fuga dæmoniorum*, "the Devil's Scourge," "the Grace of God," "the Lord God's Wonder Plant," and some other names of a like import, probably too, because found to be of curative use against insanity. Again, it used to be entitled *Hexenkraut*, and "Witch's Herb," on account of its reputed magical powers. Matthiolus said, *Scripsere quidam Hypericum adeo odisse dæmones, ut ejus suffitu statim avolent*, "Certain writers have said that the St. John's Wort is so detested by evil spirits that they fly off at a whiff of its odour."

Further names of the herb are "Amber," "Hundred Holes," and *Sol terrestris*, the "Terrestrial Sun," because it was believed that all the spirits of darkness vanish in its presence, as at the rising of the sun.

For children troubled with incontinence of urine at night, and who wet their beds, an infusion, or tea, of the St. John's Wort is an admirable preventive medicine, which will stop this untoward infirmity.

The title St. John's Wort is given, either because the plant blossoms about St. John's day, June 24th, or because the red-coloured sap which it furnishes was thought to resemble and signalise the blood of St. John the Baptist. Ancient writers certainly attributed a host of virtues to this plant, especially for the cure of hypochondriasis, and insanity. The red juice, or "red oil," of *Hypericum* made effective by hanging for some months in a glass vessel exposed to the sun, is esteemed as one of the most popular and curative applications in Europe for excoriations, wounds, and bruises.

The flowers also when rubbed together between the fingers yield a red juice, so that the plant has obtained the title of *Sanguis hominis*, human blood. Furthermore, this herb is *Medicamentum in mansâ intus sumptum*, "to be chewed for its curative effects."

And for making a medicinal infusion, an ounce of the herb should be used to a pint of boiling water. This may be given beneficially for chronic catarrhs of the lungs, the bowels, or the urinary passages. Dr. Tuthill Massy considered the St. John's Wort, by virtue of its healing properties for injuries of the spinal cord, and its dependencies, the vulnerary "arnica" of the organic nervous system. On the doctrine of signatures, because of its perforated leaves, and because of the blood-red juice contained in the capsules which it bears, this plant was formerly deemed a most excellent specific for healing wounds, and for stopping a flow of blood :—

"Hypericon was there—the herb of war,
Pierced through with wounds, and seamed with many a scar."

For lacerated nerves, and injuries by violence to the spinal cord, a warm lotion should be employed, made with one part of the tincture to twenty parts of water, comfortably hot. A salve compounded from the flowers, and known as St. John's Wort Salve, is still much used and valued in English villages. And in several countries the dew which has fallen on vegetation before daybreak on St. John's morning, is gathered with great care. It is thought to protect the eyes from all harm throughout the ensuing year, and the Venetians say it renews the roots of the hair on the baldest of heads. Peasants in the Isle of Man, are wont to think that if anyone treads on the St. John's Wort after sunset, a fairy horse will arise from the earth, and will carry him about all night, leaving him at sunrise wherever he may chance to be.

The plant has a somewhat aromatic odour; and from the leaves and flowers, when crushed, a lemon-like scent is exhaled, whilst their taste is bitter and astringent. The flowers furnish for fabrics of silk or wool a dye of deep yellow. These parts of the plant were alone ordered by the London *Pharmacopœia* to be used for supplying in chief the medicinal, oily, resinous extractive of the plant.

The juice gives a red colour to the spirit of wine with which it is mixed, and to expressed oils, being then known as the *Hypericum* "red oil" mentioned above. The flowers contain tannin, and "*Hypericum* red."

Moreover, this *Hypericum* oil made from the tops is highly useful for healing bed sores, and is commended as excellent for ulcers. A medicinal tincture (H.) is prepared with spirit of wine from the entire fresh plant, collected when flowering, or in seed, and this proves of capital service for remedying injuries to the spinal cord, both by being given internally, and by its external use. It has been employed in like manner with benefit for lock-jaw. The dose of the tincture is from five to eight drops with a spoonful of water two or three times a day.

This plant may be readily distinguished from others of the Hypericaceous order by its decidedly two edged stem. Sprigs of it are stuck at the present time in Wales over every outer door on the eve of St. John's day;

and in Scotland, milking is done on the herb to dispel the malignant enchantments which cause ropy milk.

Among the Christian saints St. John represents light; and the flowers of this plant were taken as a reminder of the beneficent sun.

Tutsan is a large flowered variety (*Hypericum androsæmum*) of the St. John's Wort, named from the French *toute saine*, or "heal all," because of its many curative virtues; and is common in Devon and Cornwall. It possesses the same properties as the perforate sort, but yields a stronger and more camphoraceous odour when the flowers and the seed vessels are bruised. A tincture made from this plant, as well as that made from the perforate St. John's Wort, has been used with success to cure melancholia, and its allied forms of insanity. The seed-capsules of the Tutsan are glossy and berry-like; the leaves retain their strong resinous odour after being dried.

Tutsan is called also provincially "Woman's Tongue," once set g(r)owing it never stops; and by country folk in Ireland the "Rose of Sharon." Its botanical name Androsœmum, *andros aima*, man's blood, derived from the red juice and oil, probably suggested the popular title of Tutsan, "heal all," often corrupted to "Touchen leaf."

Gerard gives a receipt, as a great secret, for making a compound oil of *Hypericum*, "than which," he says, "I know that in the world there is no better; no, not the natural balsam itself." "The plant," he adds, "is a singular remedy for the sciatica, provided that the patient drink water for a day or two after purging." "The leaves laid upon broken shins and scabbed legs do heal them."

The whole plant is of a special value for healing

punctured wounds; and its leaves are diuretic. It is handsome and shrubby, growing to a height of two or three feet.

JUNIPER.

THE Juniper shrub (Arkenthos of the ancients), which is widely distributed about the world, grows not uncommonly in England as a stiff evergreen conifer on heathy ground, and bears bluish purple berries. These have a sweet, juicy, and, presently, bitter, brown pulp, containing three seeds, and they do not ripen until the second year. The flowers blossom in May and June. Probably the shrub gets its name from the Celtic *jeneprus*, "rude or rough." Gerard notes that "it grows most commonly very low, like unto our ground furzes." Gum Sandarach, or Pounce, is the product of this tree.

Medicinally, the berries and the fragrant tops are employed. They contain "juniperin," sugar, resins, wax, fat, formic and acetic acids, and malates. The fresh tops have a balsamic odour, and a carminative, bitterish taste. The berries afford a yellow aromatic oil, which acts on the kidneys, and gives cordial warmth to the stomach. Forty berries should yield an ounce of the oil. Steeped in alcohol the berries make a capital *ratafia*; they are used in several confections, as well as for flavouring gin, being put into a spirit more common than the true geneva of Holland. The French obtain from these berries the *Genièvre* (*Anglice* "geneva"), from which we have taken our English word "gin." In France, Savoy, and Italy, the berries are largely collected, and are sometimes eaten as such, fifteen or twenty at a time, to stimulate the kidneys; or they are taken in powder for the same purpose. Being fragrant of smell, they have a warm, sweet, pungent flavour, which becomes bitter on further mastication.

Our British *Pharmacopœia* orders a spirit of Juniper to be made for producing the like diuretic action in some forms of dropsy, so as to carry off the effused fluid by the kidneys. A teaspoonful of this spirit may be taken, well diluted with water, several times in the day. Of the essential oil the dose is from two to three drops on sugar, or with a tablespoonful of milk. These remedies are of service also in catarrh of the urinary passages; and if applied externally to painful local swellings, whether rheumatic, or neuralgic, the bruised berries afford prompt and lasting relief.

An infusion or decoction of the Juniper wood is sometimes given for the same affections, but less usefully, because the volatile oil becomes dissipated by the boiling heat. A "rob," or inspissated juice of the berries, is likewise often employed. Gerard said: "A decoction thereof is singular against an old cough." Gin is an ordinary malt spirit distilled a second time, with the addition of some Juniper berries. Formerly these berries were added to the malt in grinding, so that the spirit obtained therefrom was flavoured with the berries from the first, and surpassed all that could be made by any other method. At present gin is cheaply manufactured by leaving out the berries altogether, and giving the spirit a flavour by distilling it with a proportion of oil of turpentine, which resembles the Juniper berries in taste; and as this sophistication is less practised in Holland than elsewhere, it is best to order "Hollands," with water, as a drink for dropsical persons. By the use of Juniper berries Dr. Mayern cured some patients who were deplorably ill with epilepsy when all other remedies had failed. "Let the patient carry a bag of these berries about with him, and eat from ten to twenty every morning for a month or more, whilst fasting." Similarly for flatulent indigestion the berries may be most usefully given; on the first day, four berries; on the second, five; on the third, six; on the fourth, seven; and so on until twelve days, and fifteen berries are reached; after this the daily dose should be reduced by one berry until only five are taken in the day; which makes an admirable 'berry-cure.'" The berries are to be well masticated, and the husks may be afterwards either rejected or swallowed.

Juniper oil, used officinally, is distilled from the full-grown, unripe, green fruit. The Laplanders almost adore the tree, and they make a decoction of its ripe berries, when dried, to be drunk as tea, or coffee; whilst the Swedish peasantry prepare from the fresh berries a fermented beverage, which they drink cold, and an extract, which they eat with their bread for breakfast as we do butter.

Simon Pauli assures us these berries have performed wonders in curing the stone, he having personally treated cases thus, with incredible success. Schroder knew a nobleman of Germany, who freed himself from the intolerable symptoms of stone, by a constant use of these berries. Evelyn called them the "Forester's Panacea," "one of the most universal remedies in the world to our crazy Forester." Astrological botanists advise to pull the berries when the sun is in Virgo.

We read in an old tract (London, 1682) on *The use of Juniper and Elder berries in our Publick Houses*: "The simple decoction of these berries, sweetened with a little sugar candy, will afford liquors so pleasant to the eye, so grateful to the palate, and so beneficial to the body, that the wonder is they have not been courted and ushered into our Publick Houses, so great are the extraordinary beauty and vertues of these berries." "One ounce, well cleansed, bruised, and mashed, will be enough for almost a pint of water. When they are boiled together the vessel must be carefully stopt, and after the boiling is over one tablespoonful of sugar candy must be put in."

From rifts which occur spontaneously in the bark of the shrubs in warm countries issues a gum resembling frankincense. This gum, as Gerard teaches, "drieth ulcers which are hollow, and filleth them with flesh if they be cast thereon." "Being mixed with oil of roses, it healeth chaps of the hands and feet." Bergius said the *lignum* (wood) of Juniper is *diureticum, sudorificum, mundificans;* the *bacca* (berry), *diuretica, nutriens, diaphoretica.*" In Germany the berries are added to *sauerkraut* for flavouring it.

Virgil thought the odour exhaled by the Juniper tree noxious, and he speaks of the *Juniperis gravis umbra*:—

> "Surgamus! solet esse gravis cantantibus umbra;
> Juniperis gravis umbra; nocent et frugibus umbræ."
>
> *Eclog. X. v. 75.*

But it is more scientific to suppose that the growth of Juniper trees should be encouraged near dwellings, because of the balsamic and antiseptic odours which they constantly exhale. The smoke of the leaves and wood was formerly believed to drive away "all infection and corruption of the aire which bringeth the plague, and such like contagious diseases."

Sprays of Juniper are frequently strewn over floors of apartments, so as to give out when trodden down, their agreeable odour which is supposed to promote sleep. Queen Elizabeth's bedchamber was sweetened with their fumes. In the French hospitals it is customary to burn Juniper berries with Rosemary for correcting vitiated air, and to prevent infection.

On the Continent the Juniper is regarded with much veneration, because it is thought to have saved the life of the Madonna, and of the infant Jesus, whom she hid under a Juniper bush when flying into Egypt from the assassins of Herod.

Virgil alludes to the Juniper as Cedar:—

> "Disce et odoratam stabulis accendere cedrum."
>
> *Georgic.*

> "But learn to burn within your sheltering rooms
> Sweet Juniper."

Its powerful odour is thought to defeat the keen scent of the hound; and a hunted hare when put to extremities will seek a safe retreat under cover of its branches. Elijah was sheltered from the persecutions of King Ahab by the Juniper tree; since which time it has been always regarded as an asylum, and a symbol of succour.

From the wood of the *Juniperus oxycœdrus*, an empyreumatic oil resembling liquid pitch, is obtained by dry distillation, this being named officinally, *Huile de cade*, or *Oleum cadinum*, otherwise "Juniper tar." It is found to be most useful as an external stimulant for curing psoriasis and chronic eczema of the skin. A recognised ointment is made with this and yellow wax, *Unguentum olei cadini.*

In Italy stables are popularly thought to be protected by a sprig of Juniper from demons and thunderbolts, just as we suppose the magic horseshoe to be protective to our houses and offices.

KNAPWEED (The Lesser).

BLACK Knapweed, the *Centaurea nigra*, is a common tough-stemmed composite weed growing in our meadows and cornfields, being well known by its heads of dull purple flowers, with brown, or almost black scales of the outer floral encasement. It is popularly called Hard heads, Loggerheads, Iron heads, Horse knob, and Bull weed.

Dr. Withering relates that a decoction made from these hard heads has afforded at least a temporary relief in cases of diabetes mellitus, "by diminishing the quantity of urine, and dispelling the sweetness."

Its chief chemical constituent *enicin*, is identical with that of the Blessed thistle, and the Blue-bottle, and closely resembles that of the Dandelion. It has been found useful in strengthless indigestion, especially when this is complicated with sluggish torpor of the liver. From half to one ounce of the herb may be boiled in eight fluid ounces of water, and a small wineglassful be taken for a dose twice or three times a day. In Bucks young women make use of this Knapweed for love divination :—

"They pull the little blossom threads
From out the Knotweed's button beads,
And put the husk with many a smile
In their white bosoms for a while ;
Then, if they guess aright, the swain
Their love's sweet fancies try to gain.
'Tis said that ere it lies an hour
'Twill blossom with a second flower."

LAVENDER.

THE Lavender of our gardens, called also Lavender Spike, is a well-known sweet-smelling shrub, of the Labiate order. It grows wild in Spain, Piedmont, and the south of France, on waysides, mountains, and in barren places. The plant was propagated by slips, or cuttings, and has been cultivated in England since about 1568. It is produced largely for commercial purposes in Surrey, Hertfordshire, and Lincoln. The shrub is set in long rows occupying fields, and yields a profitable fragrant essential oil from the flowering tops, about one ounce of the oil from sixty terminal flowering spikes. From these tops also the popular cosmetic lavender water is distilled. They contain tannin, and a resinous camphire, which is common to most of the mints affording essential oils. If a hank of cotton is steeped in the oil of Lavender, and drained off so as to be hung dry about the neck, it will prevent bugs and other noxious insects from attacking that part. When mixed with three-fourths of spirit of turpentine, or spirit of wine, this oil makes the famous *Oleum spicæ*, formerly much celebrated for curing old sprains and stiff joints. Lavender oil is likewise of service when rubbed in externally, for stimulating paralysed limbs—preferring the sort distilled from the flowering tops to that which is obtained from the stalks. Internally, the essential oil, or a spirit of Lavender made therefrom, proves admirably restorative and tonic against faintness, palpitations of a nervous sort, weak giddiness, spasms, and colic. It is agreeable to the taste and smell, provokes appetite, raises the spirits, and dispels flatulence; but the infusion of Lavender tops, if taken too freely, will cause griping, and colic. In hysteria, palsy, and similar disorders of debility, and lack of nerve power, the spirit of Lavender will act as a powerful stimulant; and fomentations with Lavender in bags, applied hot, will speedily relieve local pains. "It profiteth them much," says Gerard, "that have the palsy if they be washed with the distilled water from the Lavender flowers; or are anointed with the oil made from the flowers and olive oil, in such manner as oil of roses is used." A dose of the oil is from one to four drops on sugar, or on a small piece of bread crumb, or in a spoonful or two of milk. And of the spirit, from half to one teaspoonful may be taken with two table-spoonfuls of water, hot or cold, or of milk. The spirit of Lavender is made with one part of the essential oil to forty-nine parts of spirit of wine. For preparing distilled Lavender water, the addition of a small quantity of musk does much to develop the strength of the Lavender's odour and fragrance. The essential oil of *Lavandula latifolia*, admirably promotes the growth of the hair when weakly, or falling off.

By the Greeks the name Nardus is given to Lavender, from Naarda, a city of Syria, near the Euphrates; and many persons call the plant "Nard." St. Mark mentions this as Spikenard, a thing of great value The woman who came to Christ having an alabaster box of ointment of Spikenard, very precious "brake the box, and poured it on His head." In Pliny's time blossoms of the nardus sold for a hundred Roman denarii (or £3 2s. 6d.) the pound. This Lavender or *Nardus*, was likewise called Asarum by the Romans, because not used in garlands or chaplets. It was formerly believed that the asp, a dangerous kind of viper, made Lavender its habitual place of abode, so that the plant had to be approached with great caution.

Conserves of Lavender were much used in the time of Gerard, and desserts may be most pleasantly brought to the table on a service of Lavender spikes. It is said, on good authority, that the lions and tigers in our Zoological gardens, are powerfully affected by the smell of Lavender-water and become docile under its influence.

The Lavender shrub takes its name from the Latin *lavare*, "to wash," because the ancients employed it as a perfume. Lavender tops, when dried, and placed with linen, will preserve it from moths and other insects.

The whole plant was at one time considered indispensable in Africa, *ubi lavandis corporibus Lybes eâ utuntur ; nec nisi decocto ejus abluti mane domo egrediuntur*, "where the Libyans make use of it for washing their bodies, nor ever leave their houses of a morning until purified by a decoction of the plant."

In this country the sweet-smelling herb is often introduced for scenting newly washed linen when it is put by; from which custom has arisen the expression, "To be laid up in Lavender." During the twelfth century a washerwoman was called "Lavender," in the North of England.

A tea brewed from the flowers is an excellent remedy for headache from fatigue, or weakness. But Lavender oil is, in too large a dose, a narcotic poison, and causes death by convulsions. The tincture of red Lavender is a popular medicinal cordial; and is composed of the oils of Lavender and rosemary, with cinnamon bark, nutmeg, and red sandal wood, macerated in spirit of wine for seven days; then a teaspoonful may be given for a dose in a little water, with excellent effect, after an indigestible meal, taking the dose immediately when feeling uneasy, and repeating it after half-an-hour if needed. An old form of this compound tincture was formerly famous as "Palsy Drops," it being made from the Lavender, with rosemary, cinnamon, nutmeg, red sandal wood, and spirit. In some cases of mental depression and delusions the oil of Lavender proves of real service; and a few drops of it rubbed on the temples will cure nervous headache.

Shakespeare makes Perdita (*Winter's Tale*) class Lavender among the flowers denoting middle age:

> "Here's flowers for you,
> Hot Lavender: Mints: Savory: Marjoram;
> The Marigold that goes to bed with the sun,
> And with him rises, weeping: these are the flowers
> Of middle summer, and I think they are given
> To men of middle age."

There is a broad-leaved variety of the Lavender shrub in France, which yields three times as much of the essential oil as can be got from our narrow-leaved plant, but of a second rate quality.

The Sea Lavender, or Thrift (*Statice limonium*) grows near the sea, or in salt marshes. It gets its name *Statice* from the Greek word *isteemi* (to stop, or stay), because of its medicinal power to arrest bleeding. This is the marsh Rosemary, or Ink Root, which contains (if the root be dried in the air) from fourteen to fifteen per cent. of tannin. Therefore, its infusion or tincture will prove highly useful to control bleeding from the lungs or kidneys, as also against dysentery; and when made into a gargle, for curing an ulcerated sore throat.

LEMON.

THE Lemon *(Citrus Limonum)* is so common of use in admixing refreshing drinks, and for its fragrancy of peel, whether for culinary flavour, or as a delightful perfume, that it may well find a place among the Simples of a sagacious housewife. Moreover, the imported fruit, which abounds in our markets, as if to the manner born, is endowed with valuable medicinal properties which additionally qualify it for the domestic *Herbarium*. The Lemons brought to England come chiefly from Sicily, through Messina and Palermo. Flowers may be found on the lemon tree all the year round.

In making lemonade it is a mistake to pour boiling water upon sliced Lemons, because thus brewing an infusion of the peel, which is medicinal. The juice should be squeezed into cold water (previously boiled), adding to a quart of the same the juice of three lemons, a few crushed strawberries, and the cut up rind of one Lemon.

This fruit grows specially at Mentone, in the south of France ; and a legend runs that Eve carried two or three Lemons with her away from Paradise, wandering about until she came to Mentone, which she found to be so like the Garden of Eden that she settled there, and planted her fruit.

The special dietetic value of Lemons consists in their potash salts, the citrate, malate, and tartrate, which are respectively antiscorbutic, and of assistance in promoting biliary digestion. Each fluid ounce of the fresh juice contains about forty-four grains of citric acid, with gum, sugar, and a residuum, which yields, when incinerated, potash, lime, and phosphoric acid. But the citric acid of the shops is not nearly so preventive or curative of scurvy as the juice itself.

The exterior rind furnishes a grateful aromatic bitter ; and our word "zest" signifies really a chip of lemon peel or orange peel used for giving flavour to liquor. It comes from the Greek verb, "*skizein,*" to divide, or cut up.

The juice has certain sedative properties whereby it allays hysterical palpitation of the heart, and alleviates pain caused by cancerous ulceration of the tongue. Dr. Brandini, of Florence, discovered this latter property of fresh Lemon juice, through a patient who, when suffering grievously from that dire disease, found marvellous relief to the part by casually sucking a lemon to slake his feverish thirst. But it is a remarkable fact that the acid of Lemons is harmful and obnoxious to cats, rabbits, and other small animals, because it lowers the heart's action in these creatures, and liquifies the blood; whereas, in man it does not diminish the coagulability of the blood, but proves more useful than any other agent in correcting that thin impoverished liquidity thereof which constitutes scurvy. Rapin extols lemons, or citrons, for discomfort of the heart :—

> "Into an oval form the citrons rolled
> Beneath thick coats their juicy pulp unfold:
> From some the palate feels a poignant smart,
> Which, though they wound the tongue, yet *heal the heart*."

Throughout Italy, and at Rome, a decoction of fresh Lemons is extolled as a specific against intermittent fever; for which purpose a fresh unpeeled Lemon is cut into thin slices, and put into an earthenware jar with three breakfastcupfuls of cold water, and boiled down to one cupful, which is strained, the lemon being squeezed, and the decoction being given shortly before the access of fever is expected.

For a restless person of ardent temperament and active plethoric circulation, a Lemon squash (unsweetened) of not more than half a tumblerful is a capital sedative; or, a whole lemon may be made hot on the oven top, being turned from time to time, and being put presently when soft and moist into a teacup, then by stabbing it about the juice will be made to escape, and should be drunk hot. If bruised together with a sufficient quantity of sugar the pips of a fresh Lemon or Orange will serve admirably against worms in children. Cut in slices and put into the morning bath, a Lemon makes it fragrant and doubly refreshing.

Professor Wilhelm Schmole, a German doctor, has published a work of some note, in which he advances the theory that fresh Lemon juice is a kind of *elixir vitæ;* and that if a sufficient number of Lemons be taken daily, life may be indefinitely prolonged. Lemon juice is decidedly beneficial against jaundice from passive sluggishness of the biliary functions; it will often serve to stay bleedings, when ice and astringent styptics have failed; it will prove useful when swallowed freely against immoderately active monthly fluxes in women; and when applied externally it signally relieves cutaneous itching, especially of the genitals.

Prize-fighters refresh themselves with a fresh cut Lemon between the rounds when competing in the Ring. Hence has arisen the common saying, "Take a suck of the Lemon, and at him again."

For a relaxed sore throat, Lemon juice will help to make a serviceable gargle. By the heat of the sun it may be reduced to a solid state. For a cold in the head, if the juice of a ripe Lemon be squeezed into the palm of the hand, and strongly sniffed into the nostrils at two or three separate times, a cure will be promoted. Roast fillet of veal, with stuffing and lemon juice, was beloved by Oliver Cromwell.

For heartburn which comes on without having eaten sweet things, it is helpful to suck a thin slice of fresh Lemon dipped in salt just after each meal.

The Chinese practice of rubbing parts severely neuralgic with the wet surface of a cut Lemon is highly useful. This fruit has been sold within present recollection at half-a-crown each, and during the American war at five shillings.

The hands may be made white, soft, and supple by daily sponging them with fresh Lemon juice, which further keeps the nails in good order; and the same may be usefully applied to the roots of the hair for removing dandriff from the scalp.

The Candied Peel which we employ as a confection is got from one of the citrons (a variety of the lemon); whilst another of this tribe is esteemed for religious purposes in Jewish synagogues. These citrons are imported into England from the East; and for unblemished specimens of the latter which reach London, high prices are paid. One pound sterling is a common sum, and not infrequently as much as seventy shillings are given for a single "Citron of Law." The fruit is used at the Feast of Tabernacles according to a command given in the Book of the Law; it is not of an edible nature, but is handed round and smelt by the worshippers as they go out, when they "thank God for all good things, and for the sweet odours He has given to men." This citron is considered to be almost miraculously restorative, especially by those who regard it as the "tappñach," intended in the text, "Comfort me with apples." Ladies of the Orient, even now, carry a piece of its rind about them in a vinaigrette.

The citron which furnishes Candied Peel resembles a large juicy lemon, but without a nipple.

Virgil said of the fruit generally :—

> "Media fert tristes succos, tardumque saporem
> Felicis mali."

Fresh Lemon juice will not keep because of its mucilage, which soon ferments.

Sidney Smith, in writing about Foston, his remote Country Cure in Yorkshire, said it is "twelve miles from a Lemon."

LENTIL.

AMONG the leguminous plants which supply food for the invalid, and are endowed with certain qualifications for correcting the health, may be justly placed the Lentil, though we have to import it because our moist, cold climate is not favourable for its growth. Nevertheless, it closely resembles the small purple vetch of our summer hedgerows at home. In France its pulse is much eaten during Lent—which season takes its name, as some authors suppose, from this penitential plant. Men become under its subduing dietary influence, "*lenti et lenes.*" The plant is cultivated freely in Egypt for the sake of the seeds, which are flat on both sides, growing in numerous pods.

The botanical name is *Ervum lens*; and about the year 1840 a Mr. Wharton sold the flour of Lentils under the name of Ervalenta, this being then of a primrose colour. He failed in his enterprise, and Du Barry took up the business, but substituting the red Arabian Lentil for the yellow German pulse.

Joseph's mess of pottage which he sold to Esau for his birthright was a preparation of the red Lentil: and the same food was the bread of Ezekiel.

The legumin contained in this vegetable is very light and sustaining, but it is apt to form unwholesome combinations with any earthy salts taken in other articles of food, or in the water used in cooking; therefore Lemon juice or vinegar is a desirable addition to Lentils at table. This is because of the phosphates contained so abundantly, and liable to become deposited in the urine. "Lentils," says Gerard, "are singular good to stay the menses." They are traditionally regarded as funeral plants, and formerly they were forbidden at sacrifices and feasts.

Parkinson said, "The country people sow it in the fields as food for their cattle, and call it 'tills', leaving out the 'lent', as thinking that word agreeth not with the matter." "*Ita sus Minervam.*" In Hampshire the plant is known as "tils," and in Oxfordshire as "dills." The Romans supposed it made people indolent and torpid, therefore they named the plant from *lentus*, slow.

Allied to the Lentil as likewise a leguminous plant is the LUPINE, grown now only as an ornament to our flower beds, but formerly cultivated by the Romans as an article of food, and still capable of usefulness in this capacity for the invalid. Pliny said, "No kind of fodder is more wholesome and light of digestion than the white Lupine when eaten dry." If taken commonly at meals it will contribute a fresh colour and a cheerful countenance. When thus formerly used neither trouble nor expense was needed in sowing the seed, since it had merely to be scattered over the ground without ploughing or digging. But Virgil designated it *tristis Lupinus*, "the sad Lupine," probably because when the pulse of this plant was eaten without being first cooked in any way so as to modify its bitter taste, it had a tendency to contract the muscles of the face, and to give a sorrowful appearance to the countenance. It was said the Lupine was cursed by the Virgin Mary, because when she fled with the child Christ from the assassins of Herod, plants of this species by the noise they made attracted the attention of the soldiers.

The Lupine was originally named from *lupus*, a wolf, because of its voracious nature. The seeds were used as pieces of money by Roman actors in their plays and comedies, whence came the saying, "*nummus lupinus*," "a spurious bit of money."

LETTUCE.

OUR garden Lettuce is a cultivated variety of the wild, or strong-scented Lettuce (*Lactuca virosa*), which grows, with prickly leaves, on banks and waysides in chalky districts throughout England and Wales. It belongs to the Composite order of plants, and contains the medicinal properties of the plant more actively than does the Lettuce produced for the kitchen. An older form of the name is *Lettouce*, which is still retained in Scotland.

Chemically the wild Lettuce contains lactucin, lactucopricin, asparagin, mannite, albumen, gum, and resin, together with oxalic, malic, and citric acids; thus possessing virtues for easing pain, and inducing sleep. The cultivated Lettuce which comes to our tables retains these same properties, but in a very modified degree, since the formidable principles have become as completely toned down and guileless in the garden product as were the child-like manners and the pensive smile of Bret Harte's Heathen Chinee.

Each plant derives its name, *lactuca*, from its milky juice; in Latin *lactis;* and in Greek, *galaktos* (taking the genitive case). This juice, when withdrawn from the cut or incised stalks and stems of the wild Lettuce, is milky at first, and afterwards becomes brown, like opium, being then known (when dried into a kind of gum) as *lactucarium*. From three to eight grains of this gum, if taken at bedtime, will allay the wakefulness which follows over-excitement of brain. A similar *lactucarium*, got from the dried milk of the cultivated garden Lettuce, is so mild a sedative as to be suitable for restless infants; and two grains thereof may be safely given to a young child for soothing it to sleep.

The wild Lettuce is rather laxative; with which view a decoction of the leaves is sometimes taken as a drink to remedy. constipation, and intestinal difficulties, as also to allay feverish pains. The plant was mentioned as acting thus in an epigram by Martial (*Libr. VI., Sq.*).

> "Prima tibi dabitur ventre lactuca movendo
> Utilis, et porris fila resecta suis."

Gerard said: "Being in some degree laxative and aperient, the cultivated Lettuce is very proper for hot bilious dispositions;" and Parkinson adds (1640): "Lettuce eaten raw or boyled, helpeth to loosen the belly, and the boyled more than the raw." It was known as the "Milk Plant" to Dioscorides and Theophrastus, and was much esteemed by the Romans to be eaten after a debauch of wine, or as a sedative for inducing sleep. But a prejudice against it was entertained for a time as *venerem enervans*, and therefore *mortuorum cibi*, "food for the dead."

Apuleius says, that when the eagle desires to fly to a great height, and to get a clear view of the extensive prospect below him, he first plucks a leaf of the wild Lettuce and touches his eyes with the juice thereof, by which means he obtains the widest perspicuity of vision. "Dicunt aquilam quum in altum volare voluerit ut prospiciat rerum naturas lactucœ sylvaticœ folium evellere et succo ejus sibi oculos tangere, et maximam inde claritudinem accipere."

After the death of Adonis, Venus is related to have thrown herself on a bed of lettuces to assuage her grief. "In lactucâ occultatum a Venere Adonin —cecinit Callimachus—quod allegoricé interpretatus Athenœus illuc referendum putat quod in venerem hebetiores fiunt lactucas vescentes assidue."

The Pythagoreans called this plant "the Eunuch"; and there is a saying in Surrey, "O'er much Lettuce in the garden will stop a young wife's bearing." During the middle ages it was thought an evil spirit lurked among the Lettuces adverse to mothers, and causing grievous ills to new-born infants.

The Romans, in the reign of Domitian, had the lettuce prepared with eggs, and served with the last course at their tables, so as to stimulate their appetites afresh. Martial wonders that it had since then become customary to take it rather at the beginning of the meal:—

> "Claudere quæ cænas lactuca solebat avorum
> Dic mihi cur nostras inchoat illa dapes."

Antoninus Musa cured Cæsar Augustus of hypochondriasis by means of this plant.

The most common variety of the wild Lettuce, improved by frequent cultivation, is the Cabbage Lettuce, or Roman, "which is the best to boil, stew, or put into hodge-podge." Different sorts of the Cos Lettuce follow next onwards. The *Lactuca sylvatica* is a variety of the wild Lettuce producing similar effects. From this a medicinal tincture (H.) is prepared, and an extract from the flowering herb is given in doses of from five to fifteen grains. No attempt was made to cultivate the Lettuce in this country until the fourth year of Elizabeth's reign.

When bleached by gardeners the lettuce becomes tender, sweet, and succulent, being easily digested, even by dyspeptic persons, as to its crisp, leafy parts, but not its hard stalk. It now contains but little nutriment of any sort, but supplies some mineral salts, especially nitre. In the stem there still lingers a small quantity of the sleep-inducing principle, "lactucarin," particularly when the plant is flowering. Galen, when sleepless from advanced age and infirmities, with hard study, took decoction of the Lettuce at night; and Pope says, with reference to our garden sort:—

> "If you want rest,
> Lettuce, and cowslip wine:—'probatum est.'"

But if Lettuces are taken at supper with this view of promoting sleep, they should be had without any vinegar, which neutralises their soporific qualities. "Sleep," said Sir Thomas Brown, "is so like death that I dare not trust it without my prayers."

Some persons suppose that when artificially blanched the plant is less wholesome than if left to grow naturally in the garden, especially if its ready digestibility by those of sensitive stomachs be correctly attributed to the slightly narcotic principle. It was taken uncooked by the Hebrews with the Paschal lamb.

John Evelyn writes enthusiastically about it in his *Book of Sallets:* "So harmless is it that it may safely be eaten raw in fevers; it allays heat, bridles choler, extinguishes thirst, excites appetite, kindly nourishes, and, above all, represses vapours, conciliates sleep, and mitigates pain, besides the effect it has upon the morals—temperance and chastity."

"Galen (whose beloved sallet it was) says it breeds the most laudable blood. No marvel, then, that Lettuces were by the ancients called *sanæ* by way of eminency, and were so highly valued by the great Augustus that, attributing to them his recovery from a dangerous sickness, it is reported he erected a statue and built an altar to this noble plant." Likewise, "Tacitus, spending almost nothing at his frugal table in other dainties, was yet so great a friend to the Lettuce that he used to say of his prodigality in its purchase, *Summi se mercari illas sumitûs effusione.*" Probably the Lettuce of Greece was more active than our indigenous, or cultivated plant.

By way of admonition as to care in preparing the Lettuce for table, Dr. King Chambers has said (*Diet in Health and Disease*), "The consumption of Lettuce by the working man with his tea is an increasing habit worthy of all encouragement. But the said working man must be warned of the importance of washing the material of his meal. This hint is given in view of the frequent occurrence of the large round worm in the labouring population of some agricultural counties, Oxfordshire for instance, where unwashed Lettuce is largely eaten." Young Lettuces may be raised in forty-eight hours by first steeping the seed in brandy and then sowing it in a hot-house.

The seeds of the garden Lettuce are emollient, and when rubbed up with water make a pleasant emulsion, which contains nothing of the milky, laxative bitterness furnished by the leaves and stalk. This emulsion resembles that of almonds, but is even more cooling, and therefore a better medicine in disorders arising from acrimony and irritation.

From the *Lactuca virosa*, or strong-scented wild Lettuce, a medicinal tincture (H.) is prepared, using the whole plant. On the principle of treating with this tincture, when diluted, such toxic effects as too large doses of the juice would bring about, a slow pulse, with a disposition to stupor, and sleepy weakness, are successfully met by its use. Also a medicinal extract is made by druggists from the wild Lettuce, and given in doses of from three to ten grains for the medicinal purposes which have been particularised, and to remove a dull, heavy headache.

"The garden Lettuce is good," as Pliny said, "for

burnings and scaldings if the leaves be laid thereon, with salt (*sic*), before the blisters do appear." "By reason," concludes Evelyn, "too, of its soporiferous quality, the Lettuce ever was, and still continues, the principal foundation of the universal tribe of sallets, which cools and refreshes, besides its other properties, and therefore was held in such high esteem by the ancients, that divers of the Valerian family dignified and ennobled their name with that of *Lactucinii*." It is botanically distinguished as the *Lactuca sativa*, "from the plenty of milk," says "Adam in Eden" (W. Coles), "that it hath, and *causeth*."

Lambs' Lettuce, or Corn Salad, is a distinct plant, one of the Valerian tribe, which was formerly classed as a Lettuce, by name, *Lactuca agnina*, either because it appears about the time when lambs (*agni*) are dropped, or because it is a favourite food of lambs."

The French call this *salade de Prètre*, "monks' salad," and in reference thereto an old writer has said: "It certainly deserves a place among the *penitential* herbs, for the stomach that admits it is apt to cry *peccavi*.

The same plant is also known by the title of the White Pot Herb, in contrast to the *Olus atrum*, or Black Pot Herb. It grows wild in the banks of hedges and waste cornfields, and is cultivated in our kitchen gardens as a salad herb, the Milk Grass, being called botanically the *Valerianella olitoria*, and having been in request as a spring medicine among country folk in former days. By genus it is a *Fedia*, and bears diminutive white flowers resembling glass. Gerard says: "We know the Lambs' Lettuce as *Loblollie;* and it serves in winter as a salad herb, among others none of the worst." In France it goes by the names *manche* and *broussette*. A medicinal tincture is made (H.) from the fresh root.

The black pot-herb—so called from the dark colour of its fruit—is an umbelliferous plant, *Smyrnium olus-atrum*, or Alexanders, often found in the vicinity of abbeys, and probably therefore held in former repute by the Monks. Its names are derived from *Smyrna*, myrrh, in allusion to the odour of the plant; and from *Macedonicum*, or the parsley of Macedon, Alexander's country. The herb was also known as Stanmarch. It grows on waste places by rivers near the sea, having been formerly cultivated like celery, which has now supplanted it. When boiled it is eaten with avidity by sailors returning from long voyages, who happen to land at the South Western corner of Anglesea.

LILY OF THE VALLEY.

THE Lily of the Valley grows wild in many of our English woods, and possesses special curative virtues, which give it, according to modern knowledge, a just place among Herbal Simples of repute. This is the parent flower of our graceful, sweet-scented scape of pendent, milk-white little floral bells, enshrined within two broad leafy blades of dark green, and finding general favour for the *jardinière*, or the button-hole.

Its name *Convallaria majalis* is derived from *convallis*, "a valley," and *majalis*, "belonging to the month of May," when this Lily comes into flower.

Rustics corrupt the double title to "Liry Confancy," and provincially the plant is known as "Wood Lily," "May Lily," and "May Blossom." Also it bears the name of Mugget, and is said to have grown up after the bloody combat of St. Leonard with the Dragon. The French call it *Muguet*, or "little musk." The taste of the flowers is acrid and bitter; they have been employed with benefit, when dried and powdered, as snuff, for headache, and giddiness arising from weakness. A tincture of the plant is made, and can be procured from any leading druggist. The active medicinal principle is "convallarin," which slows the disturbed action of a weak, irritable heart, whilst at the same time increasing its power. Happily the remedy is a perfectly safe one, and no harm has been known to occur from taking it experimentally in full and frequent doses; so that, in this respect, it is far preferable to the Fox Glove, which is apt to accumulate in the blood with poisonous results. To make the tincture of *Convallaria*, one part of the flowers is treated with eight parts of spirit of wine (proof); and the dose is from five to fifteen drops, with a tablespoonful of water, three times in the twenty-four hours.

Also an infusion may be made with boiling water poured over the whole plant—root, stems, and flowers; and this infusion may be given continuously for from five to ten days; but it should be left off for a time as soon as the irritability of the heart is subdued, and the pulse steady and stronger. If taken during an attack of palpitation and laboured breathing from a weak heart, the benefit of the infusion in tablespoonful doses is felt at once.

Ten grains of the dried flowers may be infused in six ounces of boiling water, and a tablespoonful of this be given three times a day with perfect safety, and with a most soothing effect for a weak, sensitive, palpitating heart; but it does not suit a fatty heart equally well. Nevertheless, even for insufficiency of the valves, when dangerous, or distressing symptoms of heart disease have set in, an infusion of the flowers has proved very helpful. The *rhizome*, root, exhales a pleasant odour, different from that of the flowers; it tastes sweet at first but afterwards bitter.

A fluid extract is further prepared, and may be mixed in doses of from five to twenty drops with water. The Russian peasants have long employed the Lily of the Valley for certain forms of dropsy, when proceeding from a faulty heart.

In the summer, when the flowers are in bloom, two drachms, by weight, of the leaves should be steeped in a pint of water, either cold or boiling; and the whole of this may be taken, if needed, during the twenty-four hours. It will promote a free flow of urine. Culpeper commended the Lily of the Valley for weak memory, loss of speech, and apoplexy; whilst Gerard advised it for gout. In Devonshire it is thought unlucky to plant a bed of these Lilies, as the person who does so will probably die within the next twelve months.

In the *Apocrypha*, Canticles ii, 1, "I am the Lily of the Valley," this flower is apparently brought under notice, but some other plant must be intended here, because the Lily Convally does not grow in Palestine. The word Lily is used in Oriental languages for a flower in general.

Distilled water from the flowers was formerly in great repute against nervous affections, and for many troubles of the head, insomuch that it was treasured in vessels of gold and silver. Matthiolus named it *Aqua aurea*, "golden water"; and Etmuller said of the virtues of the plant, *Quod specifice armabit impotentes maritos ad bellum veneris.*

A spirit made from the petals is excellent as an outward embrocation for rheumatism and sprains; and in some parts of Germany, a wine is prepared from the flowers mixed with raisins. Old Gerard adopted an unaccountable method for extracting these virtues of the Lilies. He ordered that, "The flowers being close stopped up in a glass vessel, should be put into an ant hill, and taken away again a month after, when ye shall find a liquor in the glass which, being outwardly applied, will help the cure of the gout."

After the blossom has fallen off a berry is formed, which assumes in the autumn a bright scarlet colour, and proves attractive to birds.

LIME TREE, Flowers of (*Tiliaceæ*).

THOUGH not a native of Great Britain, yet, because of its common growth in our roadways and along the front of terraced houses, and in suburban avenues, the Lime Tree has become almost indigenous.

In the old *Herbals* it is called Lyne or Line, Tillet, Till tree, and Tilia, each of these names bearing reference to the bast or inner bark of the tree, which is used in the North for cordage. Others say the name is an alteration of Telia, from *telum*, a dart, alluding to the use of the wood. Tilia is more probably derived from *ptilon*, a feather, because of the feathery appearance of the floral leaves.

Shakespeare says :—

> "Now, tell me thy name, good fellow," said he,
> "Under the leaves of lyne."

The "n" in later writers has been changed into "m."

Its sweet-smelling and highly fragrant flowers blossom in May, and are much sought after by bees, because abounding with honied nectar. A medicinal tincture (H.) is made from them with spirit of wine; and when given in doses of from five to ten drops with water, three times in the day, it serves to relieve sick bilious giddiness, with depression of spirits, and a tendency to loose bowels, with nervous headache. The sap of the Lime Tree *(Tilia Europæa)* abounds in mucilage, from which sugar can be elaborated. A tea made from the blossoms and leaves with boiling water, is admirable for promoting perspiration. It is because of a long established reputation for giving relief in chronic epilepsy or the falling sickness, and of curing epileptiform headaches, whilst proving of indisputable usefulness in allied nervous disorders, that the flowers and leaves of the Lime or Linden Tree occupy a true place among modern medicinal Simples. Gilbert White made some Lime-blossom tea, and pronounced it a very soft, well-flavoured, pleasant saccharine julep, much resembling the juice of liquorice. This tea has been found efficacious for quieting hard coughs and for relieving hoarseness.

The flowers easily ferment, and being so fragrant may be used for making wine : likewise a fine flavoured brandy has been distilled from them. The fruit contains an oily substance, and has been proposed, when roasted, as a domestic substitute for chocolate. The sap may be procured by making incisions in the trunk, and branches. The flowers are sedative, and anti-spasmodic. Fenelon decorates his enchanted Isle of Calypso with flowering Lime trees. Hoffman says *Tiliæ ad mille usus petendæ.*

The inner bark furnishes a soft mucilage, which may be applied externally with healing effect to burns, scalds, and inflammatory swellings. Gerard taught, "that the flowers are commended by divers persons against pain of the head proceeding from a cold cause ; against dizziness, apoplexy, and the falling sickness ; and not only the flowers, but the distilled water thereof."

Hoffman knew a case of chronic epilepsy recovered by a use of the flowers in infusion drunk as tea. Such, indeed, was the former exalted anti-epileptic reputation of the Lime Tree, that epileptic persons sitting under its shade were reported to be cured.

A famous "Lind" or Lime Tree, which grew in his ancestral place, gave to the celebrated Linnæus his significant name. The well-known street, *unter den Linden* in Berlin, is a favourite resort, because of its pleasant, balmy shade; and when Heine lay beneath the Lindens, he "thought his own sweet nothing-at-all thoughts." The wood of the Lime Tree is preferred before every other wood for masterly carving. Grinling Gibbons executed his best and most noted work in this material; and the finely-cut details still remain sharp, delicate, and beautiful.

Chemically, the Linden flowers contain a particular light, fragrant, volatile oil, which is soluble in alcohol. They are used in warm baths with much success to allay nervous irritability; or a strong infusion of them is administered by enema for the same purpose.

LIQUORICE, English (*Leguminous*).

THE common Liquorice plant, a native of the warmer European countries, was first cultivated in Britain about 1562, in Turner's time. It has been chiefly grown at Pontefract (Pomfret) in Yorkshire, Worksop in Nottinghamshire, and Godalming in Surrey; whilst at the present time it is produced abundantly at Mitcham, near London, and the roots are dug up after a three years' growth, to be supplied to the shops. The use of the Liquorice plant was first learnt by the Hellenes from the Scythians; and the root was named *adipson*, being thought from the time of Theophrastus to powerfully extinguish thirst. But Dr. Cullen says his experience has not confirmed this as a true effect of chewing the root. When lightly boiled in a little water it yields all its sweetness, together with some mucilage.

A favourite pastime of school boys at the beginning of the present century, was to carry in the pocket a small phial of water containing bits of this "Spanish juice," and to shake it continually so as to make a solution, valued the more the darker and thicker it became.

The juice is commonly employed as a pectoral in coughs or hoarseness, when thickened to the consistence of a lozenge, or to that of a solid mass, which hardens in the form of a stick. It is also added to nauseous medicines, for masking their taste. Towards obtaining this juice the underground stem or root of the plant is the part employed.

The search of Diogenes for an honest man was scarcely more difficult than would be that of an average person for genuine Liquorice; since the juice is adulterated to any extent, and there is no definite standard of purity for this article so commonly used. Potato starch, miller's sweepings mixed with sugar, and any kind of rubbish are added to it.

In China, the roots of *Glycyrrhiza echinata* and *Glycyrrhiza glabra*, are used in a variety of medicinal preparations as possessing tonic, alterative, and expectorant properties, and as a mild aperient. Thereto are attributed rejuvenating and highly nutritive qualities. English Liquorice root occurs in pieces three or four inches long, and about as thick as a finger.

The extract of Liquorice must be prepared from the *dried* root, else it cannot be strained bright, and would be liable to fermentation. Chemically, the root contains a special kind of sugar, glycyrrhizine, a demulcent starch, asparagin, phosphate and malate of lime and magnesia, a resinous oil, albumen, and woody fibre. Old Fuller says concerning Nottingham, "This county affordeth the first and best Liquorice in England: great is the use thereof in physick. A stick of the same is commonly the spoon prescribed to patients to use in any Loaches. If (as the men of Œneas were forced to eat their own trenchers), these chance to eat their spoons, their danger is none at all." The Loach, or Lingence, from *ekleigma*, a substance licked-up, has become our modern lozenge. Extract of Liquorice is largely imported as "Spanish" or "Italian" juice, the Solazzi juice being most esteemed, which comes in cylindrical or flattened rolls, enveloped in bay leaves; but the pipe Liquorice of the sweetstuff shops is adulterated. Pontefract lozenges are made of refined Liquorice, and are justly popular. The sugar of Liquorice may be safely taken by diabetic patients.

Officinally, the root and stolons (underground stems) of the *Glycyrrhiza glabra* (smooth) are variously employed; for making an extract, for mixing with linseed in a tea, for combination with powdered senna, sugar, and fennel, to form a favourite mild laxative medicine, known as "Compound Liquorice Powder," and for other uses. The solid juice is put into porter and stout, because giving sweetness, thickness, and blackness to those beverages, without making them fermentative; but Liquorice, like gum, supplies scant aliment to the body. Black Liquorice is employed in the manufacture of tobacco, for smoking and chewing.

The Rest Harrow *(Ononis arvensis)*, a troublesome weed, very common in our ploughed fields, has a root which affords a sweet viscid juice, and hence it is popularly known as "Wild Liquorice."

This is a leguminous plant, called also "Ground Furze," which is a favourite food of the donkey, and therefore gets its botanical title from the Greek word *onos*, an ass. Its long and thickly matted roots will arrest the progress of the harrow, or plough. Medicinally, the plant has been given with success to subdue delirium. It is obnoxious to snakes, and they will not come near it.

Other appellations of the herb are Cammock, Stinking Tommy, *Arrête bœuf*, *Remora aratri*, *Resta bovis*, and Land Whin (which from the Latin *guindolum*, signifies a kind of cherry). The plant was formerly much extolled for obviating stone in the bladder. It is seen to be covered with spines; and a tradition exists that it was the Rest harrow which furnished the crown of thorns plaited by the Roman soldiers at the crucifixion of our Saviour. This plant has been long used as a culinary vegetable, its young shoots being boiled, or taken in salad, or pickled.

The French know it as *Bugrane*, beloved by goats, and the chief delight of donkeys, who rejoice to roll themselves amid its prickles. Simon Pauli *ne connait pas de meilleur remède contre le calcul des reins, et de la vessie.* "*Anjourdhui l'arréte bœuf est à peu pres abandonné.*" "*On y reviendra!*" The plant contains "ononin," a chemical glucoside, which is demulcent to the urinary organs.

Its botanical name of *Glycyrrhiza* comes from the Greek words, *glukus*, "sweet," and *riza*, "a root." English Liquorice root, when dried, is commercially used in two forms, the peeled and the unpeeled. By far and away the best lozenges are those of our boyhood, still attributed to one "Smith," in the Borough of London.

MALLOWS.

ALL the Mallows (*Malvaceæ*) to the number of a thousand, agree in containing mucilage freely, and in possessing no unwholesome properties.

Their family name "Mallow" is derived from the Greek *malassein*, "to soften," as alluding to the demulcent qualities of these mucilaginous plants. The Common Mallow is a well-known roadside plant, with large downy leaves, and streaked trumpet-shaped purple flowers, which later on furnish round button-like seeds, known to the rustics as "pickcheeses" in Norfolk and elsewhere, whilst beloved by schoolboys, because of their nutty flavour, and called by them "Bread and Cheese."

Clare tells playfully of the fairies, borne by mice at a gallop :—

> "In chariots lolling at their ease,
> Made of whate'er their fancies please,
> With wheels at hand of Mallow seeds,
> Which childish sport had strung as beads."

And recalls the time when he sat as a boy :—

> "Picking from Mallows, sport to please,
> The crumpled seed we called a cheese."

Both this plant and its twin sister, the Marsh Mallow (*Althœa hibiscus*, from *altho*, to cure), possess medicinal virtues, which entitle them to take rank as curative Herbal Simples. The Sussex peasant knows the Common Mallow as "Maller," so that "aller and maller" means with him Alehoof (Ground Ivy) and Mallow. Pliny said: "Whosoever shall take a spoonful of the

Mallows shall that day be free from all diseases that may come to him."

This plant is often named "Round Dock," and was formerly called "Hock Herb": our Hollyhock being of the Mallow tribe, and first brought to us from China. Pythagoras held *Malvæ folium sanctissimum;* and we read of Epimenides in *Plato,* "at his Mallows and Asphodels." The Romans esteemed the plant *in deliciis* among their dainties, and placed it of old as the first dish at their tables. The laxative properties of the Mallow, both as regards its emollient leaves, and its *radix altheæ efficacior,* were told of by Cicero and Horace.

The *Marsh Mallow* grows wild abundantly in many parts of England, especially in marshes near the sea coast. It gets its generic name *althœa,* from the Greek *althos,* "a remedy," because exercising so many curative virtues. Its old appellations were *Vismalva, Bismalva, Malvaviscus,* being twice as medicinally efficacious as the ordinary Mallow (*Sylvestris*).

Virgil in one of his eclogues teaches how to coax goats with the Marsh Mallow:—

> "Hædorumque gregem viridi compellere hibisco."

The root is sweet and very mucilaginous when chewed, containing more than half its weight of saccharine viscous mucilage. It is, therefore, emollient, demulcent, pain-soothing, and lubricating; serving to subdue heat and irritation, whilst, if applied externally, diminishing the painful soreness of inflamed parts. It is, for these reasons, much employed in domestic poultices, and in decoction as a medicine for pulmonary catarrhs, hoarseness, and irritative diarrhœa or dysentery. Also the decoction acts well as a bland soothing collyrium for bathing inflamed eyes. Gerard says: "The leaves be with good effect mixed with fomentations and poultices against pains of the sides, of the stone, and of the bladder; also in a bath they serve to take away any manner of pain."

The mucilaginous matter with which the Marsh Mallow abounds is the medicinal part of the plant; the roots of the Common Mallow being useless to yield it for such purposes, whilst those of the Marsh Mallow are of singular efficacy. A decoction of Marsh Mallow is made by adding five pints of water to a quarter-of-a-pound of the dried root, then boiling down to three pints, and straining through calico. Also Marsh Mallow ointment is a popular remedy, especially for mollifying heat, and hence it was thought invaluable by those who had to undergo the ordeal of holding red hot iron in their hands, to rapidly test their moral integrity. The sap of the Marsh Mallow was combined together with seeds of Fleabane, and the white of an hen's egg, to make a paste which was so adhesive that the hands when coated with it were safe from harm throūgh holding for a few moments the glowing iron.

French druggists prepare a famous medicinal sweetmeat, known as *Pate de gimauve* from the root of the Marsh Mallow. In Palestine, the plant is employed by the poor to eke out their food; thus we read in the book of Job (chap. xxx. ver. 4), "Who cut up Mallows by the bushes, and juniper roots for their meat."

In France, the young tops and tender leaves of the Marsh Mallow are added to spring salads, as stimulating the kidneys healthily, for which purpose is likewise prepared a syrup of Marsh Mallows *(Syrupus Althæus)* from the roots with cold water, to which the sugar is afterwards added. The leaves, flowers, and roots, are employed for making ptisans. In Devonshire, this plant is termed by the farmers, "Meshmellish," also "Drunkards," because growing close by the water; and in the West of England, "Bulls-eyes"; whilst being known in Somerset as "Bull Flowers" (pool flowers). The root of the Marsh Mallow contains starch, mucilage, pectin, oil, sugar, asparagin, phosphate of lime, glutinous matter and cellulose. An infusion made with cold water takes up the mucilage, sugar, and asparagin, then the hot water dissolves the starch.

The flowers were used formerly on May-day by country people for strewing before their doors, and weaving into garlands.

The Geranium is said to have been originally a Mallow. Mahomet having washed his shirt while on a journey, hung it on a Mallow to dry, and the plant became therefore promoted to be a Geranium.

Most probably, the modern French *Pate de gimauve* contains actually nothing of the plant or its constituents; but the root is given in France to infants, on which they may try their teeth during dentition, much as Orris root is used elsewhere.

The laxative quality of the common Mallow was mentioned by Martial :—

> "Exoneraturas ventrem mihi villica malvas
> Attulit, et varias quas habet hortus opes."

The Musk Mallow (*Malva moschata*) is another common variety of this plant, which emits from its leaves a faint musky odour, especially in warm weather, or when they are drawn lightly through the hand. Its virtues are similar in kind, but less powerful in degree, to those of the Marsh Mallow.

MARIGOLD.

In the *Grete Herball* this plant was called Mary Gowles. Three varieties of the Marigold exercise medicinal virtues which constitute them Herbal Simples of a useful nature — the Corn Marigold (*Chrysanthemum segetum*), found in our cornfields ; the cultivated garden Marigold (*Calendula officinalis*) ; and the Marsh Marigold (*Caltha palustris*), growing in moist grass lands, and popularly known as "Mareblobs."

The Corn Marigold, a Composite flower, called also Bigold, and the Yellow Oxeye, grows freely, though locally, in English cornfields, its brilliant yellow flowers contrasting handsomely with adjacent Scarlet-hued Poppies and Bluebottles (*Centaurea cyanus*). It is also named Buddle or Boodle, from *buidel*, a purse, because it bears *gools* or *goldins*, representing gold coins, in the form of the flat, round, brightly yellow blossoms, which were formerly known, too, as *Ruddes* (red flowers). The botanical title of the species, *Chrysanthemum segetum*, signifies "golden flower."

Hill named this Marigold, "the husbandman's dyall." In common with the larger Oxeye Daisy (*Chrysanthemum leucanthemum*) it has proved of late very successful in checking the night sweats of pulmonary consumption. A tincture and an infusion of the herb have been made ; from five to ten drops of the former being given for a dose, and from two to three tablespoonfuls of the latter.

The garden Marigold, often called African Marigold, came originally from Southern France, and has been cultivated in England since 1570. It is a Composite plant, and bears the name *Calendula* from the Latin *calendæ*, the first days of each month, because it flowers all the year round. Whittier styles it "the grateful and obsequious Marigold." The leaves are somewhat thick and sapid; when chewed, they communicate straightway a viscid sweetness, which is followed by a sharp, penetrating taste, very persistent in the mouth, and not of the warm, aromatic kind, but of an acrid, saline nature. This Marigold has always been grown, chiefly for its flowers, which were esteemed of old as a cordial to cheer the spirits, and when dried were put into broths as a condiment. Charles Lamb (Elia) says, in his *Essay on Christ's Hospital*: "In lieu of our half-pickled Sundays, or quite fresh boiled beef on Tuesdays (strong as *caro equina*), with detestable Marigolds floating in the pail to poison the broth." The strap-like florets of the rays are the parts of the flowers used for such a purpose. They should be gathered on a fine day when the blossoms are fully expanded, which having been divested of their outer green leaves, should be next spread on a cloth in an airy room to become dry. After having been turned frequently for a few days, they may be put by in paper bags or in drawers.

Gerard says: "The yellow leaves of the flowers are dried and kept throughout Dutch-land against winter, to put into broths and physical potions, and for divers other purposes, in such quantity that the stores of some grocers or spice-sellers contain barrels filled with them, and to be retailed by the penny, more or less; insomuch, that no broths are well made without dried Marigolds"; and, "The herb drank after the coming forth from the bath of them that hath the yellow jaundice doth in short time make them well coloured." (This is probably conjectured on the doctrine of signatures.)

A decoction of the flowers is employed by country people as a posset drink in measles and small-pox; and the expressed fresh juice proves a useful remedy against costiveness, as well as for jaundice and suppression of the monthly flow—from one to two tablespoonfuls being taken as a dose.

The plant has been considered also of service for scrofulous children, when given to them as a salad. One of the flowers if rubbed on any part recently stung by a bee or wasp, will quickly relieve it.

Buttercups and Marigolds, when growing close to each other, are called in Devonshire, "publicans and sinners." The active, bitter principle of the Marigold is "calendulin," which is yellow and tasteless, whilst swelling in water into a transparent jelly. Druggists now make a medicinal tincture (H.) of the common Marigold, using four ounces of the dried florets to a pint of proof spirit, the dose being from half a teaspoonful to two teaspoonfuls in water, twice or three times in the day. It is advised as a sudorific stimulant in low fevers, and to relieve spasms. Also, the Marigold has been employed both as a medicine and externally in treating cancer, being thought to "dispose cancerous sores to heal." A saturated tincture of the flowers when mixed with water, promotes the cure of contusions, wounds, and simple sores or ulcers; also the extract will allay chronic vomiting, if given in doses of two grains, several times a day. One drop of the tincture with two grains of powdered borax when sprayed into the ear, is very useful if a discharge has become established therefrom.

The plant, especially its flowers, was used on a large scale by the American surgeons, to treat wounds and injuries sustained during the last civil war; and obtained their warmest commendation. It quite prevented all exhausting suppurative discharges and drainings. *Succus Calendulæ* (the fresh juice) is the best form—say American surgeons—in which the *Calendula* is obtainable for ready practice. Just sufficient alcohol should be added to the juice as will prevent fermentation. For these purposes as a vulnerary, the *Calendula* owes its introduction and first use altogether to homœopathic methods, as signally valuable for healing wounds, ulcers, burns, and other breaches of the skin surface. Dr. Hughes (Brighton) says: "The Marigold is a precious vulnerary. You will find it invaluable in surgical practice."

On exposure to the sun the yellow colour of the garden Marigold becomes bleached. Some writers spell the name "Marygold," as if it, and its synonyms bore reference to the Virgin Mary; but this is a mistake, though there is a fancied resemblance of the disc's florets to rays of glory. It comes into blossom about March 25th (the Annunciation of the Virgin Mary).

> "What flower is this which bears the Virgin's name,
> And richest metal joinëd with the same?"

In the chancel of Burynarbon Church, Devonshire, is an epitaph containing a quaint allusion to this old idea respecting the Marigold:—"To the pretious memory of Mary, ye dear, and only daughter of George Westwood. January 31st, 1648."

> "This Mary Gold, lo! here doth show
> Mari's worth gold lies here below;
> The Marigold in sunshine spread,
> When cloudie closed doth bow the head."

Margaret of Orleans had for her device a Marigold turning towards the sun, with the motto, "*je ne veux suivre que lui seul.*"

Dairy women used to churn the petals of the Marigold with their cream for giving to their butter a yellow colour.

The Marsh Marigold (*Caltha poetarum*) or the Marsh

Horsegowl of old writers, grows commonly in our wet meadows, and resembles a gigantic buttercup, being of the same order of plants (*Ranunculaceæ*). The term, Marsh Marigold, is a pleonasm for Marigold, which means of itself the Marsh Gowl or Marsh Golden Flower, being an abbreviation of the old Saxon *mear-gealla*. So that the term "Marsh" has become prefixed unnecessarily. Presently, the name "Marigold," "Marsh Gowl," was passed on to the *Calendula* of the corn fields of Southern Europe, and to the garden Marigold. Furthermore, the botanical title, *Caltha*, of the Mare Blob, is got from *calathus*, a small round basket of twigs or osiers made two thousand years and more ago, which the concave golden bowl of the Marsh Marigold was thought to resemble. Persephone was collecting wild flowers in a *Calathus* when carried off by the admiring Pluto. The earliest use of the floral name *Caltha* occurs in Virgil's second Pastoral, "*Mollia luteolâ pingit vaccinia Calthâ.*" The title Mare Blob comes from the Anglo-Saxon, "*mere*" (a marsh), and "*bleb*" or "*blob*" (a bladder). These flowers were the *flaventia lumina Calthæ* of Columella, described by Shakespeare in the *Winter's Tale*. They are also known as "Bublicans," "Meadowbrights," "Crazies," "Christ's Eyes," "Bull's Eyes," "May Blobs," "Drunkards," "Water Caltrops," and wild "Batchelor's Buttons." A tincture is made (H.) from the whole plant when in flower, and may be given with success for that form of bloodlessness with great impairment of the whole health, known as pernicious anæmia. In toxic quantities the marsh Marigold has produced in its provers, a pallid, yellow, swollen state of the face, constant headache and giddiness, a thickly-coated tongue, diarrhœa, a small rapid pulse sometimes intermittent, heaviness of the limbs, and an unhealthy, eruptive state of the skin; so that the tincture of the plant in small, well-diluted doses will slowly overcome this totality of symptoms, and serve to establish a sound state of restored health. Five drops of the tincture diluted to the third strength should be given three times a day with water. Dr. Withering tells that on a large quantity of the flowers being put in the bed-room of a girl subject to fits, the attacks ceased; and an infusion of the flowers has been since given with success for similar fits.

The Marsh Marigold has been called *Verrucaria*, because efficacious in curing warts; also *Solsequia*, or *Solsequium*; and *Sponsa Solis*, since the flower opens at the rising, and shuts at the setting of the sun.

MARJORAM.

THE common Marjoram (*Origanum*) grows frequently as a wild labiate plant on dry, bushy places, especially in chalky districts throughout Britain, the whole herb being fragrantly aromatic, and bearing flowers of a deep red colour. When cultivated in our kitchen gardens it becomes a favourite pot herb, as "Sweet Marjoram," with thin compact spikes, and more elliptical leaves than the wild Marjoram. Its generic title, *Origanum*, means in Greek, the joy of the mountains (*oros-ganos*) on which it grows.

This plant and the Pennyroyal are often called "Organ." Its dried leaves are put as a pleasant condiment into soups and stuffings, being also sometimes substituted for tea. Together with the flowering tops they contain an essential volatile fragrant oil, which is carminative, warming, and tonic. An infusion made from the fresh plant will excellently relieve nervous headaches by virtue of the camphoraceous principle contained in the oil; and externally the herb may be applied with benefit in bags as a hot fomentation to painful swellings and rheumatism, as likewise for colic. "Organy," says Gerard, "is very good against the wambling of the stomacke, and stayeth the desire to vomit, especially at sea. It may be used to good purpose for such as cannot brooke their meate."

The sweet Marjoram has also been successfully employed externally for healing scirrhous tumours of the breast. Murray says: "Tumores mammarum dolentes scirrhosos herba recens, viridis, per tempus applicata feliciter dissipavit." The essential oil, when long kept, assumes a solid form, and was at one time much esteemed for being rubbed into stiff joints. The Greeks and Romans crowned young couples with Marjoram, which is in some countries the symbol of honour. Probably the name was originally, "Majoram," in Latin, *Majorana*. Our forefathers scoured their furniture with its odorous juice. In the *Merry Wives of Windsor*, Act v, Scene 5, we read:—

> "The several chairs of order look you scour
> With juice of balm, and every precious flower."

MERCURY—DOG'S (*Euphorbiaceæ*).

THE *Mercuriallis perennis* (Dog's Mercury) grows commonly in our hedges and ditches, occurring in large patches, with egg-shaped pointed leaves, square stems, and light green flowers, developed in spikes. The old herbalists called it Smerewort, and gave it for agues, as well as to cure melancholy humours. It has been eaten in mistake for Good King Henry, which is sometimes called Mercury Goosefoot; but it is decidedly poisonous, even when cooked. Some persons style it "Kentish Balsam."

The name Dog's Mercury or Dog's Cole was given either because of its supposed worthlessness, or to distinguish it from the Mercury Goosefoot aforesaid. A medicinal tincture is made (H.) from the whole plant freshly collected when in flower and fruit, with spirit of wine; and the dose of this in a diluted form is from five to ten drops, of the third decimal strength, two or three times a day, with a spoonful of water. The condition which indicates its medicinal use, is that of a severe catarrh, with chilliness, a heavy head, sneezing, a dry mouth, and general aching, lassitude, with stupor, and heat of face. Its chemical constituents have not been ascertained. In the Isle of Skye it is used for causing salivation as a vegetable mercury; and *per contra* for curing a sore mouth.

Such virtues as the herb possesses were thought to have been taught by the god Mercury. The Greeks called it Mercury's Grass (*Ermou poa*). When boiled and eaten with fried bacon in error for the English spinach, Good King Henry, it has produced sickness, drowsiness, and convulsive twitchings. The root affords both a blue and a crimson colour for dyeing.

MINTS.

(Pennyroyal, Peppermint, and Spearmint).

SEVERAL kinds of the Mints have been used medicinally from the earliest times, such as Balm, Basil, Ground Ivy, Horehound, Marjoram, Pennyroyal, Peppermint, Rosemary, Sage, Savory, Spearmint, and Thyme, some being esteemed rather as pot herbs, than as exercising positive medicinal effects. The most useful as Herbal Simples which have yet to be considered are Pennyroyal, Peppermint, and Spearmint. The Cat Mint (*Nepeta cataria*) and Horse Mint are of minor importance.

All the Mints are severally provided with leaves of a familiar fragrant character, it having been observed that this aromatic vegetation is a feature of deserts, and of other hot, dry places, all over the world. Tyndall showed the power exercised by a spray of perfume when diffused through a room to cool it, or in other words to exclude the passage of the heat rays; and it has been suggested that the presence of essential oils in the leaves of these plants serves to protect them against the intense dry heat of a desert sun as effectively as if they were partly under shelter. Nevertheless Mints, with the exception of "Arvensis," are the inhabitants of wet and marshy wastes.

They have acquired their common name *Mentha* from Minthes (according to Ovid) who was changed into a plant of this sort by Proserpina, the wife of Pluto, in a fit of jealousy. Their flowering tops are all found to contain a certain portion of camphor. Pliny said: "As for the garden Mint, the very smell of it alone recovers and refreshes the spirits, as the taste stirs up the appetite for meat, which is the reason that it is so general in our acid sauces, wherein we are accustomed to dip our meat." The Mints for paying tithes, with respect to which the Pharisees were condemned for their extravagance by our Saviour, included the Horse Mint (*Sylvestris*), the round-leaved Mint, the hairy Mint (*Aquatica*), the Corn Mint (*Arvensis*), the Bergamot Mint, and some others, besides the "Mint, Rue, and Anise," specially mentioned. "Woe unto you Pharisees; for ye tithe Mint and Rue, and all manner of herbs. Ye pay tithe of Mint, and Anise, and Cummin."

The Mint Pennyroyal (*Mentha Pulegiūm*) gets its name from the Latin *puleium regium*, because of its royal efficacy in destroying fleas *(pulices)*. The French call this similarly, *Pouliot.* It grows on moist heaths and pastures, and by the margins of brooks, being cultivated further in our herb gardens, for kitchen and market uses. Also, it is produced largely about Mitcham, and is mostly sold in a dry state. The herb was formerly named Pudding Grass, from its being used to make the stuffing for meat, in days when this was termed a pudding. Thus we read in an old play, *The Ordinary*:—

> "Let the corporal
> "Come sweating under a breast of mutton stuffed with
> [pudding."

The Pennyroyal was named by the Greeks *Bleekon* and *Gleekon*, being often used by them as a condiment for seasoning different viands. Formerly it was known in England as "Lurk in ditch," and "Run by the ground," from its creeping nature, and love of a damp soil. Its first titles were "Puliall Royall," and "Hop Marjoram." A chaplet of Pennyroyal was considered admirable for clearing the brain. Treadwell says, the Pennyroyal was especially put into hog's puddings, which were made of flour, currants, and spice, and stuffed into the entrail of a hog.

The oil of Pennyroyal is used commercially in France and Germany. Its distilled water is carminative and anti-spasmodic; whilst the whole plant is essentially stimulating. The fresh herb yields about one per cent. of a volatile oil containing oxygen, but of which the exact composition has not been ascertained. From two to eight drops may be given as a dose in suitable cases, but not where feverish or inflammatory symptoms are present.

If added to an ordinary embrocation the oil of

Pennyroyal increases the reddening and the benumbing (anodyne) effects, acting in the same way as menthol (oil of Peppermint) for promptly dispelling severe neuralgic pain. With respect to the Pennyroyal, folk speak in Devonshire of "Organs," "Organ Tea," and "Organ Broth." An essence is made of the oil, mixed and diluted with spirit of wine. The Pennyroyal has proved useful in whooping cough; but the chief purpose to which it has long been devoted, is that of promoting the monthly flow with women. Haller says he never knew an infusion of the herb in white wine, with steel, to fail of success; *Quod me nunquam fefellit.* It is certain that in some parts of England preparations of Pennyroyal are in considerable demand, and a great number of women ascribe *emmenagogue* properties to it, that is, the power of inducing the periodical monthly flux. Many married women of intelligence and close observation, assert as a positive fact, that Pennyroyal will bring on the periodical flow when suppressed; and yet the eminent jurisprudist, Dr. Taylor, was explicit in declaring that Pennyroyal has no such properties. He stated that it has no more effect on the womb than peppermint or camphor water. So there is difficulty in collecting evidence as regards the real action of Pennyroyal in such respect. Chemists supply the medicine in the full belief of this eminent opinion just quoted: at the same time they know it is not wanted for "catarrh of the chest," as alleged. The purchaser keeps her secret to herself, and does not communicate her experience to anyone. Dr. Taylor evidently supposed Peppermint water and Camphor water to be almost inert, especially as exercising any toxical effect on the womb. The medicinal basis of the latter is certainly a powerful agent, and its stimulating volatile principles are found to exist in most of the aromatic herbs; in fact, Camphor is a concrete volatile vegetable oil, and camphoraceous properties signalise all the essences derived from carminative Herbal Simples.

The Camphor of commerce is secreted by trees of the laurel sort native to China and Japan, whilst coming also from the West Indies. Everyone knows by sight and smell the white crystalline granular semi-translucent gum, strongly odorous, and having a warm pungent characteristic taste. Branches, leaves, and chips of the trees are soaked in water until it is saturated with the extract, which is then turned out into an earthen basin to coagulate. This is completely soluble in spirit of wine, but scarcely at all in water; nevertheless, if a lump of the Camphor be kept in a bottle of fresh water, to be drawn off from time to time as required, it will constitute Camphor julep. A wineglassful of it serves to relieve nervous headache and hysterical depression.

The domestic uses of Camphor are multiple, and within moderate limits perfectly safe; but a measure of caution should be exercised, as was shown a while ago by the school-boy, whom his mother furnished affectionately after the holidays with a bottle of supersaturated pilules to be taken one or two at a time against any incipient catarrh or cold. The whole bottleful was devoured at once as a sweetmeat, and the lad's life was rescued with difficulty because of intense nervous shock occasioned thereby.

An old Latin adage declares that *Camphora per nares emasculat mares*, "Camphor in excess makes men eunuchs," even when imbibed only through the air as a continuous practice. And, therefore, as a "similar" the odorous gum, in small repeated doses, is an excellent sexual restorative. Likewise, persons who have taken poisonous, or large probative quantities of Camphor found themselves quickly affected by exhausting choleraic diarrhœa; and Hahnemann therefore advised, with much success, to give (in doses of from one to three or four drops on sugar), repeatedly for cholera, a tincture of Camphor (Rubini's) made with spirit of wine above proof. This absorbs as much as is possibly soluble of the drug.

Physiologically Camphor acts by reducing reflex nervous irritability. Externally its spirit makes an admirable warming liniment, either by itself, or when conjoined with other rubefacients. In persons poisoned by the drug, all the superficial blood vessels of the bodily skin have been found immensely dilated; acting on a knowledge of which fact anyone wishing to produce copious general sweating, may do so by sitting over a plate on which Camphor is heated, whilst a blanket envelops the body loosely, and is pinned round the neck so that the fumes do not get down the throat.

In medical books of the last century this substance was called "Camphire." To a certain extent its effluvium is noxious to insects, and it may therefore be employed for preserving specimens, as well as for protecting fabrics against moths. But its volatile odours swiftly evaporate, and become even offensively diffused about the room. In a moderate measure Camphor is antiseptic, and lessens urinary irritation. Recently a dose of ninety-six grains, taken toxically, produced giddiness, then epileptic convulsions, with dilated pupils, and stertor of breathing.

The Peppermint (*Mentha piperita*), or "Brandy Mint," so called because having a pungent smell, and taste of a peppery (*piper*) nature, is a labiate plant, found not uncommonly in moist places throughout Britain, and occurring of several varieties. Both it and the Spearmint probably escaped from cultivation at first, and then became our wild plants. Its leaves and stems exhale a powerful, refreshing, characteristic aroma, and give a taste which, whilst delicate at first, is quickly followed by a sense of numbness and coldness, increased by inspiring strongly. Preparations of Peppermint, when swallowed, diffuse warmth in the stomach and mouth, acting as a stimulating carminative, with some amount of anodyne power to allay the pain of colic, flatulence, spasm, or indigestion. This is through the powerful volatile oil, of which the herb yields one per cent.

Its bruised fresh leaves, if applied, will relieve local pains and headache. A hot infusion, taken as tea, soothes stomach ache, allays sickness, and stays colicky diarrhœa. This will also subdue menstrual colic in the female. The essential oil owes its virtues to the menthol, or mint camphor, which it contains.

The Peppermint is largely grown at Mitcham, and is distilled on the ground at a low temperature, the water which comes away with the oil not being re-distilled, but allowed for the most part to run off.

Chinese oil of Peppermint (*Po Ho Yo*) yields menthol in a solid crystalline form, which, when rubbed over the surface of a painful neuralgic part, will afford speedy and marked relief, as also for neuralgic tooth-ache, tic douloureux, and the like grievous troubles. It is sold in diminutive bottles and cases labelled with Chinese characters. An ethereal tincture of menthol is made officinally with one part of menthol to eight parts of pure ether. If some of this is inhaled by vaporisation from a mouthpiece inhaler, or is sprayed into the nostrils and hindermost throat, it will relieve acute affections thereof, and of the nose, by making the blood vessels contract, and by arresting the flow of mucous discharge, thus diminishing the congestion, and quieting the pain. This camphoraceous oil was formerly applied by the Romans to the temples for the cure of headache. In local rheumatic affections the skin may be painted beneficially with oil of Peppermint. For internal use, from one to three drops of the oil may be given as a dose on sugar, or in a spoonful of milk; but the diluted essence, made from some of the oil admixed with spirit of wine, is to be preferred. Put on cotton wool into the hollow of a carious tooth, a drop or two of the essential oil will often ease the pain speedily. The fresh plant, bruised, and applied against the pit of the stomach over the navel, will allay sickness, and is useful to stay the diarrhœic purging of young children. From half to one teaspoonful of the spirituous essence of Peppermint may be given for a dose with two tablespoonfuls of hot water; or, if Peppermint water be chosen, the dose of this should be from half to one wineglassful. Distilled Peppermint water should be preferred to that prepared by adding the essence to common water. Lozenges made of the oil, or the essence, are admirable for affording ease in colic, flatulence, and nausea. They will also prevent or relieve sea-sickness.

When Tom Hood lay a dying he turned his eyes feebly towards the window on hearing it rattle in the night, whereupon his wife, who was watching him, said softly, "It's only the wind, dear"; to which he replied, with a sense of humour indomitable to the last, "Then put a Peppermint lozenge on the sill."

Two sorts of this herb are cultivated for the market—black and white Peppermint, the first of which furnishes the most, but not the best oil. The former has purple stems, and the latter green. As an antiseptic, and destroyer of disease germs, this oil is signally efficacious, on which important account it is now used for inhalation by consumptive patients as a volatile vapour to reach remote diseased parts of the lung passages, and to heal by destroying the morbid germs which are keeping up mischief therein. Towards proving this preservative power exercised by the oil of Peppermint, pieces of meat, and of fat, wrapped in several layers of gauze medicated with the oil have been kept for seven months sweet, and free from putrescent changes. A simple respirator for inhaling the oil is made from a piece of thin perforated zinc plate adapted to the shape of the mouth and nostrils like a small open funnel, within the narrow end of which is fitted a pledget of cotton wool saturated with twenty drops of the oil, or from twenty to thirty drops of the spirituous essence. This should be renewed each night and morning, whilst the apparatus is to be worn nearly all day. At the same time the oil is agreeable of odour, and is altogether harmless. It may be serviceably admixed with liniments for use to rheumatic parts.

"Peppermint," says Dr. Hughes (Brighton), "should be more largely employed than it is in coughs, especially in a dry cough, however caused, when it seems to act specifically as a cure, just as arnica does for injuries, or aconite for febrile inflammation. It will relieve even the irritative hectic cough of consumptive patients. Eight or ten drops of the essence should be given for this purpose as a dose with a tablespoonful of water. In France continuous inhalations of Peppermint oil combined with creasote and glycerine, have become used most successfully, even when cavities exist in the lungs, with copious bacillary expectoration. The cough, the night sweats, and the heavy phlegm have been arrested, whilst the nutrition and the weight have steadily increased."

A solution of menthol one grain, spirit of wine fifty drops, and oil of cloves ten drops, if painted over the seat of pain, will relieve neuralgia of the face, or sciatica promptly. Unhealthy sores may be cleansed, and their healing promoted, by being dressed with strips of soft rag dipped in sweet oil, to each ounce of which one or two drops of the oil of Peppermint has been added. For diphtheria, Peppermint oil has been of marked use when applied freely twice or three times in the day to the ulcerated parts of the throat. This oil, or the essence, can be used of any strength, in any quantity, without the least harm to the patient. It checks suppuration when applied to a sore or wound, whilst exercising an independent antiseptic influence. "Altogether," says Dr. Braddon, "the oil of Peppermint forms the best, safest, and most agreeable of known antiseptics." Pliny tells that the Greeks and Romans crowned themselves with the Peppermint at their feasts, and adorned their *al fresco* tables with its sprays. The "chefs" introduced this herb into all their sauces, and scented their wines with its essence. The Roman housewives made a paste of the Peppermint with honey, which they esteemed highly, partaking of it to sweeten their breath, and to conceal their passion for wine at a time when the law punished with death every woman convicted of quaffing the ruby seductive liquor. Seneca perished in a bath scented with woolly mint.

The Spearmint (*Mentha viridis*) is found growing apparently wild in England, but is probably not an indigenous herb. It occurs in watery places, and on the banks of rivers, such as the Thames, and the Exe. If used externally, its strong decoction will heal chaps and indolent eruptions.

It possesses a warm, aromatic odour and taste, much

resembling those of Peppermint, but not so pungent. Its volatile oil, and its essence, made with spirit of wine, contain a similar stimulating principle, but are less intense, and therefore better adapted for children's maladies.

The Spearmint is called "Mackerel Mint," and in Germany "Lady's Mint," with a pun on the word *münze.* Its name, Spear, or Spire, indicates the spiry form of its floral blossoming. When the leaves of the herb are macerated in milk, this curdles much less quickly than it otherwise would ; and therefore the essence is to be commended for use with milk diets by delicate persons, or for young children of feeble digestive powers, though not when feverishness is present. "Spearmint," says John Evelyn, "is friendly to the weak stomach, and powerful against all nervous crudities." "This is the Spearmint that steadies giddiness," writes Alfred Austin, Poet Laureate.

Our cooks employ it with vinegar for making the mint sauce which we eat with roast lamb, because of its condimentary virtues as a spice to the immature meat, whilst the acetic acid of the vinegar serves to help dissolve the crude albuminous fibre.

The oil is less used than that of Peppermint. From two to five drops may be given on sugar ; or from half to one teaspoonful of the spirit of Spearmint with two tablespoonfuls of water. Also a distilled water of Spearmint is made, which will relieve hiccough, and flatulence, as well as the giddiness of indigestion. The tincture prepared from the dried herb looks of a bright dark green by day, but of a deep red colour by night. Martial called the Spearmint *Ructatrix mentha.* "*Nec deest ructatrix mentha.*"

The Calamint, or Basil Thyme, grows frequently in

our waysides and hedges, a labiate plant, with downy stems and leaves, whilst bearing light purple flowers. The whole herb has a sweet, aromatic odour, and makes a pleasant cordial tea. It is named from the Greek *kalos*, "excellent," because thought useful against serpents. "There is made hereof," said Galen, "an antidote marvellous good for young women that want their courses."

The stem of this pretty slender herb is seldom more than five or six inches high, and its blossoms are so inconspicuous as to be often overlooked. The flowers droop gracefully before expansion. In country places it is often called Mill Mountain, and its infusion is an old remedy for rheumatism. If bruised, and applied externally, it reddens the skin, and will sometimes even blister it. In this way it acts well when judiciously used for lumbago, and rheumatic pains. The Calamint contains a camphoraceous, volatile, stimulating oil, in common with the other mints; this is distilled by water, but its virtues are better extracted by rectified spirit. The lesser Calamint is a variety of the herb possessing almost superior virtues, with a stronger odour resembling that of Pennyroyal. "Apple Mint" is the "*Mentha rotundifolia.*"

"Many robust men and women among our peasantry," says Dr. George Moore, "from notions of their own, use infusions of Balm, Sage, or even a little Rue, or wild Thyme, as a common drink, with satisfaction to their stomachs, and advantage to their health, instead of infusing the Chinese herb." The Calamint is a favourite herb with such persons. About the Cat mint there is an old saying, "If you set it the cats will eat it: if you sow it the cats won't know it." This, the *Nepeta cataria*, or *herbe aux chats*, is as much beloved by cats as *Valerian*, and the common *Marum*, for which herbs they have a frenzied passion. They roll themselves over the plants, which they lick, tear with their teeth, and bathe with their urine. But the Cat mint is the detestation of rats, insomuch that with its leaves a small barricade may be constructed which the vermin will never pass however hungry they may be. It is sometimes called "Nep," as contracted from *Nepeta*. Hoffman said, "The root of the Cat mint, if chewed, will make the most gentle person fierce and quarrelsome"; and there is a legend of a certain hangman who could never find courage to exercise his gruesome task until he had masticated some of this aromatic root.

MISTLETOE.

THE Mistletoe, which we all associate so happily with the festivities of Christmas, is an evergreen parasite, growing on the branches of deciduous trees, and penetrating with simple roots through the bark into the wood. It belongs to the *Loranthaceæ*, and has the botanical name of *Viscum*, or "sticky," because of its glutinous juices. The Mistletoe contains mucilage, sugar, a fixed oil, resin, an odorous principle, some tannin, and various salts. Its most interesting constituent is the "viscin," or bird glue, which is mainly developed by fermentation, and becomes a yellowish, sticky, resinous mass, such as can be used with success as a bird-lime.

The dried young twigs, and the leaves, are chiefly the medicinal parts, though young children have been attacked with convulsions after eating freely of the berries.

The name (in Anglo-Saxon, *Mistiltan*) is derived, says Dr. Prior, from *mistil*, "different," and *tan*, "a twig," because so unlike the tree it grows upon; or, perhaps, *mist* may refer to excrement, and the adjective, *viscum*, bear some collateral reference to *viscera*, "entrails." Probably our *viscum* plant differs from that of the Latin writers in their accounts of the Druids, which would be the *Loranthus* growing on the *Quercus pubescens* (an oak indigenous to the south of France). They knew it by a name answering to "all-heal." It is of a larger and thicker sort than our common Mistletoe, which, however, possesses the same virtues in a lesser degree. The Germans call the plant *Vogellein*, and the French *Gui*, which is probably Celtic.

The plant is given powdered, or as an infusion, or made into a tincture (H.) with spirit of wine. From ten to sixty grains of the powder may be taken for a dose, or a decoction may be made by boiling two ounces of the bruised plant with half-a-pint of water, and giving one tablespoonful for a dose several times in the day; or from five to ten drops of the tincture (which is prepared almost exclusively by the homœopathic chemists) are a dose, with one or two tablespoonfuls of cold water.

Sir John Colebatch published in 1720 a pamphlet, on *The Treatment of Epilepsy by Mistletoe*, regarding it, and with much justice, as a specific. He procured the parasite from the lime trees at Hampton Court. The powdered leaves were ordered to be given (in black cherry water), as much of these as will lie on a sixpence every morning.

Sir John says, "This beautiful plant must have been designed by the Almighty for further and more noble purposes than barely to feed thrushes, or to be hung up superstitiously in houses to drive away evil spirits." His treatise was entitled, *A Dissertation concerning the Misseltoe—A most wonderful Specifick Remedy for the Cure of Convulsive Distempers.* The physiological effect of the plant is that of lessening, and temporarily benumbing such nervous action as is reflected to distant organs of the body from some central organ which is the actual seat of trouble. In this way the spasms of epilepsy and of other convulsive distempers, are allayed. Large doses of the plant, or of its berries, would, on the contrary, aggravate these convulsive disorders.

In a French "*Recueil de Remedes domestiques,*" 1682, *Avec privilege du Roy*, we read, de l'epilepsie: "Il est certain que contre ce deplorable mal le veritablè Guy de Chêne (Mistletoe) est un remede excellent, curatif, preservatif, et qui soulage beaucoup dans l'accident. Il le faut secher au four apres qu'on aura tiré le pain: le mettre en poudre fort subtile; passer cette poudre par un tamis de foye, et la conserver pour le besoin. Il faut prendre les poids dun ecu d'or de cette poudre chaque matin dans vin blanc tous les trois derniers jours de la lune vieille. Il est encore bon que la personne affligée de ce mal porte toujours un morceau de Guy de Chêne pendu à son col; mais ce morceau doit etre toujours frais, et sans avoir eté mis au four." The active part of the plant is its resin (*viscin*), which is yielded to spirit of wine in making a tincture. This is prepared (H.) with proof spirit from the leaves and ripe berries of our Mistletoe in equal quantities, but it is difficult of manufacture owing to the viscidity of the sap. A special process is employed of passing the material twice through a sausage machine, and then mixing the mass with powdered glass before its percolation with the spirit. A trituration made from the leaves, berries, and tender twigs, is given for epilepsy, in doses of twenty grains, twice or three times a day.

Nowadays the berries are taken by country people when finding themselves troubled with severe stitches, and they obtain almost instantaneous relief. In accordance with which experience Johnson says it was creditably reported to him, "That a few of the berries of the Misseltoe, bruised and strained into oyle and drunken, hath presently and forthwith rid a grievous and sore stitch." The tincture, moreover, is put to a modern use as a heart tonic in place of the foxglove. It lessens reflex irritability, and strengthens the heart's beat, whilst raising the frequency of a slow pulse. Dr. J. Wilde has shown that the Mistletoe possesses a high repute in rural Hampshire for the cure of St. Vitus's dance, and similar spasmodic nervous complaints. In the United States the leaves have been successfully employed as an infusion to check female fluxes, and hæmorrhages, also to hasten childbirth by stimulating the womb when labour is protracted to the exhaustion of the mother. In Scotland the plant is almost unknown, and is restricted to one locality only.

The Druids regarded the Mistletoe as the soul of their sacred tree—the oak; and they taught the people to believe that oaks on which it was seen growing were to be respected, because of the wonderful cures which the priests were then able to effect with it, particularly of the falling sickness. The parasite was cut from the tree with a golden sickle at a high and solemn festival, using much ceremonial display, it being then credited with a special power of "giving fertility to all animals." Ovid said, "Ad viscum cantare Druidœ solebant."

Shakespeare calls it "The baleful Mistletoe," in allusion to the Scandinavian legend, that Balder, the god of peace, was slain with an arrow made of Mistletoe. He was restored to life at the request of the other gods and goddesses. The mistletoe was afterwards given to be kept by the goddess of love; and it was ordained in Olympus that every one who passed under it should receive a kiss, to show that the branch was the emblem of love, and not of death.

Persons in Sweden afflicted with epilepsy carry with them a knife having a handle of oak mistletoe, which plant they call Thunder-besom, connecting it with lightning and fire. The thrush is the great disseminator of the parasite. He devours the berries eagerly, and soils, or "missels" his feet with their viscid seeds, conveying them thus from tree to tree, and getting thence the name of missel thrush.

In Brittany the plant is named *Herbe de la croix*, and, because the crucifix was made from its wood when a tree, it is thought to have become degraded to a parasite.

When Norwood, in Surrey, was really a forest the Mistletoe grew there on the oak, and, being held as medicinal, it was abstracted for apothecaries in London. But the men who meddled with it were said to become lame, or to fall blind with an eye, and a rash fellow who ventured to cut down the oak itself broke his leg very shortly afterwards. One teaspoonful of the dried leaves, in powder, from the appletree Mistletoe, taken in acidulated water twice a day, will cure chronic giddiness. Sculptured sprays and berries, with leaves of Mistletoe, fill the spandrils of the tomb of one of the Berkeleys in Bristol Cathedral—a very rare adornment, because for some unknown reason the parasite has been always excluded from the decorations of churches. In some districts it is called Devil's-fuge, also the Spectre's Wand, from a belief that with due incantations a branch held in the hand will compel the appearance of a spectre, and require it to speak.

MOUNTAIN ASH.

A somewhat common. and handsomely conspicuous tree in many parts of England, especially about high lands, is the Rowan, or Mountain Ash. In May and June it attracts attention by its bright green feathery foliage set off by cream-coloured bloom, whilst in September it bears a brilliant fruitage of berries, richly orange in colour at first, but presently of a clear ripe vermilion. Popularly this abundant fruit is supposed to be poisonous, but such is far from being the case. A most excellent and wholesome jelly may be prepared therefrom, which is slightly tonic by its salutary bitterness, and is an admirable antiseptic accompaniment to certain roast meats, such as venison and mutton. To make this jelly, boil the berries in water (cold at first) in an enamelled preserving pan; when the fruit has become sufficiently soft, run the contents of the pan through a flannel bag without pressure; tie the bag between two chairs, with a basin below, and let the juice strain leisurely through so as to come out clear. Then to each pint of the juice add a pound of sugar, and boil this from ten to twenty minutes; pour off into warm dry jars, and cover them securely when cool. After the juice has dripped off the fruit a pleasant refreshing drink may be made for children by pouring a kettleful of boiling water through the flannel bag. Some persons mix with the fruit an equal quantity of green apples when making the jelly. Birds, especially field fares, eat the berries with avidity; and a botanical designation of the tree is *aucuparia*, as signifying fruit used by the *auceps*, or bird catcher, with which to bait his snares.

"There is," says an old writer, "in every berry the exhilaration of wine, and the satisfying of old mead; and whosoever shall eat three berries of them, if he has completed a hundred years, he will return to the age of thirty years."

At the same time it must be noted that the *leaves* of the Mountain Ash are of a poisonous quality, and contain prussic acid like those of the laurel. But, as already shown, the berries, when ripe, may be eaten freely without fear. Chemically they contain tartaric acid when unripe, and both malic and citric acids when ripe. They also furnish sorbin, and parasorbic acid. The unripe fruit and the bark are extremely astringent, being useful in decoction, or infusion, to check diarrhœa; and externally in poultices or lotions, to constringe such relaxed parts as the throat, and lower bowel.

The title Rowan tree has affixed itself to the Mountain Ash, as derived from the Norse, *Runa* (a charm), because it is supposed to have the power of averting the evil eye.

> "Rowan tree and red thread
> Hold the witches a' in dread."

"Runa" was really a magician, or whisperer, from *ru*, to murmur, and in olden times *runes*, or mystical secrets, were carved exclusively on the Mountain Ash tree in Scandinavia and the British Isles.

Crosses made of the twigs, and tied with red thread were sewn by Highlandmen into their clothes. Dame Sludge fastened a piece of the wood into Flibbertigibbet's collar as a protection against Wayland Smith's sorceries.—(Kenilworth). Other folk-names of the tree are Quicken tree, Quick Beam, Wiggen, and Witcher.

The Mountain Ash is botanically a connecting link between the dog rose of our hedges and the apple tree of our orchards. Its flowers exactly resemble apple blossoms, and its thickly-clustered red berries are only small crabs dwarfed by the love of the tree for mountain heights and bleak windy situations. In the harsh cold regions of the north it is only a stunted shrub with leaves split up into many small leaflets, so as to suffer less by any breadth of resistance to the sharp driving blasts of icy winds.

Confusion has been often made between this tree and the Service tree (*Sorbus*, or *Pyrus domestica*), which is quite distinct, being more correctly called Servise tree, from *Cerevisia*, fermented beer. Formerly this Servise, or Checker-tree, was employed for making an intoxicating drink. Virgil says:—

> "Et pocula læti
> Fermento atque acidis imitantur vitea *sorbis*."
>
> "With acid juices from the Service Ash,
> And humming ale, they make their Lemon Squash."

The fruit of the Service tree (or Witten Pear-tree) resembles a small pear, and is considered in France very useful for dysentery because of its tannin; but this *Pyrus domestica* is a rare tree in England. Sometimes mistaken for it is the *wild* Service tree (the *Pyrus torminalis*), much more common in our south country hedges. Its fruit is threaded on long strings, and carried in procession at village feasts in Northamptonshire, but is worthless. Evelyn says, "Ale and beer brewed from the berries, when ripe, of the true Service tree is an incomparable drink."

MUGWORT and WORMWOOD.

THE herb Mugwort (*Artemisia vulgaris*), a Composite plant, is frequent about hedgerows and waste ground throughout Britain; and it chiefly merits a place among Herbal Simples because of a special medicinal use in certain female derangements. Its name Mugwort has been attributed to "moughte," a moth, or maggot, this title being given to the plant because Dioscorides commended it for keeping off moths. Its Anglo-Saxon synonym is *Wyrmwyrt.* Mugwort is named from Artemis, the Greek goddess of the moon, and is also called Maidenwort or Motherwort (womb wort), being a plant beneficial to the womb.

Macer says, terming it by mistake "Mother of Worts":

> "Herbarum matrem justum puto ponere primo
> Præcipue morbis mulieribus illa medetur."

A decoction of the fresh tops acts famously to correct female irregularities when employed as a bath. *Uterina est, adeoque usus est creberrimus mulierculis quæ eam adhibent externe, atque interne ut vix balnea et lotiones parent in quibus artemisia non contineatur.* Thus writes Ray, quoting from Schroder. Or it may be that the term Mugwort became popularly applied because this herb was in demand for helping to preserve ale. The plant was formerly known as *Cingulum Sancti Johannis,* since a crown made from its sprays was worn on St. John's Eve, to gain security from evil possession; also as *Zona divi Johannis,* it being believed that John the Baptist bore a girdle of it in the wilderness. In Germany and Holland it has received the name of St. John's Plant, because, if gathered on St. John's Eve, it is thought protective against diseases and misfortunes. The Mugwort is also styled "Felon wort," or "Felon herb." If placed in the shoes, it will prevent weariness. A dram of the powdered leaves taken four times a day has cured chronic hysterical fits, which were otherwise intractable. "Mugwort," says Gerard, "cureth the shakings of the joynts inclining to the palsie."

The mermaid of the Clyde is said to have exclaimed,

when she beheld the funeral of a young maiden who had died from consumption and decline:—

"If they wad drink nettles in March,
And eat muggins [Mugwort] in May,
Sae mony braw young maidens
Wad na' be gang to clay."

Portions of old dead roots are found at the base of the herb, which go by the name of "coals," and are thought to be preventive of epilepsy when taken internally, or worn around the neck as an amulet. Parkinson says: "Mugwort is of wonderful help to women in risings of the mother, or hysteria." It is also useful against gout by boiling the tender parts of the roots in weak broth, and taking this frequently; whilst at the same time the affected limbs should be bathed and fomented with a hot decoction of the herb. The plant, without doubt, is decidedly anti-epileptic, its remedial effects being straightway followed by profuse and fetid perspirations. It is similarly useful against the convulsions of children in teething. For preventing disorders, as well as for curing rheumatism, the Japanese, young and old, rich and poor, indiscriminately, are said to be singed with a "moxa" made from the Mugwort. Its dried leaves are rubbed in the hands until the downy part becomes separated, and can be moulded into little cones. One of these having been placed over the site of the disease, is ignited and burnt down to the skin surface, which it blackens and scorches in a dark circular patch. This process is repeated until a small ulcer is formed when treating chronic diseases of the joints, which sore is kept open by issue peas retained within it so that they may constantly exercise a derivative effect.

The flesh of geese is declared to be more savoury when

stuffed with this herb, which contains "absinthin" as its active principle, and other chemical constituents in common with Wormwood; but the odour of Mugwort is not fragrant or aromatic, because it does not possess a volatile essential oil like that of the *Artemisia absinthium* (Wormwood).

This Wormwood is also a Composite plant of the same tribe and character, but with an intensely bitter taste; and hence its name, *Absinthium*, has been derived from the Greek privative, *a*, and *psinthos*, "delight," because the flavour is so bitterly distasteful. It is a bushy plant, which abounds in our rural districts, having silky stems and leaves, with small heads of dull yellow flowers, the whole plant being *amara et aromatica*.

The Mugwort, as an allied Wormwood of the same genus, is taller and more slender than the *Absinthium*, and is distinguished by being scentless, its leaves being green above, and white below. The bitter taste of the true Wormwood is also due to "absinthin," and each kind contains nitrate of potash, tannin, and resin, with succinic, malic, and acetic acids.

Old Tusser says:—

> "Where chamber is swept, and wormwood is strown,
> No flea for his life dare abide to be known."

And again:—

> "What savour is better, if physic be true,
> For places infected, than wormwood and rue."

The infusion of Wormwood makes a useful fomentation for inflammatory pains, and, combined with chamomile flowers and bay leaves, it formed the anodyne fomentation of the earlier dispensatories. This infusion, with a few drops of the essential oil of Wormwood, will serve as an astringent wash to prevent the hair from falling off when it is weak and thin.

Both Mugwort and Wormwood have been highly esteemed for overcoming epilepsy in persons of a feeble constitution, and of a sensitive nervous temperament, especially in young females. Mugwort tea, and a decoction of Wormwood, may be confidently given for the purposes just named, also to correct female irregularities.

For promoting the monthly flow, Chinese women make a confection of the leaves of Mugwort mixed with rice and sugar, which, when needed to overcome arrested monthly fluxes, or hysteria, they *instar bellaria ingerunt*, "eat as a sweetmeat."

A drachm of the powdered leaves of the Mugwort, taken four times a day, has cured chronic hysterical fits otherwise irrepressible. The true Wormwood (*Artemisia absinthium*) is used for preparing absinthe, a seductive liqueur, which, when taken to excess, induces epileptic attacks. Any habitual use of alcohol flavoured with this herb singularly impairs the mental and physical powers.

"An ointment," says Meyrick, "made of the juice of Mugwort with hogs' lard, disperses hard knots and kernels about the neck and throat."

MULBERRY.

THE Mulberry tree (*Morus nigra*) has been cultivated in England since the middle of the sixteenth century, being first planted at Sion house in 1548. It is now grown commonly in the garden, orchard, or paddock, where its well-known rich syrupy fruit ripens in September. This fruit, abounding with a luscious juice of regal hue, is used in some districts, particularly in Devonshire, for mixing with cider during fermentation, giving to the beverage a pleasant taste, and a deep red colour. The juice, made into syrup, is curative of sore throats, especially of the putrid sort, if it be used in gargles; also of thrush in the mouth, if applied thereto; and the ripe fruit is gently laxative.

Horace recommends that Mulberries be gathered before sunset:—

> "Æstatis peraget qui nigris prandia moris
> Finiet ante gravem quæ legerit arbore solem."

The generic name, *Morus*, is derived from the Celtic *mor*, "black." In Germany (at Iserlohn), mothers, in order to deter their children from eating Mulberries, tell them the devil requires the juicy berries for the purpose of blacking his boots. This fruit was fabled to have become changed from white to a deep red through absorbing the blood of Pyramus and Thisbe, who were slain beneath its shade.

It is thought by some that "morus" has been derived from the Latin word *mora*, delay, as shown in a tardy expansion of the buds. Because cautious not to burst into leaf until the last frost of spring is over, the Mulberry tree, as the wisest of its fellows, was dedicated by the ancients to Minerva, and the story of Pyramus and Thisbe owed its origin to the white and black fruited varieties:—

> "The Mulberry found its former whiteness fled,
> And, ripening, saddened into dusky red."

Shakespeare's famous Mulberry tree, planted in 1609, was of the black species. It was recklessly cut down at New Place, Stratford-on-Avon, in 1759. Ten years afterwards, when the freedom of the city was presented to Garrick, the document was enclosed in a casket made from the wood of this tree. Likewise a cup was wrought therefrom, and at the Shakespeare Jubilee, Garrick, holding the cup aloft, recited the following lines, composed by himself for the occasion :—

> " Behold this fair goblet: 'twas carved from the tree
> Which, oh, my sweet Shakespeare, was planted by thee!
> As a relic I kiss it, and bow at thy shrine,
> What comes from thy hand must be ever divine."

> " All shall yield to the Mulberry tree;
> Bend to the blest Mulberry:
> Matchless was he who planted thee,
> And thou, like him, immortal shall be."

A slip of it was grown by Garrick in his garden at Hampton Court. The leaves of the Mulberry tree are known to furnish excellent food for silk worms.

Botanically, each fruit is a collection of berries on a common pulpy receptacle, being, like the Strawberry, especially wholesome for those who are liable to heartburn, because it does not undergo acetous fermentation in the stomach. In France Mulberries are served at the beginning of a meal. Among the Romans the fruit was famous for maladies of the throat and windpipe.

The tree does not bear until it is somewhat advanced in age. It contains in every part a milky juice, which will coagulate into a sort of Indian rubber, and this has been thought to give tenacity to the filament spun by the silkworm.

The juice of Mulberries contains malic and citric acids, with glucose, pectin, and gum. The bark of the root has been given to expel tapeworm; and the fruit is remarkable for its large quantity of sugar, being excelled in this respect only by the fig, the grape, and the cherry.

We are told in *Ivanhoe* that the Saxons made a favourite drink, "Morat," from the juice of Mulberries with honey. During the thirteenth century these berries were sometimes called "pynes."

In the memorable narrative of the Old Testament, 2 *Samuel*, v., 24, "When thou hearest the sound of a going in the tops of the Mulberry trees," the word used (*bekhaim*) has been mistranslated, really intending the Aspen (*Populus tremula*).

MULLEIN.

THE great Mullein (*Verbascum thapsus*) grows freely in England on dry banks and waste places, but somewhat sparingly in Scotland. It belongs to the scrofula-curing order of plants, having a thick stalk, from eighteen inches to four feet high, with large woolly mucilaginous leaves, and with a long flower-spike bearing plain yellow flowers, which are nearly sessile on the stem. The name "Molayne" is derived from the Latin, *mollis*, soft.

In most parts of Ireland, besides growing wild, it is carefully cultivated in gardens, because of a steady demand for the plant by sufferers from pulmonary consumption. Constantly in Irish newspapers there are advertisements offering it for sale, and it can be had from all the leading local druggists. The leaves are best when gathered in the late summer, just before the plant flowers. The old Irish method of administering Mullein is to put an ounce of the dried leaves, or a corresponding quantity of the fresh ones, in a pint of milk, which is boiled for ten minutes, and then strained. This is afterwards given warm to the patient twice a day, with or without sugar. The taste of the decoction is bland, mucilaginous, and cordial. Dr. Quinlan, of Dublin, treated many cases of tubercular lung disease, even when some were far advanced in pulmonary consumption, with the Mullein, and with signal success as regards palliating the cough, staying the expectoration, and increasing the weight.

Mullein leaves have a weak, sleepy sort of smell, and rather a bitter taste. In Queen Elizabeth's time they were carried about the person to prevent the falling sickness; and distilled water from the flowers was said to be curative of gout.

The leaves and flowers contain mucilage, with a yellowish volatile oil, a fatty substance, and sugar, together with some colouring matter. Fish will become stupefied by eating the seeds. Gerard says "Figs do not putrifie at all that are wrapped in the leaves of Mullein. If worn under the feet day and night in the manner of a sock they bring down in young maidens their desired sicknesse."

The plant bears also the name of Hedge Taper, and used to be called Torch, because the stalks were dipped in suet, and burnt for giving light at funerals and other gatherings. "It is a plant," says the *Grete Herball*, "whereof is made a manner of lynke if it be tallowed."

According to Dodœus the Mullein was called "Candela." *Folia siquidem habet mollia hirsuta ad lucernarum funiculos apta.* "It was named of the Latines, *Candela Regia* and *Candelaria.*" The modern Romans style it the "Plant of the Lord." Other popular English names of the plant are "Adam's flannel," "Blanket," "Shepherd's club," "Aaron's rod," "Cuddie's lungs"; and in Anglo-Saxon, "Feldwode." Gower says of Medea:—

> "Tho' toke she feldwode, and verveine,
> Of herbes ben nought better tweine."

The name *Verbascum* is an altered form of the Latin *barbascum*, from *barba*, "a beard," in allusion to the dense woolly hairs on both sides of the leaves; and the appellation, Mullein, is got from the French *molène*, signifying the "scab" in cattle, and for curing which disease the plant is famous. It has also been termed Cow's Lung Wort, Hare's Beard, Jupiter's Staff, Ladies' Foxglove, and Velvet Dock from its large soft leaves. The Mullein bears the title "Bullock's lung wort," because of its supposed curative powers in lung diseases of this animal, on the doctrine of signatures, because its leaf resembles a dewlap; and the term "Malandre" was formerly applied to the lung maladies of cattle. Also the "Malanders" meant leprosy, whence it came about that the epithet "Malandrin" was attached to a brigand, who, like the leper, was driven from society and forced to lead a lawless life.

An infusion of the flowers was used by the Roman ladies to tinge their tresses of the golden colour once so much admired in Italy; and now in Germany, a hair wash made from the Mullein is valued as highly restorative. A decoction of the root is good for cramps and against the megrims of bilious subjects, which especially beset them in the dark winter months. The dried leaves of the Mullein plant, if smoked in an ordinary tobacco pipe, will completely control the hacking cough of consumption; and they can be employed with equal benefit, when made into cigarettes, for asthma, and for spasmodic coughs in general.

By our leading English druggists are now dispensed a *succus verbasci* (Mullein juice), of which the dose is from half to one teaspoonful; a tincture of *Verbascum* (Mullein), the dose of which is from half-a-teaspoonful to two teaspoonfuls; and an infusion of Mullein, in doses of from one to four tablespoonfuls. Also a tincture (H.) is made from the fresh herb with spirit of wine, which has been proved beneficial for migraine (sick head-ache) of long standing, with oppression of the ears. From eight to ten drops of this tincture are to be given as a dose, with cold water, and repeated pretty frequently whilst needed.

Mullein oil is a most valuable destroyer of disease germs. If fresh flowers of the plant be steeped for twenty-one days in olive oil whilst exposed to the sunlight, this makes an admirable bactericide; also by simply instilling a few drops two or three times a day into the ear, all pain therein, or discharges therefrom, and consequent deafness, will be effectually cured, as well as any itching eczema of the external ear and its canal. A conserve of the flowers is employed on the Continent against ringworm. Some of the most brilliant results have been obtained in suppurative inflammation of the inner ear by a single application of Mullein oil. In acute or chronic cases of this otorrhœa, two or three drops of the oil should be made fall into the ear twice or thrice in the day. And the same oil is an admirable remedy for children who " wet the bed " at night. Five drops should be put into a small tumblerful of cold water; and a teaspoonful of the mixture, first stirred, should be taken four times in the day.

Flowers of Mullein in olive oil, when kept near the fire for several days in a corked bottle, form a remedy popular in Germany for frost-bites, bruises, and piles. Also a poultice made with the leaves is a good application to these last named troublesome evils. For the cure of piles, sit for five minutes on a chamber vessel containing live coals, with crisp dry Mullein leaves over them, and some finely powdered resin.

MUSHROOMS.

WITHOUT giving descriptive attention to those Mushrooms (*Agarics*, *Boleti*, and others) which are edible, and of which over a hundred may be enumerated, as beyond our purpose when treating of curative Herbal Simples, notice will be bestowed here on two productions of the Mushroom nature—the Puff Ball and the Fly Agaric,—because of their medicinal qualities.

It may be first briefly stated that the *Agaricus campestris*, or field Mushroom, is the kind most commonly eaten in England, being highly nitrogenous, and containing much fat. This may be readily distinguished from any harmful fungus by the pink colour of its gills, the solidity of its stem, the fragrant anise-like odour which it possesses, and the separability of its outer skin. Other edible Mushrooms which grow with us, and are even of a better quality than the above, are the *Agaricus augustus* and the *Agaricus elvensis*, not to mention the *Chanturelle*, said to be unapproachable for excellence.

The Greeks were aware of edible fungi, and knew of injurious sorts which produced a sense of choking, whilst subsequent wasting of the body occurred. Athenæus quotes an author who said: "You will be choked like those who waste after eating mushrooms." The Romans also esteemed some fungi as of so exquisite a flavour that these would be stolen sooner than silver or gold by anyone entrusted with their delivery:—

> "Argentum, atque aurum facile est lænamque togamque.
> Mittere, boletos mittere difficile est."

Mushrooms were styled by Porphry *deorum filii*, and "without seed, as produced by the midwifery of autumnal thunderstorms, and portending the mischief which these cause." "They are generally reported to have something noxious in them, and not without reason; but they were exalted to the second course of the Cæsarean tables with the noble title "bromatheon," a dainty fit for the gods, to whom they sent the Emperor Claudius, as they have many since to the other world." "So true it is he who eats Mushrooms many times, *nil amplius edit*, eats no more of anything."

The poisonous kinds may be commonly recognised by their possessing permanently white gills which do not touch the stem; and a thin ring, or frill, is borne by the stem at some distance from the top, whilst the bottom of the stem is surrounded by a loose sheath, or volva. If "phalline" is the active poisonous principle, this is not rendered inert by heat in cooking; but the helvellic acid of other sorts disappears during the process, and its fungi are thus made non-poisonous. There is a popular belief that Mushrooms which grow near iron, copper, or other metals, are deadly; the same idea obtaining in the custom of putting a coin in the water used for boiling Mushrooms in order that it may attract and detach any poison, and so serve to make them wholesome.

In Essex there is an old saying:—

> "When the moon is at the full,
> Mushrooms you may freely pull;
> But when the moon is on the wane,
> Wait till you think to pluck again."

Even the most poisonous species may be eaten with impunity after repeated maceration in salt and water, or vinegar and water—which custom is generally adopted in the South of Europe, where the diet of the poorer classes largely includes the fungi which they gather; but when so treated the several Mushrooms lose much of their soluble nutritive qualities as well as their flavour. For the most part, *Agarics* with salmon-coloured spores are injurious, likewise fungi having a rancid or fetid odour, and an acrid, pungent, peppery taste. Celsus said: "If anyone shall have eaten noxious fungi, let him take radishes with vinegar and water, or with salt and vinegar."

Wholesome Mushrooms afford nourishment which is a capital substitute for butchers' meat, and almost equally sustaining. If a poisonous fungus has been eaten, its ill-effects may nowadays be promptly met by antidotes injected beneath the skin, and by taking small doses of strychnia in coffee.

Gerard says: "I give my advice to those that love such strange and new fangled meats to beware of licking honey among thorns, lest the sweetness of the one do not countervail the sharpness and pricking of the other." With regard to Mushrooms generally, Horace said :—

> "Pratensibus optima fungis
> Natura est; aliis male creditur."

> "The meadow Mushrooms are in kind the best;
> 'Tis ill to trust in any of the rest."

The St. George's Mushroom, an early one, takes, perhaps, the highest place as an agaric for the table. Blewits (formerly sold in Covent Garden market for Catsup), and Blue Caps, each an autumnal species, are savoury fungi to be fried. They may be served with bacon on toast.

A very old test as to the safety of Mushrooms is to stew with them in the saucepan a small carefully-peeled onion. If after boiling for a few minutes this comes out white, and clean-looking, the Mushrooms may all be confidently eaten: but if it has turned blue, or black, there are dangerous ones among them, and all should be rejected.

The Puff Ball (*Lycoperdon giganteum bovista*) grows usually on the borders of fields, in orchards, or meadows, also on dry downs, and occasionally in gardens. It should be collected as a Simple in August and September. This Puff Ball is smooth, globose, and yellowish-white when young, becoming afterwards brown. It contains, when ripe, a large quantity of extremely fine brown black powder, which is a capital application for stopping bleeding from slight wounds and cuts. This also makes a good drying powder for dusting on weeping eruptive sores between parts which approximate to one another, as the fingers, toes, and armpits. The powder is very inflammable, and when propelled in a hollow cone against lighted spirit of wine on tow at the other end by a sudden jerk, its flash serves to imitate lightning for stage purposes. It was formerly used as tinder for lighting fires with the flint and steel.

When the fungus is burnt, its fumes exercise a narcotic property, and will stupify bees, so that their honey may be removed. It has been suggested that these fumes may take the place of chloroform for minor surgical operations. The gas given off during combustion is carbonic oxide.

Puff Balls vary in size from that of a moderately large turnip to the bigness of a man's head. Their form is oval, depressed a little at the top, and the colour is a pure white both without and within. The surface is smooth at first, but at length cracking, and as the fungus ripens it becomes discoloured and dry; then the interior is resolved into a yellow mass of delicate threads, mixed with a powder of minute spores, about the month of September.

When young and pulpy the Puff Ball is excellent to be eaten, and is especially esteemed in Italy; but it deteriorates very rapidly after being gathered, and should not be used at table if it has become stained with yellow marks. When purely white it may be cut into thick slices of a quarter-of-an-inch, and fried in fresh butter, with pepper, salt, and pounded herbs, and each slice should be first dipped in the yolk of an egg; the Puff Ball will also make an excellent omelette. Small Puff Balls are common on lawns, heaths, and pastures. These are harmless, and eatable as long as their flesh remains quite white. The Society of Amateur Botanists, 1863, had its origin (as described by the president, Mr. M. C. Cooke), "over a cup of tea and fried Puff Balls," in Great Turnstile.

Pieces of its dried inner woolly substance, with a profusion of minute snuff-coloured spores, have been long kept by the wise old women of villages for use to staunch wounds and incisions; whilst a ready surgical appliance to a deep cut is to bind a piece of Puff Ball over it, and leave it until healing has taken place. In Norfolk large Puff Balls found at the margins of cornfields are known as Bulfers, or Bulfists, and are regarded with aversion.

In medicine a trituration (H.) is made of this fungus, and its spores, rubbed up with inert sugar of milk powdered, and it proves an effective remedy against dull, stupid, sleepy headache, with passive itchy pimples about the skin. From five to ten grains of the trituration, diluted to the third decimal strength, should be given twice a day, with a little water, for two or three weeks.

Sir B. Richardson found that even by smelling at a strong tincture of the fungus great heaviness of the head was produced; and he has successfully employed the same tincture for relieving an analogous condition when coming on of its own accord. But the Puff Ball, whether in tincture (H.) or in trituration, is chiefly of service for curing the itchy pimply skin of "tettery" subjects, especially if this is aggravated by washing. Likewise the remedy is of essential use in some forms of eczema, especially in what is known as bakers', or grocers' itch. Five drops of the diluted tincture may be given with a spoonful of water three times in the day; and the affected parts should be sponged equally often with a lotion made of one part of the stronger tincture to four parts of water, or thin strained gruel. Sometimes when a full meal of the Puff Ball fried in butter, or stewed in milk, has been taken, undoubted evidences of its narcotic effects have shown themselves.

Gerard said: "In divers parts of England, where people dwell far from neighbours, they carry the Puff Balls kindled with fire, which lasteth long." In Latin they were named *Lupi crepitum*, or Wolfs' Fists. "The powder of them is fitly applied to merigals, kibed heels, and such like; the dust or powder thereof is very dangerous for the eyes, for it hath been observed that divers have been poreblind even after when some small quantity thereof hath been blown into their eyes." This fungus has been called Molly Puff, from its resemblance to a powder puff; also Devil's Snuff Box, Fuss Balls, and Puck Fists (from *feist*, *crepitus ani*, and *Puck*, the impish king of the fairies). In Scotland the Puff Ball is the blind man's e'en, because it has been believed that its dust will cause blindness; and in Wales it is the "bag of smoke."

The Fly Agaric, or Bug Agaric (*Agaricus muscarius*) gives the name of Mushroom to all the tribe of Fungi as used for the destruction of flies (*mousches*). Albertus Magnus describes it as *Vocatus fungus muscarum eo quidem lacte pulverisatus interficit muscas*: and this seems to be the real source of the word, which has by caprice become transmitted from a poisonous sort to the wholesome kinds exclusively. The pileus of the Fly Agaric is broad, convex, and of a rich orange scarlet colour, with a striate margin and white gills. It gets its name, as also that of Flybane, from being used in milk to kill flies; and it is called Bug Agaric from having been formerly employed to smear over bedsteads so as to destroy bugs. It inhabits dry places, especially birchwoods, and pinewoods, having a bright red upper surface studded with brown warts; and when taken as a poisonous agent it causes intoxication, delirium, and death through narcotism. It is more common in Scotland than in England. This Mushroom is highly poisonous, and therefore the remedial preparations are only to be given in a diluted form. For medicinal purposes a tincture is made (H.) from the fresh fungus: and a trituration of the dried fungus powdered and mixed with inert sugar of milk also powdered. These preparations are kept specially by the homœopathic chemists: and the use of the Fly Agaric has been adopted by the school which they represent for curatively treating an irritable spinal cord, with soreness, twitching of the limbs, dragging of the legs, unsteadiness of the head, neuralgic pains in the arms and legs (as if caused by sharp ice), some giddiness, a coating of yellow fur on the lining mucous membranes, together with a crawling, or burning, and eruptive skin. In fact for a lamentably depraved condition of all the bodily health, such as characterises advanced locomotor ataxy, and allied spinal degradations leading to general physical failure. Just such a totality of symptoms has been recorded by provers after taking the fungus for some length of time in toxical quantities. The tincture should be used of the third decimal strength, five drops for a dose twice or three times a day with a spoonful of water; or the trituration of the third decimal strength, for each dose as much of the powder as will lie on the flat surface of a sixpence. Chilblains may be mitigated by taking the tincture of this Agaric, and by applying some of the stronger tincture on cotton wool over the swollen and itching parts at night.

"Muscarin" is the leading active principle of the Fly Agaric, in conjunction with agaricin, mycose, and mannite. It stimulates, when swallowed in strong doses, certain nerves which tend to retard the action of the heart. Both our Fly Agaric and the White Agaric of the United States serve to relieve the night sweats of advanced pulmonary consumption, and they have severally proved of supreme palliative use against the cough, the sleeplessness, and the other worst symptoms of this wasting disease, as also for drying up the milk in weaning. Each of these fungi when taken by mistake will salivate profusely, and provoke both immoderate, and untimely laughter. When the action of the heart is laboured and feeble through lack of nervous power, muscarin, or the tincture of Fly Agaric, in a much diluted potency will relieve this trouble. The dose of Muscarin, or Agaricin, is from a sixth to half a grain in a pill. These medicines increase the secretion of tears, saliva, bile, and sweating, but they materially lessen the quantity of urine. Belladonna is found to be the best antidote. From the Oak Agaric, "touchwood," or "spunk,"—when cut into thin slices and beaten with a hammer until soft,—is made "Amadou," or German tinder. This is then soaked in a solution of nitre and dried; it afterwards forms an excellent elastic astringent application for staying bleedings and for bed sores. The Larch Agaric is powdered, and given in Germany as a purgative, its dose being from twenty to sixty grains.

In Belgium the *Polyporus Officinalis* is used medicinally

as an aperient, and to check profuse sweating. By the Malays the *Polyporus Sanguineus* is used outwardly for leprosy.

Truffles (*Tuber cibarium*) may receive a passing notice whilst treating of fungi, though they are really subterranean tubers of an edible sort found in the earth, especially beneath beech trees, and uprooted by dogs trained for the purpose. They somewhat resemble our English "earth nuts," which swine discover by their scent. The ancients called the Truffle *lycoperdon*, because supposing it to spring from the dung of wolves. In Athens the children of Cherips had the rights of citizenship granted them because their father had invented a choice ragout concocted of Truffles. But delicate and weak stomachs find them difficult to digest. Pliny said, "Those kinds which remain hard after cooking are injurious; whilst others, naturally harmful if they admit of being cooked thoroughly well, and if eaten with saltpetre, or, still better, dressed with meat, or with pear stalks, are safe and innocent.

In Italy these tubers are fried in oil and dusted with pepper. For epicures they are mixed with the liver of fattened geese in *paté de foie gras.* Also, greedy swine are taught to discover and root them out, "being of a chestnut colour and heavy rank hercline smell, and found not seldom in England." Black Truffles are chiefly used: but there are also red and white varieties, the best tubers being light of weight in proportion to their size, with an agreeable odour, and elastic to the touch.

They are stimulating and heating, insomuch, that for delicate children who are atrophied, and require a *multum in parvo* of fatty and nitrogenous food in a compact but light form, which is fairly easy of digestion, the *paté de foie gras* on bread is a capital prescription. Truffles grow in clusters several inches below the soil, being found commonly on the downs of Wiltshire, Hampshire and Kent; also in oak and chestnut forests. Dogs have been trained to discriminate their scent below the surface of the soil, and to assist in digging them out. There is a Garlic Truffle of a small inferior sort which is put into stews; and the best Truffles are frequently found full of perforations. The presence of the tubers beneath the ground is denoted by the appearance above of a beautiful little fly having a violet colour—this insect being never seen except in the neighbourhood of Truffles. They are subject to the depredations of certain animalcules, which excavate the tubers so that they soon become riddled with worms. These, after passing through a chrysalis state, develop into the violet flies. Gerard called Truffles "Spanish fussebals." They were not known to English epicures in Queen Elizabeth's day. Another appellation borne by them formerly was "Swines' bread," and they were supposed to be engendered by thunderbolts. In Northern France they were first popularised four hundred and fifty years ago, by John, Duke of Berry, a reprobate gambler, third son of John the Good. The Perigord Truffle has a dark skin, and smells of violets. Piedmontese truffles suggest garlic: those of Burgundy are a little resinous: the Neapolitan specimens are redolent of sulphur: and in the Gard Department (France) they have an odour of musk. The English truffle is white, and best used in salads. Dr. Warton, Poet Laureate, 1750, said "Happy the grotto'ed hermit with his pulse, who wants no truffles." A Girton girl under examination described the tuber as a "sort of sea-anemone on land." When once dug up truffles soon lose their perfume and aroma, so they are imported bedded in the very earth which produced them.

The Earth Nut (*Bunium flexuosum*) is also called Hog Nut, Pig Nut, Jur Nut, St. Anthony's Nut, Earth Chesnut, and Kipper Nut. Caliban says, in the *Tempest*, "I with my long nails will dig thee Pig Nuts." They are an excellent diuretic, serving to stimulate the kidneys.

Pliny talked of fungi in general as a great delicacy to be eaten with amber knives and a service of silver. But Seneca called them *voluptuaria venena.* The Russians take some which we think to be deleterious; but they first soak these in vinegar, which (adds Pliny), "being contrary to them neutralizes their dangerous qualities; also they are rendered still more safe if cooked with pear stalks; indeed it is good to eat pears immediately after all fungi." Almost every species except the common Mushroom is characterized by the majority of our countrymen as a toadstool; but this title really appertains to the large group bearing the subgeneric name of *Tricholoma*, which probably does not contain a single unwholesome species. Other rustic names given to this group are "Puckstools" and "Puckfists." They are further known as "Toad skeps" (toad's cap) in the Eastern counties.

Puck, the mischievous king of the fairies, has been commonly identified with *pogge*, the toad, which was believed to sit upon most of the unwholesome fungi; and the *Champignon* (or Paddock Stool) was said to owe its growth to "those wanton elves whose pastime is to make midnight mushrooms." One of the "toad stools" (the *Clathrus cancellatus*) is said to produce cancerous sores if handled too freely. It has an abominably disgusting odour, and is therefore named the "lattice stinkhorn." The toad was popularly thought to impersonate the devil; and the toad-stool, pixie stool, or paddock stool was believed to spring from the devil's droppings.

The word Mushroom may have been derived from the French *Moucheron*, or *Mousseron*, because of its growing among moss. The chief chemical constituents of wholesome Mushrooms are albuminoids, carbo-hydrates, fat, mineral matters, and water. When salted they yield what is known as catsup, or ketchup (from the Japanese *kitchap*). The second most edible fungus of this nature is the Parasol Mushroom (*Lepcota procera*).

Edible Mushrooms, if kept uncooked, become dangerous: they cannot be sent to table too soon. In Rome our favourite *Pratiola* is held in very small esteem, and the worst wish an Italian can express against his foe is "that he may die of a *Pratiola*." If this species were exposed for sale in the Roman markets it would be certainly condemned by the inspector of fungi.

Fairy rings are produced by the spawn, or *mycelium*, beginning to germinate where dropped by a bird or a beast, and exhausting the soil of carbon, nitrogen, phosphorus and potash, from the centre continuously outwards; whilst immediately within the enlarging ring there is constantly a band of coarse rank grass fed by the manure of the penultimate dead spawn. The innermost starved ground remains poor and barren. In this duplicate way the rings grow larger and larger.

Our edible Mushroom is a *Pratella* of the subgenus *Psalliota*, and the *Agaricus campestris* of English botanists. In common with the esculent Mushrooms of France it contains phosphate of potassium—a cell salt essentially reparative of exhausted nerve tissue and energy.

The old practice of testing Mushrooms with a silver

spoon, which is supposed to become tarnished only when the juices are of an injurious quality (*i.e.*, when sulphur is developed therein under decomposition) is not to be trusted. In cases of poisoning by injurious fungi after the most violent symptoms may have been relieved, and the patient rescued from immediate danger, yet great emaciation will often follow from the subsequent effects of the poison: and the skin may exhibit an abundant outbreak of a vesicular eruption, whilst the health will remain perhaps permanently injured. Strong alcoholic drinks should never be taken together with, or immediately after eating Mushrooms, or other innocent fungi. Experienced fungus eaters (mycophagists) have found themselves suffering from severe pains, and some swellings through taking whiskey and water shortly after the meal: whereas precisely the same fungus, minus the whiskey, could be eaten with impunity by these identical experimentalists.

MUSTARD.

THE wild Mustard (*Brassica Sinapistrum*), a Cruciferous herb commonly called Chedlock, from *leac*, a weed, and *kiede*, to annoy, grows abundantly as a product of waste places, and in newly disturbed ground.

The Field Mustard (*Arvensis*) is Charlock, or Brassock; its botanical term, *Sinapis*, being referable to the Celtic *nap*, as a general name for plants of the rape kind. Mustard was formerly known as "senvie" in English. It has been long cultivated and improved, especially in Durham.

Now we have for commercial and officinal purposes two varieties of the cultivated plant, the black Mustard (*Sinapis nigra*), and the white Mustard (*Brassica*, or *Sinapis alba*). There is also a plain plant of the hedges,

Hedge Mustard (*Sisymbrium officinale*) which is a mere rustic Simple.

It is the black Mustard which yields by its seeds the condiment of our tables, and the pungent yellow flour which we employ for the familiar stimulating poultice, or sinapism. This black Mustard is a tall smooth plant, having entire leaves, and smooth seed pods, being now grown for the market on rich alluvial soil chiefly in Lincolnshire and Yorkshire. In common with its kindred plants it gets its name from *mustum*, the "must," or newly fermented grape juice, and *ardens*, burning, because as a condiment, Mustard flour was formerly mixed with home-made wine and sugar. The virtues of black Mustard depend on the acrid volatile oil contained in its seeds. These when unbruised and macerated in boiling water yield only a tasteless mucilage which resides in their skin. But when bruised they develop a very active, pungent, and highly stimulative principle with a powerful penetrating odour which makes the eyes water. From thence is perhaps derived the generic name of the herb *Sinapis* (*Para tou sinesthai tous hopous*, "because it irritates the eyes"). This active principle contains sulphur abundantly, as is proved by the discoloration of a silver spoon when left in the mustard-pot, the black sulphuret of silver being formed. The chemical basis of black Mustard is "sinnigrin" and its acid myronic. The acridity of its oil is modified in the seeds by combination with another fixed oil of a bland nature which can be readily separated by pressure, then the cake left after the expression of this fixed oil is far more pungent than the seeds. The bland oil expressed from the hulls of the black seeds after the flour has been sifted away, promotes the growth of the hair, and may be used with benefit externally for rheumatism. Whitehead's noted Essence of Mustard is made with spirits of turpentine and rosemary, with which camphor and the farina of black Mustard seed are mixed. This oil is very little affected by frost or the atmosphere ; and it is therefore specially prized by clock makers, and for instruments of precision.

A Mustard poultice from the farina of black Mustard made into a paste with, or without wheaten flour commingled, constitutes one of the most powerful external stimulating applications we can employ. It quickly induces a sharp burning pain, and it excites a destructive outward inflammation which enters much more into the true skin than that which is caused by an old fashioned blister of Spanish fly. This has therefore superseded the latter as more promptly and reliably effective for the speedy relief of all active internal congestions. If the application of Mustard has caused sores, these may be best soothed and healed by lime-water liniment.

Mustard flour is an infallible antiseptic and sterilising agent. It is a capital deodoriser; and if rubbed thoroughly into the hands and nails will take away all offensive stink when corrupt or dead tissues have been manipulated.

If a tablespoonful of Mustard flour is added to a pint of tepid water, and taken at a draught it operates briskly as a stimulating and sure emetic. Hot water poured on bruised seeds of black Mustard makes a good stimulating footbath for helping to throw off a cold, or to dispel a headache ; and meantime the volatile oil given out as an aroma, if not too strong, proves soporific. This oil contains erucic, and sinapoleic acids. When properly mixed with spirit of wine, twenty-four drops of the oil to an ounce of spirit, the essential oil forms, by reason of its stimulating properties and its contained sulphur, a capital liniment for use in rheumatism, or for determining blood to the surface from deeper parts. Caution should be used not to apply a plaster made altogether of Mustard flour to the delicate skin of young children, or females, because ulcers difficult to heal may be the result, or even gangrenous destruction of the deeper skin may follow. The effects of a Mustard bath, at about ninety degrees, are singular ; decided chills are felt at first throughout the whole body, with some twitchings at times of the limbs ; and later on, even after the skin surface has become generally red, this sense of coldness persists, until the person leaves the water, when reaction becomes quickly established, with a glowing heat and redness of the whole skin.

For obstinate hiccough a teacupful of boiling water should be poured on a teaspoonful of Mustard flour, and taken when sufficiently cool, half at first, and the other half in ten minutes if still needed. For congestive headache a small roll of Mustard paper or Mustard leaf may be introduced into one or both nostrils, and left there for a minute or more. It will relieve the headache promptly, and may perhaps induce some nose bleeding.

Admixture with vinegar checks the development of the pungent principles of Mustard. This used to be practised for the table in England, but is now discontinued, though some housewives add a little salt to their made Mustard.

Claims for the introduction of Mustard at Durham in 1720, have been raised in favour of a Mrs. Clements, but they cannot be substantiated. Shakespeare in the *Taming of the Shrew* makes Grumio ask Katherine "What say you to a piece of beef and Mustard?" and speaks, in *Henry IV.*, of Poins' wit being "as thick as Tewkesbury Mustard"; whilst Fuller in his *Worthies of England*, written only a very few years after Shakespeare's death, says "the best Mustard in England is made at Tewkesbury in the county of Gloucester." Coles observes (1657), "in Gloucestershire about Teuxbury they grind Mustard seed and make it up into balls, which are brought to London and other remote places as being the best that the world affords." George the First restored the popularity of Mustard by his approval of it. Prior to 1720 no such condiment as Mustard in its present form was used at table in this country. It is not improbable that the Romans, who were great eaters of Mustard-seed pounded and steeped in new wine, brought the condiment with them to our shores, and taught the ancient Britons how to prepare it. At Dijon in France where the best mixed continental Mustard is made, the condiment is seasoned with various spices and savouries, such as Anchovies, Capers, Tarragon, Catsup of Walnuts, or Mushrooms, and the liquors of other pickles. Philip the Bold granted armorial ensigns (1382) to Dijon, with the motto *moult me tarde* (I wish for ardently). The merchants of Sinapi copied this on their wares, the middle word of the motto being accidentally effaced. A well-known couplet of lines supposed to occur in *Hudibras* (but not to be found there), has long baffled the research of quotation hunters:

> "Sympathy without relief
> Is like to Mustard without beef."

Mustard flour moistened with a little water into a paste has the singular property of dispelling the odours of musk, camphor, and the fetid gum resins. For deodorising vessels which have contained the essences of turpentine, creasote, assafetida, or other such drugs, it will answer to introduce some bruised Mustard seed, and then a little water, shaking the vessel well for a minute or more, and afterwards rinsing it out with plenty of water.

The white Mustard grows when uncultivated on waste ground with large yellow flowers, and does not yield under any circumstances a pungent oil like the black Mustard. It is a hirsute plant, with stalked leaves and hairy seed pods ; and when produced in our gardens its young leaves are eaten as a salad, or as "Mustard, with Cress."

"When in the leaf," says John Evelyn in his *Acetaria*, "Mustard, especially in young seedling plants, is of incomparable effect to quicken and revive the spirits, strengthening the memory, expelling heaviness, preventing the vertiginous palsy, and a laudable cephalic, besides being an approved antiscorbutic." He tells further that the Italians, in making Mustard as a condiment, mingle lemon and orange peel with the (black) seeds. "In the composition of a sallet the Mustard (a noble ingredient) should be of the best Tewkesbury or else of the soundest and weightiest Yorkshire seed, tempered a little by the fire to the consistence of a pap with vinegar, in which some shavings of the horse-radish have been steeped. Then, cutting an onion, and putting it into a small earthen gally-pot, pour the Mustard over it and close it very well with a cork. *Note.*—The seeds should have been pounded in a mortar, or bruised with a polished cannon bullet in a large wooden bowl dish."

The active principle of white Mustard is "Sinapin," and the seed germinates so rapidly that it has been said a salad of this may be grown while the joint of meat is being roasted for dinner. Seeds of the white Mustard have been employed medicinally from early times.

Hippocrates advised their use both internally, and as a counter-irritating poultice made with vinegar. When swallowed whole in teaspoonful doses three or four times a day, they exercise a laxative effect mechanically, and are voided without undergoing any perceptible change, only the outer skin being a little softened and mucilaginous. An infusion of the seed taken medicinally will relieve chronic bronchitis, and confirmed rheumatism: also for a relaxed sore throat a gargle of Mustard seed tea will be found of service.

A French expression for trifling one's time away is *s'amuser à la moutarde.* The essential oil is an admirable deodorant and disinfectant, especially on an emergency.

But the "grain of Mustard seed, the smallest of all seeds" (*Mark* iv., 31), "which when it is grown up is the greatest among herbs," was a tree of the East, very different from our Mustard, and bearing branches of real wood.

The Hedge Mustard (*Sisymbrium,* or *Erisymum*) grows by our roadsides, and on waste grounds, where it seems to possess a peculiar aptitude for collecting and retaining dust. The pods are downy, close pressed to the stem, and the leaves hairy with their points turned backwards. It is named by the French "St. Barbara's Hedge Mustard," and the Singer's Plant, "*herbe au chantre,*" or "*herbe au chanteur.*" Up to the time of Louis XIV. it was considered an infallible remedy for loss of the voice. Racine writing to Boileau recommended the syrup of *Erysimum* to him when visiting the waters of Bourbonne in order to be cured of voicelessness. "Si les eaux de Bourbonne ne vous guerissent pas de votre extinction de voix, le sirop d'Erysimum vous guerirait infalliblement. Ne l'oubliez pas, et ā l'occasion vingt grammes par litre d'eau en tisane matin et soir." It used to be called Flix, or Flux weed from being given with benefit in dysentery, a disease formerly known as the Flix. This herb has been commended for chronic coughs and hoarseness, using the juice mixed with an equal quantity of honey, or sugar. It has been designated "the most excellent of all remedies for diseases of the throat, especially in ulcerated sore throats, which it will serve to cure when all the advice of physicians and surgeons has proved ineffectual." A strong infusion of the herb is excellent in asthmas, and it may be made with sugar into a syrup which will keep all the year round. The Hedge Mustard contains chemically a soft resin, and a sulphuretted volatile oil. This herb with the vervain is supposed to form Count Mattæi's noted nostrum *Febrifugo*.

NETTLE.

No plant is more commonplace and plentiful in our fields and hedges throughout an English summer than the familiar stinging Nettle. And yet most persons unknowingly include under this single appellation several distinct herbs. Actually as Nettles are to be found: the annual *Urtica dioica*, or true Stinging Nettle; the perennial *Urtica urens* (burning); the White Dead Nettle; the Archangel, or Yellow Weasel Snout, and the Purple Hedge Nettle. This title "Urtica" comes *ab urendo*, "from burning."

The plant which stings has a round hairy stalk, and carries only a dull colourless bloom, whereas the others are labiate herbs with square stems, and conspicuous lipped flowers. As Simples only the great Stinging Nettle, the lesser Stinging Nettle, and the white Dead Nettle call for observation. Also another variety of our Stinging Nettle is the *Urtica pilulifera*, called by corruption the Roman Nettle, really because found abundantly at Romney in Kent. But a legend obtains belief with some that Roman soldiers first brought with them to England the seeds of this plant, and sowed it about for their personal uses. They heard before coming that the climate here was so cold that it might not be endured without some friction to warm the blood, and to stir up the natural heat; and they therefore bethought them to provide Nettles wherewith to chafe their limbs when "stiffe and much benummed." Or, again, Lyte says, "They do call al such strange herbes as be unknown of the common people Romish, or Romayne herbes, although the same be brought direct from Sweden or Norweigh." The cure for Nettle stings has been from early times to rub the part with a dock leaf. The dead Nettles are so named as having no sting, but possessing nettle-like leaves. The stinging effect of the true Nettle is caused by an acrid secretion contained in minute vesicles at the base of each of the stiff hairs; and *urtication*, or flogging with Nettles, is an old external remedy, which was long practised for chronic rheumatism, and loss of muscular power. *Tacta quod exurat digitos urtica tenentis.*—Macer. Tea made from the young tops is a Devonshire cure for Nettle-rash. Gerard says, "the Nettle is a good medicine for them that cannot breathe unless they hold their necks upright: and being eaten boiled with periwinkles it makes the body soluble."

The word Nettle is derived from *net*, meaning something spun, or sewn; and it indicates the thread made from the hairs of the plant, and formerly used among Scandinavian nations. This was likewise employed by Scotch weavers in the seventeenth century. Westmacott, the historian, says, "Scotch cloth is only the housewifery of the Nettle." And the poet Campbell writes in one of his letters, "I have slept in Nettle sheets, and dined off a Nettle table cloth: and I have heard my mother say she thought Nettle cloth more durable than any other linen." Goldsmith has recorded the "rubbing of a cock's heart with stinging Nettles to make it hatch hen's eggs." Some think the word "Nettle" an alteration of the Anglo-Saxon "Needl," with reference to the needle-like stings. Spun silk is now made in England from "Ramie" the decorticated fibre of Nettles after washing away the glutinous juice from under their bark.

The seeds (*dioica*) contain a fine oil, and powerfully stimulate the sexual functions.

In Russia, as a recent mode of treatment, *urtication* is now enthusiastically commended, that is, slapping, or pricking with a bundle of fresh Nettle twigs for one or more minutes, once, or several times in the day. It is a superlative method of cure because harmless (neither irritating the kidneys nor disfiguring the skin), cleanly, simple in application, rapid in its effects, and cheap, though perhaps somewhat rude.

For sciatica, for incipient wasting, for the difficult breathing of some heart troubles (where such stimulation along the backbone affords more prompt and complete relief than any other treatment), for some coughs palsy, suppression of the monthly flow in women, rheumatism, and for lack of muscular energy, this *urtication* is said to be an invaluable resuscitating measure which has been successfully resorted to by the peasantry of Russia from time immemorial. It will sometimes produce a crop of small harmless blisters.

The analysis of the fresh Nettle shows a presence of formic acid (the irritating principle of the stinging hairs), with mucilage, salts, ammonia, carbonic acid, and water. A strong decoction of Nettles drunk too freely by mistake has produced severe burning over the whole body, with general redness, and a sense of being stung. The features became swollen, and minute vesicles appeared on the skin, which burst, and discharged a limpid fluid. No fever accompanied the attack, and after five or six days the eruption dried up. A medicinal tincture (H.) is made from the entire plant with spirit of wine: and this, as taught by the principle of similars, may be confidently given in small diluted doses to mitigate such a totality of symptoms as now described, whether coming on as an attack of severe Nettle rash, or assuming some more pronounced eruptive aspect, such as chicken pox. The same tincture also acts admirably in cases of burns, when the deep skin is not destructively involved. And again for relieving the itching of the fundament caused by the presence of threadworms.

"Burns," says Lucomsky, "may be rapidly cured by applying over them linen cloths well wetted with an alcoholic tincture of the Stinging Nettle prepared from the fresh plant, this being diluted with an equal, or a double quantity of cold water. The cloths should be frequently re-wetted, but without removing them, so as to prevent pain from exposure." Dr. Burnett has shown conclusively that Nettle tea, and Nettle tincture (ten drops for a dose in water), are curative of feverish gout, as well as of intermittent fever and ague. Either remedy will promote a speedy extrication of gravel through the kidneys. Again the Nettle was a favourite old English remedy for consumption, as already mentioned (see *Mugwort*), with reference to the mermaid of the Clyde, when she beheld with regret the untimely funeral of a young Glasgow maiden.

Fresh Nettle juice given in doses of from one to two tablespoonfuls is a most serviceable remedy for all sorts of bleeding, whether from the nose, the lungs, or some internal organ. Also the decoction of the leaves and stalks taken in moderate quantities is capital for many of the minor skin maladies.

An alcoholic extract is made officinally from the entire young plant gathered in the spring, and some of this if applied on cotton wool will arrest bleeding from the nose, or after the extraction of a tooth, when persistent. If a leaf of the plant be put upon the tongue and pressed against the roof of the mouth, it will stop a bleeding from the nose. Taken as a fresh young vegetable in the spring, or early summer, Nettle tops make a very wholesome and succulent dish of greens, which is slightly laxative; but during Autumn they are hurtful. In Italy where herb soups are in high favour, "herb knodel" (or round balls made like a dumpling in size and consistency) of Nettles are esteemed as nourishing and medicinal. The greater Nettle (*Urtica dioica*), and the lesser Nettle (*Urtica urens*) possess stinging properties in common.

A crystalline alkaloid which is fatal to frogs in a dose of one centigramme, has been isolated from the common Stinging Nettle. The watery extract has but little effect on mammals: but in the frog it causes paralysis, beginning in the great nervous centres and finally stopping the action of the heart. If planted in the neighbourhood of beehives, the Nettle will serve to drive away frogs.

The expressed seeds yield an oil which may be used for burning in lamps. Nettle leaves, rubbed into wooden vessels, such as tubs, &c., will prevent their leaking. The juice of the leaves coagulates, and fills up the interstices of the wood. When dried the leaves will often relieve asthma and similar bronchial troubles by inhalation, although other means have failed. Eight or ten grains should be burnt, and the fumes inspired at bedtime.

The *Lamium album* (white dead Nettle), a labiate plant, though not of the stinging Nettle order, is likewise of special use for arresting hæmorrhage, as in spitting of blood, dysentery, and female fluxes. Its name *Lamium* is got from the Greek *laimos*, the throat, because of the shape of its corollæ. If the plant be macerated in alcohol for a week, then cotton wool dipped in the liquid is as efficacious for staying bleeding, when applied to the spot, as the strongly astringent muriate of iron. Also, a tincture of the flowers is made (H.) for internal use in similar cases. From five to ten drops of this tincture should be given for a dose with a tablespoonful of cold water. The Red Nettle, another *Lamium*, is also called Archangel, because it blossoms on St. Michael's day, May 8th. If made into a tea and sweetened with honey, it promotes perspiration, and acts on the kidneys. The white dead Nettle is a degenerate form of this purple herb as shown by still possessing on its petals the same brown markings. Nevertheless, having disobeyed the laws of its growth, it has lost its original colour, and, like the Lady of Shalott, it is fain to complain "the curse has come upon me." Count Mattæi's nostrum *Pettorale* is thought to be got from the *Galeopsis* (hemp Nettle), another of the labiate herbs, with Nettle-like leaves, but no stinging hairs, named from *galee*, a cat, or weazel, and *opsis*, a countenance, because supposed to have a blossom resembling the face of the animal specified.

NIGHT SHADE, DEADLY (*Belladonna*).

THIS is a Solanaceous plant found native in Great Britain, and growing generally on chalky soil under hedges, or about waste grounds. It bears the botanical name of *Atropa*, being so called from one of the classic Fates,—she who held the shears to cut the thread of human life:—

"Clotho velum retinet, Lachesis net, et atropos occit."

Its second title, *Belladonna*, was bestowed because the Spanish ladies made use of the plant to dilate the pupils of their brilliant black eyes. In this way their orbs appeared more attractively lustrous: and the *donna* became *bella* (beautiful). The plant is distinguished by a large leaf growing beside a small one about its stems, whilst the solitary flowers, which droop, have a dark full purple border, being paler downwards, and without scent. The berries (in size like small cherries) are of a rich purplish black hue, and possess most dangerously narcotic properties. They are medicinally useful, but so deadly that only the skilled hands of the apothecary should attempt to manipulate them; and they should not be prescribed for a patient except by the competent physician. When taken by accident their mischievous effects may be prevented by swallowing as soon as possible a large glass of warm vinegar.

A tincture of allied berries was used of old by ladies of fashion in the land of the Pharaohs, as discovered among the mummy graves by Professor Baeyer, of Munich. This had the property of imparting a verdant sheen to the human iris; and, perhaps by the quaint colour-effect it produced on the transparent cornea of some wily Egyptian belle, it gave rise to the saying, "Do you see any green in the white of my eye?"

At one time *Belladonna* leaves were held to be curative of cancer when applied externally as a poultice, either fresh, or dried, and powdered. It is remarkable that sheep, rabbits, goats, and swine can eat these leaves with impunity, though (as Boerhaave tells) a single berry has been known to prove fatal to the human subject; and a gardener was once hanged for neglecting to remove plants of the deadly Night Shade from certain grounds which he knew. A peculiar symptom in those poisoned by *Belladonna* berries is the complete loss of voice, together with frequent bending forward of the trunk, and continual movements of the hands and fingers. The Scotch under Macbeth sent bread and wine treacherously impregnated with this poison to the troops of Sweno.

The plant bears other titles, as "Dwale" (death's herb), "Great Morel," and "Naughty Man's Cherry." The term "Morel" is applied to the plant as a diminutive of *mora*, a Moor, on account of the black-skinned berries. The *Belladonna* grows especially near the ruins of monasteries, and is so abundant around Furness Abbey that this locality has been styled the "Vale of Night Shade."

Hahnemann taught that, acting on the law of similars, *Belladonna* given in very small doses of its tincture will protect from the infection of scarlet fever. He confirmed this fact by experiments on one hundred and sixty children. When taken by provers in actual toxic doses the tincture, or the fresh juice, has induced sore throat, feverishness, and a dry, red, hot skin, just as if symptomatic of scarlet fever. The plant yields atropine and hyoscyamine from all its parts. As a drug it specially affects the brain and the bladder. The berries are known in Buckinghamshire as "Devil's cherries."

NUTMEG, CINNAMON, GINGER, and CLOVES.

THE spice box is such a constant source of ready domestic comforts of a medicinal sort in every household that the more important, and best known of its contents may well receive some consideration when treating of Herbal Simples; though it will, of course, be understood these spices are of foreign growth, and not indigenous products.

Cinnamon, Nutmeg, Ginger, and Cloves, claim particular notice in this respect.

> "Sinament, Ginger, Nutmeg, and Cloves,
> And that gave me my jolly red nose."
>
> *Beaumont and Fletcher.*

Cinnamon possesses positive medicinal as well as aromatic virtues. What we employ as this spice consists of the inner bark of shoots from the stocks of a Ceylon tree, first cultivated here in 1768.

Such bark chemically contains cinnamic acid, tannin, a resin, and sugar, so that its continued use will induce constipation. The aromatic and stimulating effects of Cinnamon have been long known. It was freely given in England during the epidemic scourges of the early and middle centuries, nearly every monastery keeping a store of the cordial for ready use. The monks administered it in fever, dysentery, and contagious diseases. And recent discovery in the laboratory of M. Pasteur, the noted French bacteriologist, has shown that Cinnamon possesses the power of absolutely destroying all disease germs. Our ancestors, it would appear, had hit upon a valuable preservative against microbes, when they infused Cinnamon with other spices in their mulled drinks. Mr. Chamberland says, "no disease germ can long resist the antiseptic powder of essence of Cinnamon, which is as effective to destroy microbes as corrosive sublimate."

By its warming astringency, it exercises cordial properties which are most useful in arresting passive diarrhœa, and in relieving flatulent indigestion.

Its volatile oil is procured from the bark, and likewise a tincture, as well as an aromatic water of Cinnamon. For a sick qualmish stomach either preparation is an excellent remedy, as the virtue of the bark rests in this essential volatile oil. When obtained from the *fruit* it is extremely fragrant, of thick consistence, and sometimes made into candles at Ceylon, for the sole use of the king. The doses are of the powdered bark from ten to twenty grains; of the oil from one to five drops; of the tincture from half to one teaspoonful, and of the distilled water from one to two tablespoonfuls. Our Queen is known to be partial to the use of Cinnamon. Keats, the poet, wrote of "lucent syrups tinct. with Cinnamon." And Saint Francis of Sales says in his *Devout Life*: "With respect to the labour of teaching, it refreshes and revives the heart by the sweetness it brings to those who are engaged in it, as the Cinnamon does in *Arabia Felix* to them who are laden with it." In toxic quantities of an injurious amount, Cinnamon bark has produced hæmorrhage from the bowels, and nose bleeding. Therefore small doses of the diluted tincture are well calculated to obviate these symptoms when presenting themselves through illness.

The bark was formerly thought to stimulate the functions of the womb, and of late it has come again into medical use for this purpose. To check fluxes from that organ, a teaspoonful of the bruised bark should be infused in half a pint of boiling water, and a tablespoonful given frequently when cool. Lozenges made with the essential oil are also medicinally available for the speedy relief of sickness, and as highly useful against influenza. It is well known that persons who live in Cinnamon districts have an immunity from malaria.

Ginger (*Zingiberis radix*) is the root-stock of a plant grown in the East and West Indies, and is scraped before importation. Its odour is due to an essential oil, and its pungent hot taste to a resin. It was known in Queen Elizabeth's reign, having been introduced by the Dutch about 1566. "Grene Gynger of almondes" is mentioned in the Paston Letters, 1444. "When condited," says Gerard, "it provoketh veneric."

This Green Ginger, which consists of the young shoots of the *rhizome*, when boiled in syrup makes an excellent preserve. Officinally from the dried and scraped rhizome are prepared a tincture, and a syrup. If a piece of the root is chewed it causes a considerable flow of saliva, and an application of powdered Ginger, made with water into paste, against the skin will produce intense tingling and heat. To which end it may be spread on paper and applied to the forehead as a means for relieving a headache from passive fulness. In India, Europeans who suffer from languid indigestion drink an infusion of Ginger as a substitute for tea. For gouty dyspepsia the root may be powdered in a mortar: and a heaped teaspoonful of it should be then infused in boiling milk; to be taken when sufficiently cool, for supper or at breakfast.

The dose of the powder is from ten to twenty grains; of the tincture from a third of a teaspoonful to a teaspoonful, in water hot or cold; of the syrup from one to two teaspoonfuls in water. Either preparation is of service to correct diarrhœa, and to relieve weakly chronic bronchitis. Also as admirably corrective of chronic constipation through general intestinal sluggish ness, a vespertine slice of good, old-fashioned Ginger-bread made with brown treacle and grated ginger may be eaten with zest, and reliance. There is a street in Hull called "The land of Ginger."

The habitat of the tree from which our Nutmeg comes is the Molucca Islands, and the part of the nut which constitutes the Spice is the kernel. This is called generically *Nux moschata*, or Mugget (French *Musqué*) a diminutive of musk, from its aromatic odour, and properties. The Nutmeg is oval, or nearly round, of a brown wrinkled aspect, with an aromatic smell, and a bitter fragrant taste. Officinally the tree is named *Myristica officinalis*, and the oil distilled from the Nutmeg in Britain is much superior to foreign oil.

Ordinarily as a condiment of a warming character the Nutmeg is employed to correct cold indigestible food, or as a cordial addition to negus: and medicinally for languid digestion, with giddiness and flatulence, causing oppressed breathing. Its activity depends on the volatile oil, contained in the proportion of six per cent. in the nut. This when given at all largely is essentially narcotic. Four Nutmegs have been known to completely paralyse all nervous sensibility, and have produced a sort of wakeful unconsciousness for three entire days, with loss of memory afterwards, and with more or less paralysis until after eight days.

The Banda, or Nutmeg Islands in the Indian Ocean, are twelve in number, and the strength of the Nutmeg in its season is said to overcome birds of Paradise so that they fall helplessly intoxicated.

When taken to any excess, whether as a spice, or as a medicine, the Nutmeg and its preparations are apt to cause giddiness, oppression of the chest, stupor, and delirium. A moderate dose of the powdered Nutmeg is from five to twenty grains, but persons with a tendency to apoplexy should abstain from any free use of this spice. From two to six drops of the essential oil may be taken on sugar to relieve flatulent oppression and dyspepsia, or from half to one teaspoonful of the spirit of Nutmeg made by mixing one part of the oil with forty parts of spirit of wine; this dose being had with one or two tablespoonfuls of hot water, sweetened if desired.

A medicinal tincture is prepared (H.) from the kernel with spirit of wine (not using the oil, nor the essence). This in small diluted doses is highly useful for drowsiness connected with flatulent indigestion, and a disposition to faintness: also for gout retrocedent to the stomach. The dose is from five to ten drops with a spoonful of water every half hour, or every hour until the symptoms are adequately relieved. Against diarrhœa Nutmeg grated into warm water is very helpful, and will prove an efficient substitute for opium in mild cases. Externally the spirit of Nutmeg is a capital application to be rubbed in for chronic rheumatism, and for paralysed limbs. The "butter of Nutmegs," or their concrete oil, is used in making plasters of a warming, and stimulating kind. A drink that was concocted by our grandmothers was Nutmeg tea. One Nutmeg would make a pint of this tea, two or three cupfuls of which would produce a sleep of many hours' duration. The worthy old ladies were wont to carry a silver grater and Nutmeg case suspended from the waist on their chatelaines. But in any large quantity the Nutmeg may produce sleep of such a profundity as to prove really dangerous. Two drachms of the powder have brought on a comatose sleep with some delirium.

The Nutmeg contains starch, protein, and other simple constituents, in addition to its stimulating principles. Mace is the aromatic envelope of the Nutmeg, and possesses the same qualities in a minor degree. Its infusion is a good warming medicine against chronic cough, and moist bronchial asthma in an old person. Mace is a membranaceous structure enveloping the Nutmeg, having a fleshy texture, and being of a light yellowish-brown colour. It supplies an allied essential volatile principle, which is fragrant and cordial. If given three or four times during the twenty-four hours, in a dose of from eight to twelve grains, crushed, or powdered Mace will prove serviceable against long-continued looseness of the bowels; but this dose should not be exceeded for fear of inducing narcotism.

Cloves (from *clavus*, a nail), also found in the kitchen spice box, and owning certain medicinal resources of a cordial sort, which are quickly available, belong to the Myrtle family of plants, and are the unexpanded flower buds of an aromatic tree (*Caryophyllus*), cultivated at Penang and elsewhere. They contain a volatile oil which, like that of Chamomile, although cordial, lowers nervous sensibility, or irritability: also tannin, a gum resin, and woody fibre. This volatile oil consists principally of "eugenin" with a camphor, "caryophyllin." The "eugenic acid," with a strong odour of cloves, is powerfully antiseptic and anti-putrescent. It reduces the sensibility of the skin: and therefore the oil with lanolin is a useful application for eczema.

Dr Burnett has lately taught (1895) that a too free use of Cloves will bring on albuminuria; and that when this disease has supervened from other causes, the dilute tincture of Cloves, third decimal strength, will frequently do much to lessen the quantity of albumen excreted by the kidneys. From five to ten drops of this tincture should be given with water three times a day.

Used in small quantities as a spice the Clove stimulates digestion, but when taken more freely it deadens the susceptibility of the stomach, lessens the appetite, and induces constipation. An infusion of Cloves, made with half an ounce to a pint of water, and drank in doses of a small wineglassful, will relieve the nausea and coldness of flatulent indigestion. The oil put on cotton wool into the hollow of a decayed tooth is a useful means for giving ease to toothache. The dose of the oil is from one to five drops, on sugar, or in a spoonful of milk. The odour of Cloves is aromatic, and the taste pleasantly hot, but acrid. Half a tumbler of quite hot water poured over half a dozen Cloves (which are to brew for a few minutes on the hob, and then to be taken out), will often secure a good night to a restless dyspeptic patient, if taken just before getting into bed. Or if given cold before breakfast this dose will obviate constipation. In Holland the oil of Cloves is prescribed with cinchona bark for ague. Arthur Cecil's German medico in the Play advises his patient to "rub your pelly mit a Clove."

All-Spice (*Pimento*) is another common occupant of the domestic spice box. It is popular as a warming cordial, of a sweet odour, and a grateful aromatic taste; but being a native of South America, grows with us only as a stove plant. The leaves and bark are full of inflammable particles, whilst walks between Pimento trees are odorous with a delicious scent. The name All-Spice is given because the berries afford in smell and taste a combination of Cloves, Juniper berries, Cinnamon and Pepper. The special qualities of the Pimento reside in the rind of these berries; and this tree is the *Bromelia ananas*, named in Brazil *Nana*. An extract made from the crushed berries by boiling them down to a thick liquor, is, when spread on linen, a capital stimulating plaster for neuralgic or rheumatic parts. About the physician in "les Francais" it was said admiringly "c'est lui qui a inventé la salade d'Ananas." The essential oil, as well as the spirit and the distilled water of Pimento, are useful against flatulent indigestion and for hysterical paroxysms. This Spice was formerly added to our syrup of buckthorn to prevent it from griping. The berries are put into curry powder, and added to mulled wines.

OAT.

THE Oat is a native of Britain in its wild and uncultivated form, and is distinguished by the spikelets of its ears hanging on slender pedicels. This is the *Avena fatua*, found in our cornfields, but not indigenous in Scotland. When cultivated it is named *Avena sativa*. As it needs less sunshine and solar warmth to ripen the grain than wheat, it furnishes the principal grain food of cold Northern Europe. With the addition of some fat this grain is capable of supporting life for an indefinite period. Physicians formerly recommended highly a diet-drink made from Oats, about which Hoffman wrote a treatise at the end of the seventeenth century; and Johannis dé St. Catherine, who introduced the drink, lived by its use to a hundred years free from any disease. Nevertheless the Oat did not enjoy a good reputation among the old Romans; and Pliny said "Primum omnis frumenti vitium avena est."

American doctors have taken of late to extol the Oat (*Avena sativa*) when made into a strong medicinal tincture with spirit of wine, as a remarkable nervine stimulant and restorative: this being "especially valuable in all cases where there is a deficiency of nervous power, for instance, among over-worked lawyers, public speakers, and writers."

The tincture is ordered to be given in a dose of from ten to twenty drops, once or twice during the day, in hot water to act speedily; and a somewhat increased dose in cold water at bedtime so as to produce its beneficial effects more slowly then. It proves an admirable remedy for sleeplessness from nervous exhaustion, and as prepared in New York may be procured from any good druggist in England. Oatmeal contains two per cent. of protein compounds, the largest portion of which is avenin. A yeast poultice made by stirring Oatmeal into the grounds of strong beer is a capital cleansing and healing application to languid sloughing sores.

Oatmeal supplies very little saccharine matter ready formed. It cannot be made into light bread, and is therefore prepared when baked in cakes; or, its more popular form for eating is that of porridge, where the ground meal becomes thoroughly soft by boiling, and is improved in taste by the addition of milk and salt. "The halesome parritch, chief of Scotia's food," said Burns, with fervid eloquence. Scotch people actually revel in their parritch and bannocks. "We defy your wheaten bread," says one of their favourite writers, "your home-made bread, your bakers' bread, your baps, rolls, scones, muffins, crumpets, and cookies, your bath buns, and your sally luns, your tea cakes, and slim cakes, your saffron cakes, and girdle cakes, your shortbread, and singing hinnies: we swear by the Oat cake, and the parritch, the bannock, and the brose." Scotch beef brose is made by boiling Oatmeal in meat liquor, and kail brose by cooking Oatmeal in cabbage-water.

Crushed Oatmeal, from which the husk has been removed, is known as "groats," and is employed for making gruel. At the latter end of the seventeenth century this was a drink asked-for eagerly by the public at London taverns. "Grantham gruel," says quaint old Fuller, in his *History of the Worthies of England*, "consists of nine grits and a gallon of water." When "thus made, it is wash rather, which one will have little heart to eat, and yet as little heart by eating." But the better gruel concocted elsewhere was "a wholesome spoon meat, though homely; physic for the sick, and food for persons in health; grits the form thereof: and giving the being thereunto." In the border forays of the twelfth and thirteenth centuries all the provision carried by the Scotch was simply a bag of Oatmeal. But as a food it is apt to undergo some fermentation in the stomach, and to provoke sour eructations. Furthermore, it is somewhat laxative, because containing a certain proportion of bran which mechanically stimulates the intestinal membranes: and this insoluble bran is rather apt to accumulate. Oatmeal gruel may be made by boiling from one to two ounces of the meal with three pints of water down to two pints, then straining the decoction, and pouring off the supernatant liquid when cool. Its flavour may be improved by adding raisins towards the end of boiling, or by means of sugar and nutmeg. Because animals of speed use up, by the lungs, much heat-forming material, Oats (which abound in carbonaceous constituents) are specially suitable as food for the horse.

ONION (*see* Garlic, *page* 209).

ORANGE.

THOUGH not of native British growth, except by way of a luxury in the gardens of the wealthy, yet the Orange is of such common use amongst all classes of our people as a dietetic fruit, when of the sweet China sort, and for tonic medicinal purposes when of the bitter Seville kind, that some consideration may be fairly accorded to it as a Curative Simple in these pages.

The *Citrus aurantium*, or popular Orange, came originally from India, and got its distinctive title of *Aurantium*, either (*ab aureo colore corticis*) from the golden colour of its peel, or (*ab oppido Achæiæ Arantium*) from Arantium, a town of Achaia. It now comes to us chiefly from Portugal and Spain. This fruit is essentially a product of cultivation extending over many years. It began in Hindustan as a small bitter berry with seeds; then about the eighth century it was imported into Persia, though held somewhat accursed. During the tenth century it bore the name "Bigarade," and became better known. But not until the sixteenth century was it freely grown by the Spaniards, and brought into Mexico. Even at that time the legend still prevailed that whoever partook of the luscious juice was compelled to embrace the faith of the prophet. Spenser and Milton tell of the orange as the veritable golden apple presented by Jupiter to Juno on the day of their nuptials: and hence perhaps arose its more modern association with marriage rites.

Of the varieties the China Orange is the most juicy, being now grown in the South of Europe; whilst the St. Michael Orange (a descendant of the China sort, first produced in Syria), is now got abundantly from the Azores, whence it derives its name.

John Evelyn says the first China Orange which appeared in Europe, was sent as a present to the old Condé Mellor, then Prime Minister to the King of Portugal, when only one plant escaped sound and useful of the whole case which reached Lisbon, and this became the parent of all the Orange trees cultivated by our gardeners, though not without greatly degenerating.

The Seville Orange is that which contains the medicinal properties, more especially in its leaves, flowers, and fruit, though the China sort possesses the same virtues in a minor degree. The leaves and the flowers have been esteemed as beneficial against epilepsy, and other convulsive disorders ; and a tea is infused from the former for hysterical sufferers.

Two delicious perfumes are distilled from the flowers—oil of neroli, and napha water,—of which the chemical hydro-carbon "hesperidin," is mainly the active principle. This is secreted also as an aromatic attribute of the leaves through their minute glands, causing them to emit a fragrant odour when bruised. A scented water is largely prepared in France from the flowers, *l'eau de fieur d'oranger*, which is frequently taken by ladies as a gentle sedative at night, when sufficiently diluted with sugared water. Thousands of gallons are drunk in this way every year. As a pleasant and safely effective help towards wooing sleep, from one to two teaspoonfuls of the French *Eau de fleur d'oranger*, if taken at bedtime in a teacupful of hot water, are to be highly commended for a nervous, or excitably wakeful person.

Orange buds are picked green from the trees in the gardens of the Riviera, and when dried they retain the sweet smell of the flowers. A teaspoonful of these buds is ordered to be infused in a teacupful of quite hot water, and the liquid to be drunk shortly before going to bed. The effect is to induce a refreshing sleep, without any subsequent headache or nausea. The dried berries may be had from an English druggist.

A peeled Orange contains some citric acid, with citrate of potash; also albumen, cellulose, water, and about eight per cent. of sugar. The white lining pith of the peel possesses likewise the crystalline principle "hesperidin." Dr. Cullen showed that the acid juice of oranges, by uniting with the bile, diminishes the bitterness of that secretion; and hence it is that this fruit is of particular service in illnesses which arise from a redundancy of bile, chiefly in dark persons of a fibrous, or bilious temperament. But if the acids of the Orange are greater in quantity than can be properly corrected by the bile (as in persons with a small liver, and feeble digestive powers), they seem, by some prejudicial union with that liquid, to acquire a purgative quality, and to provoke diarrhœa, with colicky pains.

The rind or peel of the Seville Orange is darker in colour, and more bitter of taste than that of the sweet China fruit. It affords a considerable quantity of fragrant, aromatic oil, which partakes of the characters exercised by the leaves and the flowers as affecting the nervous system. Pereira records the death of a child which resulted from eating the rind of a sweet China Orange.

The small green fruits (windfalls) from the Orange trees of each sort, which become blown off, or shaken down during the heats of the summer, are collected and dried, forming the "orange berries" of the shops. They are used for flavouring curacoa, and for making issue peas. These berries furnish a fragrant oil, the *essence de petit grain*, and contain citrates, and malates of lime and potash, with "hesperidin," sulphur, and mineral salts. The Orange flowers yield a volatile, odorous oil, acetic acid, and acetate of lime. The juice of the Orange consists of citric and malic acids, with sugar, citrate of lime, and water. The peel furnishes hesperidin, a volatile oil, gallic acid, and a bitter principle.

By druggists, a confection of bitter orange peel is sold; also a syrup of this orange peel, and a tincture of the same, made with spirit of wine, to be given in doses of from one to two teaspoonfuls with water, as an agreeable stomachic bitter. *Eau de Cologne* contains oil of neroli, oil of citron, and oil of orange.

The fresh juice of Oranges is antiseptic, and will prevent scurvy if taken in moderation daily. Common Oranges cut through the middle while green, and dried in the air, being afterwards steeped for forty days in oil, are used by the Arabs for preparing an essence famous among their old women because it will restore a fresh dark, or black colour to grey hair. The custom of a bride wearing Orange blossoms, is probably due to the fact that flowers and fruit appear together on the tree, in token of a wish that the bride may retain the graces of maidenhood amid the cares of married life. This custom has been derived from the Saracens, and was originally suggested also by the fertility of the Orange tree.

The rind of the Seville Orange has proved curative of ague, and powerfully remedial to restrain the monthly flux of women when in excess. Its infusion is of service also against flatulency. A drachm of the powdered leaves may be given for a dose in nervous and hysterical ailments. Finally, "the Orange," adds John Evelyn, "sharpens appetite, exceedingly refreshes, and resists putrefaction."

With respect to the fruit, it is said that workpeople engaged in the orange trade enjoy a special immunity from influenza, whilst a free partaking of the juice given largely, has been found preventive of pneumonia as complicating this epidemic. The benefit is said to occur through lessening the fibrin of the blood.

In the time of Shakespeare, it was the fashion to carry "pomanders," these being oranges from which all the pulp had been scooped out, whilst a circular hole was made at the top. Then after the peel had become dry, the fruit was filled with spices, so as to make a sort of scent-box. Orange lilies, Orangemen, and William of Orange, are all more or less associated with this fruit. The Dutch Government had no love for the House of Orange: and many a grave burgomaster went so far as to banish from his garden the Orange lily, and Marigold; also the sale of Oranges and Carrots was prohibited in the markets on account of their aristocratic colour.

There exists at Brighton a curious custom of bowling or throwing Oranges along the high road on Boxing day. He whose Orange is hit by that of another, forfeits the fruit to the successful hitter.

In Henry the Eighth's reign Oranges were made into pies, or the juice was squeezed out, and mixed with wine. This fruit when peeled, and torn into sections, after removing the white pith, and the pips, and sprinkling over it two or three spoonfuls of powdered loaf sugar, makes a most wholesome salad. A few candied orange-flower petals will impart a fine flavour to tea when infused with it.

ORCHIDS.

OUR common English Orchids are the "Early Purple," which is abundant in our woods and pastures; the "Meadow Orchis"; and the "Spotted Orchis" of our heaths and commons. Less frequent are the "Bee Orchis," the "Butterfly Orchis," "Lady's Tresses," and the "Tway blade."

Two roundish tubers form the root of an Orchid, and give its name to the plant from the Greek *orchis*, testicle. A nutritive starchy product named Salep, or Saloop, is prepared from the roots of the common Male Orchis, and its infusion or decoction was taken generally in this country as a beverage before the introduction of tea and coffee. Sassafras chips were sometimes added for giving the drink a flavour. Salep obtained from the tubers of foreign Orchids was specially esteemed; and even now that sold in Indian bazaars is so highly valued for its fine qualities that most extravagant prices are paid for it by wealthy Orientals. Also in Persia and Turkey it is in great repute for recruiting the exhausted vitality of aged, and enervated persons. In this country it may be purchased as a powder, but not readily miscible with water, so that many persons fail in making the decoction. The powder should be first stirred with a little spirit of wine: then the water should be added suddenly, and the mixture boiled. One dram by weight of the salep powder in a fluid dram and a half of the spirit, to half-a-pint of water, are the proper proportions. Sometimes amber, cloves, cinnamon, and ginger are added.

Dr. Lind, in the middle of the last century, strongly advised that ships, and soldiers on long marches, should be provided with Salep made into a paste or cake. This (with a little portable soup added) will allay hunger and thirst if made liquid. An ounce in two quarts of boiling water will sufficiently sustain a man for one day, being a combination of animal and vegetable foods. Among the early Romans the Orchis was often called "Satyrion," because it was thought to be the food of the Satyrs, exciting them to their sexual orgies. Hence the Orchis root became famous as an aphrodisiac medicine, and has been so described by all herbalists from the time of Dioscorides.

A tradition is ascribed to the English Orchis Mascula (early Purple), of which the leaves are usually marked with purple spots. It is said that these are stains of the precious blood which flowed from our Lord's body on the cross at Calvary, where this species of Orchis is reputed to have grown. Similarly in Cheshire, the plant bears the name of Gethsemane. This early Orchis is the "long Purples," mentioned by Shakespeare in Hamlet: and it is sometimes named "Dead men's fingers," from the pale colour, and the hand-like shape of its tubers.

> "That liberal shepherds give a grosser name,
> But our cold maids do 'dead men's fingers' call them."

It is further styled "Cain and Abel" and "Rams' horns," the odour being offensive, especially in the evening. It thrives wherever the wild hyacinth flourishes, and is believed by some to grow best where the earth below is rich in metal. Country people in Yorkshire call it "Crake feet," and in Kent "Keat legs," or "Neat legs." The roots of this Orchis abound with a glutinous sweetish juice, of which a Salep may be made which is quite equal to any brought from the Levant. The new root should be washed in hot water, and its thin brown skin rubbed off with a linen cloth. Having thus prepared a sufficient number of roots, the operator should spread them on a tin plate in a hot oven for eight or ten minutes, until they get to look horny, but without shrinking in size: and being then withdrawn, they may be dried with more gentle heat, or by exposure to the air. Their concocted juice can be employed with the same intentions and in the same complaints as gum arabic,—about which we read that not only has it served to sustain whole negro towns during a scarcity of other provisions, but the Arabs who collect it by the river Niger have nothing else to live upon for months together.

Salep is a most useful article of diet for those who suffer from chronic diarrhœa.

PARSLEY.

PARSLEY is found in this country only as a cultivated plant, having been introduced into England from Sardinia in the sixteenth century. It is an umbelliferous herb, which has been long of garden growth for kitchen uses. The name was formerly spelt "Percely," and the herb was known as March, or Merich (in Anglo-Saxon, Merici). Its adjective title, *Petro-selinum*, signifies "growing on a rock." The Greeks held Parsley in high esteem, making therewith the victor's crown of dried and withered Parsley, at their Isthmian games, and the wreath for adorning the tombs of their dead. Hence the proverb, *Deeisthai selinon* (to need only Parsley) was applied to persons dangerously ill, and not expected to live. The herb was never brought to table of old, being held sacred to oblivion and the defunct.

It is reputed to have sprung from the blood of a Greek hero, Archemorus, the fore-runner of death; and Homer relates that chariot horses were fed by warriors with this herb. Greek gardens were often bordered with Parsley and Rue: and hence arose the saying when an undertaking was in contemplation but not yet commenced, "Oh! we are only at the Parsley and Rue."

Garden Parsley was not cultivated in England until the second year of Edward the Sixth's reign, 1548. In our modern times the domestic herb is associated rather with those who come into the world than with those who go out of it. Proverbially the Parsley-bed is propounded to our little people who ask awkward questions, as the fruitful source of new-born brothers and sisters when suddenly appearing within the limits of the family circle. In Suffolk there is an old belief that to ensure the herb coming up "double," Parsley seed must be sown on Good Friday.

The root is faintly aromatic, and has a sweetish taste. It contains a chemical principle, "apiin," sugar, starch, and a volatile oil. Likewise the fruit furnishes the same volatile oil in larger abundance, this oil comprising parsley-camphor, and "apiol," the true essential oil of parsley, which may be now had from all leading druggists. Apiol exercises all the virtues of the entire plant, and is especially beneficial for women who are irregular as to their monthly courses because of ovarian debility. From three to six drops should be given on sugar, or in milk (or as a prepared capsule) twice or three times in the day for some days together, at the times indicated, beginning early at the expected date of each period. If too large a dose of apiol be taken it will cause headache, giddiness, staggering, and deafness; and if going still further, it will induce epileptiform convulsions. For which reason, in small diluted doses, the same medicament will curatively meet this train of symptoms when occurring as a morbid state. And it is most likely on such account Parsley has been popularly said to be "poison to men, and salvation to women." Apiol was first obtained in 1849, by Drs. Joret and Homolle, of Brittany, and proved an excellent remedy there for a prevailing ague. It exercises a singular influence on the great nervous centres within the head and spine. Bruised Parsley seeds make a decoction which is likewise beneficial against ague and intermittent fever. They have gained a reputation in America as having a special tendency to regulate the reproductive functions in either sex. Country folk in many places think it unlucky to sow Parsley, or to move its roots; and a rustic adage runs thus: "Fried parsley brings a man to his saddle, and a woman to her grave." Taking Parsley in excess at table will impair the eyesight, especially the tall Parsley; for which reason it was forbidden by Chrysippus and Dionysius.

The root acts more readily on the kidneys than other parts of the herb; therefore its decoction is useful when the urine becomes difficult through a chill, or because of gravel. The bruised leaves applied externally will serve to soften hard breasts early in lactation, and to resolve the glands in nursing, when they become knotty and painful, with a threatened abscess. Sheep are fond of the plant, which protects them from foot-rot; but it acts as a deadly poison to parrots.

In France a rustic application to scrofulous swellings is successfully used, which consists of Parsley and snails pounded together in a mortar to the thickness of an ointment. This is spread on coarse linen and applied freely every day. Also on the Continent, and in some parts of England, snails as well as slugs are thought to be efficacious medicinally in consumption of the lungs, even more so than cod-liver oil. The *Helix pomatia* (or Apple Snail) is specially used in France, being kept for the purpose in a snaillery, or boarded-in space of which the floor is covered half-a-foot deep with herbs.

The Romans were very partial to these Apple Snails, and fattened them for the table with bran soaked in wine until the creatures attained almost a fabulous size. Even in this country shells of Apple Snails have been found which would hold a pound's worth of silver. The large Snail was brought to England in the sixteenth century, to the South downs of Surrey, and Sussex, and to Box Hill by an Earl of Arundel for his Countess, who had them dressed, and ate them because of her consumptive disease. Likewise in Pliny's time Snails beaten up with warm water were commended for the cure of coughs. Gipsies are great Snail eaters, but they first starve the creatures, which are given to devour the deadly Night Shade, and other poisonous plants. It is certain that Snails retain the flavour and odour of the vegetables which they consume.

The chalky downs of the South of England are literally covered with small snails, and many persons suppose that the superior flavour of South Down mutton is due to the thousands of these snails which the sheep consume together with the pasture on which they feed. In 1854 a medical writer set forth the curative virtues of *Helicin*, a glutinous constituent principle derived from the Snail, and to be given in broth as a remedy for pulmonary consumption. In France the Apple Snail is known as the "great Escargot"; and the Snail gardens in which the gasteropods are fattened, and reared, go by the name of "Escargotoires." Throughout the winter the creatures hybernate, shutting themselves up by their operculum whilst lying among dead leaves, or having fixed themselves by their glutinous secretion to a wall or tree. They are only taken for use whilst in this state. According to a gipsy, the common English Snail is quite as good to be eaten, and quite as beneficial as an Apple Snail, but there is less of him. In Wiltshire, when collected whilst hybernating, snails are soaked in salted water, and then grilled on the bars of the grate. About France the Escargots are dried, and prepared as a lozenge for coughs. Our common garden Snail is the *Helix aspersa.* On the Continent for many years past the large Apple Snail, together with a reddish-brown slug, the Arion Rufus, has been employed in medicine for colds, sore throats, and a tendency to consumption of the lungs. These contain "limacine," and eight per cent. of emollient mucilage, together with "helicin," and uric acid just under the shell. Many quarts of cooked garden snails are sold every week to the labouring classes in Bristol; and an annual Feast of Snails is held in the neighbourhood of Newcastle. Mrs. Delaney in 1758, recommended that "two or three snails should be boiled in the barley-water which Mary takes who coughs at night. She must know nothing of it; they give no manner of taste. Six or eight boiled in water, and strained off, and put in a bottle would be a good way of adding a spoonful of the same to every liquid thing she takes. They must be fresh done every two or three days, otherwise they grow too thick." The *London Gazette,* of March 23rd, 1739, tells that Mrs. Joanna Stephens received from the Government five thousand pounds for revealing the secret of her famous cure against stone in the bladder, and gravel. This consisted chiefly of eggshells, and snails, mixed with soap, honey and herbs. It was given in powders, decoctions, and pills. To help weak eyes in South Hampshire, snails and bread crust are made into a poultice.

A moderate dose of Parsley oil when taken in health, induces a sense of warmth at the pit of the stomach, and of general well-being. The powdered seeds may be taken in doses of from ten to fifteen grains. The bruised leaves have successfully resolved tumours of hard (scirrhous) cancer when cicuta, and mercury had failed.

Though used so commonly at table, facts have proved

that the herb, especially when uncooked, may bring on epilepsy in certain constitutions, or at least aggravate the fits in those who are subject to them. Alston says: "I have observed after eating plentifully of raw Parsley, a fulness of the vessels about the head, and a tenderness of the eyes (somewhat inflamed) and face, as if the cravat were too tight."

The victors at the old Grecian games were crowned with chaplets of Parsley leaves; and it is more than probable our present custom of encircling a joint, and garnishing a dish with the herb had its origin in this practice. The Romans named Parsley *Apium*, either because their bee (*apis*) was specially fond of the herb, or from *apex*, the head of a conqueror, who was crowned with it. The tincture has a decided action on the lining membrane of the urinary passages, and may be given usefully when this is inflamed, or congested through catarrh, in doses of from five to ten drops three times in the day with a spoonful or two of cold water.

Wild Parsley is probably identical with our garden herb. It is called in the Western counties Eltrot, perhaps because associated with the gambols of the elves.

The Fool's Parsley (*Œthusa cynapium*) is a very common wayside weed, and grows wild in our gardens. It differs botanically from all other parsleys in having no bracts, but three narrow leaves at the base of each umbel. This is a more or less poisonous herb, producing, when eaten in a harmful quantity, convulsive and epileptic symptoms; also an inflamed state of the eyelids, just such as is seen in the scrofulous ophthalmia of children, the condition being accompanied with swelling of glands and eruptions on the skin. Therefore the tincture which is made (H.) of Fool's Parsley, when given in small doses, and diluted, proves very useful for such ophthalmia, and for obviating the convulsive attacks of young children, especially if connected with derangement of the digestive organs. Also as a medicine it has done much good in some cases of mental imbecility. And this tincture will correct the Summer diarrhœa of infants, when the stools are watery, greenish, and without smell. From three to ten drops of the tincture diluted to the third decimal strength, should be given as a dose, and repeated at intervals, for the symptoms just recited.

This variety is named Œthusa, because of its acridity, from the Greek verb *aitho* (to burn). "It has faculties," says Gerard, "answerable to the common Hemlock," the poisonous effects being inflamed stomach and bowels, giddiness, delirium, convulsions, and insensibility. It is called also "Dog's Parsley" and "Kicks."

The leaves of the Fool's Parsley are glossy beneath, with lanceolate lobes, whereas the leaflets of other parsleys are woolly below. Gerard calls it Dog's Parsley, and says: "The whole plant is of a naughty smell." It contains a peculiar alkaloid "cynapina." The tincture, third decimal strength, in half-drop doses, with a teaspoonful of water, will prevent an infant from vomiting the breast milk in thick curds.

Another variety which grows in chalky districts, the Stone Parsley, *Sison*, or breakstone, was formerly known as the "Hone-wort," from curing a "hone," or boil, on the cheek. It was believed at one time to break a glass goblet or tumbler if rubbed against this article.

PARSNIP.

THE Wild Parsnip (*Pastinaca sativa*) grows on the borders of ploughed fields and about hedgerows, being generally hairy, whilst the Garden Parsnip is smooth, with taller stems, and leaves of a yellowish-green colour. This cultivated Parsnip has been produced as a vegetable since Roman times. The roots furnish a good deal of starch, and are very nutritious for warming and fattening, but when long in the ground they are called in some places "Madnip," and are said to cause insanity.

Chemically, they contain also albumen, sugar, pectose, dextrin, fat, cellulose, mineral matters, and water, but less sugar than turnips or carrots. The volatile oil with which the cultivated root is furnished causes it to disagree with persons of delicate stomach; otherwise it is highly nutritive, and makes a capital supplement to salt fish, in Lent. The seeds of the wild Parsnip (quite a common plant) are aromatic, and are kept by druggists. They have been found curative in ague, and for intermittent fever, by their volatile oil, or by its essence given as a medicine. But the seeds of the garden Parsnip, which are easier to get, though not nearly so efficacious, are often substituted at the shops. A decoction of the wild root is good for a sluggish liver, and in passive jaundice.

In Gerard's time, Parsnips were known as Mypes. Marmalade made with the roots, and a small quantity of sugar, will improve the appetite, and serve as a restorative to invalids.

From the mashed roots of the wild Parsnip in some parts of Ireland, when boiled with hops, the peasants brew a beer. In Scotland a good dish is prepared from Parsnips and potatoes, cooked and beaten together, with butter. Parsnip wine, when properly concocted, is particularly exhilarating and refreshing.

The Water Parsnip (spelt also in old *Herbals*, Pasnep, and Pastnip, and called Sium) is an umbelliferous plant, common by the sides of rivers, lakes, and ditches, with tender leaves which are "a sovereign remedy against gravel in the kidney, and stone in the bladder." It is known also as *Apium nodiflorum*, from *apon*, water, and contains "pastinacina," in common with the wild Parsnip. This is a volatile alkaloid which is not poisonous, and is thought to be almost identical with ammonia. The fresh juice, in doses of one, two, or three tablespoonfuls, twice a day, is of curative effect for scrofulous eruptions on the face, neck, and other parts of children. Dr. Withering tells of a child, aged six years, who was thus cured of an obstinate and otherwise intractable skin disease. The juice may be readily mixed with milk, and does not disagree in any way.

PEA and BEAN.

TYPICAL of leguminous plants (so called because they furnish legumin, or vegetable cheese), whilst furthermore possessing certain medicinal properties, the Bean and the Pea have a claim to be classed with Herbal Simples.

The common Kidney Bean (*Phaseolus vulgaris*) is a native of the Indies, but widely cultivated all over Europe, and so well known as not to need any detailed description as a plant. Because of the seed's close resemblance to the kidney, as well as to the male testis, the Egyptians made it an object of sacred worship, and would not partake of it as food. They feared lest by so doing they should eat what was human remaining after death in the Bean, or should consume a soul. The Romans celebrated feasts (Lemuria) in honour of their departed, when Beans were cast into the fire on the altar; and the people threw black Beans on the graves of the deceased, because the smell was thought disagreeable to any hostile Manes. In Italy at the present day it is customary to eat Beans, and to distribute them among the poor, on the anniversary of a death. Because of its decided tendency to cause sleepiness the Jewish High Priest was forbidden to partake of Beans on the day of Atonement; and there is now a common saying in Leicestershire that for bad dreams, or to be driven crazy, one has only to sleep all night in a Bean field. The philosopher, Pythagoras, warned his pupils against eating Beans, the black spot thereon being typical of death; and the disciples were ever mindful: "*Jurare in verba magistri.*" When bruised and boiled with garlic, Beans have been known to cure coughs which were past other remedies. But the roots of the Kidney Bean have proved themselves dangerously narcotic.

The Pea (*Pisum sativum*) is a native of England, first taking its botanical name from Pisa, a town of Elis, where Peas grew in plenty. The English appellation was formerly Peason, or Pease, and the plant has been cultivated in this country from time immemorial; though not commonly, even in Elizabeth's day, when (as Fuller informs us) "Peas were brought from Holland, and were fit dainties for ladies, they came so far, and cost so dear." In Germany Peas are thought good for many complaints, especially for wounds and bruises; children affected with measles are washed there systematically with water in which peas have been boiled. These, together with Beans and lentils, etc., are included under the general name of pulse, about which Cowper wrote thus:—

> "Daniel ate pulse by choice: example rare!
> Heaven blest the youth, and made him fresh and fair."

Grey Peas were provided in the pits of the Greek and Roman theatres, as we supply oranges and a bill of the Play.

"Hot Grey Pease and a suck of bacon" (tied to a string of which the stall-keeper held the other end), was a popular street cry in the London of James the First.

Peas and Beans contain sulphur, and are richer in mineral salts, such as potash and lime, than wheat, barley, or oats; but their constituents are apt to provoke indigestion, whilst engendering flatulence through sulphuretted hydrogen. They best suit persons who take plenty of out-door exercise, but not those of sedentary habits. The skins of parched Peas remain undigested when eaten cooked, and are found in the excrements. These leguminous plants are less easily assimilated than light animal food by persons who are not robust, or laboriously employed, though vegetarians assert to the contrary. Lord Tennyson wrote to such effect as the result of his personal experience (in his dedication of *Tiresias* to E. Fitzgerald):—

> "Who live on meal, and milk, and grass:—
>   And once for ten long weeks I tried
> Your table of Pythagoras,
>   And seem'd at first 'a thing enskied'
> (As Shakespeare has it)—airylight,
>   To float above the ways of men:
> Then fell from that half spiritual height,
>   Until I tasted flesh again.
> One night when earth was winter black,
>   And all the heavens were flashed in frost,
> And on me—half asleep—came back
>   That wholesome heat the blood had lost."

But none the less does a simple diet foster spirituality of mind. "In milk"—says one of the oldest Vedas—"the finer part of the curds, when shaken, rises and becomes butter. Just so, my child, the finer part of food rises when it is eaten, and becomes mind."

Old Fuller relates "In a general dearth all over

England (1555), plenty of Pease did grow on the sea-shore, near Dunwich (Suffolk), never set or sown by human industry, which being gathered in full ripeness much abated the high prices in the markets, and preserved many hungry families from famishing." "They do not grow" says he, "among the bare stones, neither did they owe their original to shipwrecks, or Pease cast out of ships." The Sea-side Pea *(pisum maritimum)* is a rare plant.

PEACH.

THE Peach (*Amygdalus Persica*), the apple of Persia, began to be cultivated in England about 1562, or perhaps before then. Columella tells of this fatal gift conveyed treacherously to Egypt in the first century :—

> "Apples, which most barbarous Persia sent,
> With native poison armed."

The Peach tree is so well known by its general characteristics as not to need any particular description. Its young branches, flowers, and seeds, after maceration in water, yield a volatile oil which is chemically identical with that of the bitter almond. The flowers are laxative, and have been used instead of manna. When distilled, they furnish a white liquor which communicates a flavour resembling the kernels of fruits. An infusion made from one drachm of the dried flowers, or from half an ounce of the fresh flowers, has a purgative effect. The fruit is wholesome, and seldom disagrees if eaten when ripe and sound. Its quantity of sugar is only small, but the skin is indigestible.

The leaves possess the power of expelling worms if applied outside a child's belly as a poultice, but in any medicinal form they must be used with caution, as they contain some of the properties of prussic acid, as found also in the leaves of the laurel. A syrup of Peach flowers was formerly a preparation recognised by apothecaries. The leaves infused in white brandy, sweetened with barley sugar, make a fine cordial similar to noyeau. Soyer says the old Romans gave as much for their peaches as eighteen or nineteen shillings each.

Peach pie, owing to the abundance of the fruit, is as common fare in an American farm-house, as apple pie in an English homestead. Our English King John died at Swinestead Abbey from a surfeit of peaches, and new ale.

A tincture made from the flowers will allay the pain of colic caused by gravel; but the kernels of the fruit, which yield an oil identical with that of bitter almonds, have produced poisonous effects with children.

Gerard teaches "that 'a syrup or strong infusion of Peach flowers doth singularly well purge the belly, and yet without grief or trouble." Two tablespoonfuls of the infusion for a dose.

In Sicily there is a belief that any one afflicted with goitre, who eats a Peach on the night of St. John, or the Ascension, will be cured, provided only that the Peach tree dies at the same time. In Italy Peach leaves are applied to a wart, and then buried, so that they and the wart may perish simultaneously.

Thackeray one day at dessert was taken to task by his colleague on the *Punch* staff, Angus B. Reach, whom he addressed as Mr. Reach, instead of as Mr. (*Scotticé*) Re-ack. With ready promptitude, Thackeray replied: "Be good enough Mr. Rē-ack to pass me a pē-ack."

PEAR.

The Pear, also called Pyrrie, belongs to the same natural order of plants (the *Rosaceæ*) as the Apple. It is sometimes called the Pyerie, and when wild is so hard and austere as to bear the name of Choke-pear. It grows wild in Britain, and abundantly in France and Germany. The Barland Pear, which was chiefly cultivated in the seventeenth century, still retains its health and vigour, "the identical trees in Herefordshire which then supplied excellent liquor, continuing to do so in this, the nineteenth century."

This fruit caused the death of Drusus, a son of the Roman Emperor Claudius, who caught in his mouth a Pear thrown into the air, and by mischance attempted to swallow it, but the Pear was so extremely hard that it stuck in his throat, and choked him.

Pears gathered from gardens near old monasteries were formerly held in the highest repute for flavour, and it was noted that the trees which bore them continued fruitful for a great number of years. The secret cause seems to have been, not the holy water with which the trees were formally christened, but the fact that the sagacious monks had planted them upon a layer of stones so as to prevent the roots from penetrating deep into the ground, and so as thus to ensure their proper drainage.

The cellular tissue of which a Pear is composed differs from that of the apple in containing minute stony concretions which make it, in many varieties of the fruit, bite short and crisp; and its specific gravity is therefore greater than that of the apple, so much so that by taking a cube of each of equal size, that of the Pear will sink when thrown into a vessel of water, while that of the apple will float. The wood of the wild Pear is strong, and readily stained black, so as to look like ebony. It is much employed by wood-engravers. Gerard says "it serveth to be cut up into many kinds of moulds: not only such fruits as those seen in my Herbal are made of, but also many sorts of pretty toies for coifes, breast plates, and such like; used among our English gentlewomen."

The good old black Pear of Worcester is represented in the civic arms, or rather in the second of the two shields belonging to the faithful city: Argent, a fesse between three Pears, sable. The date of this shield coincides with that of the visit of Queen Elizabeth to Worcester.

Virgil names three kinds of Pears which he received as a present from Cato:—

> "Nec surculus idem,
> Crustaneis, Syriisque pyris, gravibusque volemis."

The two first of these were Bergamots and Pounder Pears, whilst the last-named was called *a volemus*, because large enough to fill the hollow of the hand, (*vola*).

Mural paintings which have been disclosed at Pompeii represent the Pear tree and its fruit. In Pliny's time there were "proud" Pears, so called because they ripened early, and would not keep; and "winter" pears for baking, etc. Again, in the time of Henry the Eighth, a "warden" Pear, so named (Anglo-Saxon "wearden") from its property of long keeping, was commonly cultivated.

> "Her cheek was like the Catherine Pear,
> The side that's next the sun,"

says one of our old poets concerning a small fruit seen often now-a-days in our London streets, handsome, but hard, and ill-flavoured.

The special taste of Pears is chemically due for the most part to their containing amylacetate; and a solution of this substance in spirit is artificially prepared for making essence of Jargonelle Pears, as used for flavouring Pear drops and other sweetmeats. The acetate amyl is a compound ether got from vinegar and potato oil. Pears contain also malic acid, pectose, gum, sugar, and albumen, with mineral matter, cellulose, and water. Gerard says wine made of the juice of Pears, called in English, Perry, purgeth those that are not accustomed to drinke thereof, especially when it is new; notwithstanding, it is as wholesome a drink (being taken in small quantity) as wine; it comforteth and warmeth the stomacke, and causeth good digestion."

Perry contains about one per cent. alcohol over cider, and a slightly larger proportion of malic acid, so that it is rather more stimulating, and somewhat better calculated to produce the healthful effects of vegetable acids in the economy. How eminently beneficial fruits of such sort are when ripe and sound, even to persons out of health, is but little understood, though happily the British public is growing wiser to-day in this respect. For instance, it has been lately discovered that there is present in the juice of the Pine-apple a vegetable digestive ferment, which, in its action, imitates almost identically the gastric juices of the stomach; and a demand for Bananas is developing rapidly in London since their wholesome virtues have become generally recognised. It is a remarkable fact that the epidemics of yellow fever in New Orleans have declined in virulence almost incredibly since the Banana began to be eaten there in considerable quantities. If a paste of its ripe pulp dried in the sun be made with spice, and sugar, this will keep well for years.

At Godstone, as is related in *Bray's Survey*, the water

from a well sunk close to a wild Pear tree (which bore fruit as hard as iron) proved so curative of gout, that large quantities of it were sent to London and sold there at the rate of sixpence a quart. Pears were deemed by the Romans an antidote to poisonous fungi; and for this reason, which subsequent experience has confirmed, Perry is still reckoned the best thing to be taken after eating freely of mushrooms, as also Pear stalks cooked therewith.

There is an old Continental saying: *Pome, pere, ed noce guastano la voce*—"Apples, pears, and nuts spoil the voice." And an ancient rhymed distich says:—

"For the cough take Judas eare,
With the paryngе of a pear;
And drynke them without feare,
If ye will have remedy."

All Pears are cold, and have a binding quality, with an earthy substance in their composition.

It should be noted that Pears dried in the oven, and kept without syrup, will remain quite good, and eatable for a year or more.

Most Pears depend on birds for the dispersion of their seeds, but one striking variety prefers to attract bees, and the larger insects for cross-fertilization, and it has therefore assumed brilliant crimson petals of a broadly expanded sort, instead of bearing a succulent edible fruit. This is the highly ornamental *Pyrus Japonica*, which may so often be seen trained on the sunny walls of cottages.

PELLITORY.

A PLANT belonging to the order of Nettles, the Pellitory of the Wall, or Paritory—*Parietaria*, from the Latin *parietes*, walls—is a favourite Herbal Simple in many rural districts. It grows commonly on dry walls, and is in flower all the summer. The leaves are narrow, hairy, and reddish ; the stems are brittle, and the small blossoms hairy, in clusters. Their filaments are so elastic that if touched before the flower has expanded, they suddenly spring from their incurved position, and scatter the pollen broadcast.

An infusion of the plant is a popular medicine to stimulate the kidneys, and promote a large flow of watery urine. The juice of the herb acts in the same way when made into a thin syrup with sugar, and given in doses of two tablespoonfuls three times in the day. Dropsical effusions caused by an obstructed liver, or by a weak dilated heart, may be thus carried off with marked relief. The decoction of *Parietaria*, says Gerard, "helpeth such as are troubled with an old cough." All parts of the plant contain nitre abundantly. The leaves may be usefully applied as poultices.

But another Pellitory, which is more widely used because of its pungent efficacy in relieving toothache, and in provoking a free flow of saliva, is a distinct plant, the *Pyrethrum*, or Spanish Chamomile of the shops, and not a native of Great Britain, though sometimes cultivated in our gardens. The title "Purethron" is from *pur*, fire, because of its burning ardent taste. Its root is scentless, but when chewed causes a pricking sensation (with heat, and some numbness) in the mouth and tongue. Then an abundant flow of saliva, and of mucus within the cheeks quickly ensues. These effects are due to "pyrethrin" contained in the plant, which is an acid fixed resin ; also there are present a second resin, and a yellow, acrid oil, whilst the root contains inulin, tannin, and other substances. When sliced and applied to the skin it induces heat, tingling, and redness. A patient seeking relief from rheumatic or neuralgic affections of the head and face, or for palsy of the tongue, should chew the root of this *Pyrethrum* for several minutes.

The "Pelleter of Spain" (*Pyrethrum Anacyclus*), was so styled, not because of being brought from Spain, but because it is grown there.

A gargle of *Pyrethrum* infusion is prescribed for relaxed uvula, and for a partial paralysis of the tongue and lips. The tincture made from the dried root may be most helpfully applied on cotton wool to the interior of a decayed tooth which is aching, or the milder tincture of the wall Pellitory may be employed for the same purpose. To make a gargle, two or three teaspoonfuls of the tincture of *Pyrethrum*, which can be had from any druggist, should be mixed with a pint of cold water, and sweetened with honey, if desired. The powdered root forms a good snuff to cure chronic catarrh of the head and nostrils, and to clear the brain by exciting a free flow of nasal mucus and tears—*Purgatur cerebrum mansâ radice Pyrethri.*

Incidentally, as a quaint but effective remedy for carious toothache, may be mentioned the common lady bird insect, Coccinella, which when captured secretes from its legs a yellow acrid fluid having a disagreeable odour. This fluid will serve to ease the most violent toothache, if the creature be placed alive in the cavity of the hollow tooth.

Gerard says this *Pyrethrum* (Pellitory of Spain, or Pelletor) "is most singular for the surgeons of the hospitals to put into their unctions *contra Neapolitanum morbum*, and such other diseases that are cousin germanes thereunto." The *Parietaria*, or Pellitory of the wall, is named Lichwort, from growing on stones.

Sir William Roberts, of Manchester, has advised jujubes, made of gum arabic and pyrethrum, to be slowly masticated by persons who suffer from acid fermentation in the stomach, a copious flow of alkaline saliva being stimulated thereby in the mouth, which is repeatedly swallowed during the sucking of one or more of the jujubes, and which serves to neutralise the acid generated within the stomach. Distressing heartburn is thus effectively relieved without taking injurious alkalies, such as potash and soda.

PENNYROYAL, *see* MINT.

PERIWINKLE.

THERE are two British Periwinkles growing wild; the one *Vinca major*, or greater, a doubtful native, and found only in the neighbourhood of dwelling-houses; the other *Vinca minor*, lesser, abounding in English woods, particularly in the Western counties, and often entirely covering the ground with its prostrate evergreen leaves. The common name of each is derived from *vincio*, to bind, as it were by its stems resembling cord; or because bound in olden times into festive garlands and funeral chaplets. Their title used also to be Pervinca, and Pervinkle, Pervenkle, and Pucellage (or virgin flower).

This generic name has been derived either from *pervincire*, to bind closely, or from *pervincere*, to overcome. Lord Bacon observes that it was common in his time for persons to wear bands of green Periwinkle about the calf of the leg to prevent cramp. Now-a-days we use for the same purpose a garter of small new corks strung on worsted. In Germany this plant is the emblem of immortality. It bears the name "Penny-winkles" in Hampshire, probably by an inland confusion with the shell fish "winkles."

Each of the two kinds possesses acrid astringent properties, but the lesser Periwinkle, *Vinca minor* or Winter-green, is the Herbal Simple best known of the pair, for its medicinal virtues in domestic use. The Periwinkle order is called *Apocynaceæ*, from the Greek *apo*, against, and *kunos*, a dog; or dog's bane.

The flowers of the greater Periwinkle are gently purgative, but lose their effect by drying. If gathered in the Spring, and made into a syrup, they will impart all their virtues, and this is excellent to keep the bowels of children gently open, as well as to overcome habitual constipation in grown persons. But the leaves are astringent, contracting and strengthening the genitals if applied thereto either as a decoction, or as the bruised leaves themselves. An infusion of the greater Periwinkle, one part of the fresh plant to ten of water, may be used for staying female fluxes, by giving a wine-glassful thereof when cool, frequently; or of the liquid extract, half a teaspoonful for a dose in water. On account of its striking colour, and its use for magical purposes, the plant, when in bloom, has been named the Sorcerer's Violet, and in some parts of Devon the flowers are known as Cut Finger or Blue Buttons. The Italians use it in making garlands for their dead infants, and so call it Death's flower.

Simon Fraser, whose father was a faithful adherent of Sir William Wallace, when on his way to be executed (in 1306) was crowned in mockery with the Periwinkle, as he passed through the City of London, with his legs tied under the horse's belly. In Gloucestershire, the flowers of the greater Periwinkle are called Cockles.

The lesser Periwinkle is perennial, and is sometimes

cultivated in gardens, where it has acquired variegated leaves. It has no odour, but gives a bitterish taste which lasts in the mouth. Its leaves are strongly astringent, and therefore very useful to be applied for staying bleedings. If bruised and put into the nostrils, they will arrest fluxes from the nose, and a decoction made from them is of service for the diarrhœa of a weak subject, as well as for chronic looseness of the bowels; likewise for bleeding piles, by being applied externally, and by being taken internally. Again, the decoction makes a capital gargle for relaxed sore throat, and for sponginess of the mouth, of the tonsils, and the gums.

This plant was also a noted Simple for increasing the milk of wet nurses, and was advised for such purpose by physicians of repute. Culpeper gravely says: "The leaves of the lesser Periwinkle, if eaten by man and wife together, will cause love between them."

A tincture is made (H.) from the said plant, the *Vinca minor*, with spirit of wine. It is given medicinally for the milk-crust of infants, as well as for internal hæmorrhages, the dose being from two to ten drops three or four times in the day, with a spoonful of water.

PIMPERNEL.

THE "Poor Man's Weather Glass" or "Shepherd's Dial," is a very well-known and favourite little flower, of brilliant scarlet hue, expanding only in bright weather, and closing its petals at two o'clock in the day. It occurs quite commonly in gardens and open fields, being the scarlet Pimpernel, or *Anagallis arvensis*, and belonging to the Primrose tribe of plants. Old authors called it Burnet; which is quite a distinct herb, cultivated now for kitchen use, the *Pimpinella Saxifraga*, of so cheery and exhilarating a quality, and so generally commended, that its excellence has passed into a proverb, "*l'insolata non buon, ne betta ove non é Pimpinella.*" But this Burnet Pimpinella is of a different (Umbelliferous) order, though similarly styled because its leaves are likewise bipennate.

The Scarlet Pimpernel is named *Anagallis*, from the Greek *anagelao*, to laugh ; either because, as Pliny says, the plant removes obstructions of the liver, and spleen, which would engender sadness, or because of the graceful beauty of its flowers :—

> "No ear hath heard, no tongue can tell
> The virtues of the Pimpernell."

The little plant has no odour, but possesses a bitter taste, which is rather astringent. Doctors used to consider the herb remedial in melancholy, and in the allied forms of mental disease, the decoction, or a tincture being employed. It was also prescribed for hydrophobia, and linen cloths saturated with a decoction were kept applied to the bitten part.

Narcotic effects were certainly produced in animals by giving considerable doses of an extract made from the herb. The flowers have been found useful in epilepsy, twenty grains dried being given four times a day. A medicinal tincture (H.) is prepared with spirit of wine. It is of approved utility for irritability of the main urinary passage, with genital congestion, erotism, and dragging of the loins, this tincture being then ordered of the third decimal strength, in doses of from five to ten drops every three or four hours, with a spoonful of water.

A decoction of the plant is held in esteem by country-folk as checking pulmonary consumption in its early stages. Hill says there are many authenticated cases of this dire disease being absolutely cured by the herb.

The infusion is best made by pouring boiling water on the fresh plant. It contains "saponin," such as the Soapwort also specially furnishes.

In France the Pimpernel (*Anagallis*) is thought to be a noxious plant of drastic narcotico-acrid properties, and called *Mouron—qui tue les petits oiseaux, et est un violent drastique pour l'homme, et les grands animaux ; à dose tres elevée le mouron peut meme leur donner la mort.* In California a fluid extract of the herb is given for rheumatism, in doses of one teaspoonful with water three times a day.

The *Burnet Pimpinella* is more correctly the Burnet Saxifrage, getting its first name because the leaves are brown, and the second because supposed to break up stone in the bladder. It grows abundantly in our dry chalky pastures, bearing terminal umbels of white flowers. It contains an essential oil and a bitter resin, which are useful as warmly carminative to relieve flatulent indigestion, and to promote the monthly flow in women. An infusion of the herb is made, and given in two tablespoonfuls for a dose. Cows which feed on this plant have their flow of milk increased thereby. Small bunches of the leaves and shoots when tied together and suspended in a cask of beer impart to it an agreeable aromatic flavour, and are thought to correct tart, or spoiled wines. The root, when fresh, has a hot pungent bitterish taste, and may be usefully chewed for toothache, or to obviate paralysis of the tongue. In Germany a variety of this Burnet yields a blue essential oil which is used for colouring brandy. Again the herb is allied to the Anise (*Pimpinella Anisum*). The term Burnet was formerly applied to a brown cloth. Smaller than this Common Burnet is the Salad Burnet, *Poterium sanguisorba, quod sanguineos fluxus sistat,* a useful styptic, which is also cordial, and promotes perspiration. It has the smell of cucumber, and is, therefore, an ingredient of the salad bowl, or often put into a cool tankard, whereto, says Gerard, "it gives a grace in the drynkynge." Another larger sort of the Burnet Pimpinella (*Magna*), which has broad upper leaves less divided, grows in our woods and shady places.

A bright blue variety of the true Scarlet Pimpernel (*Anagallis*) is less frequent, and is thought by many to be a distinct species. Gerard says, "the Pimpernel with the blue flower helpeth the fundament that is fallen down: and, contrariwise, red Pimpernel being applied bringeth it down."

The Water Pimpernel (*Anagallis aquatica*) is more commonly known as Brooklime, or Beccabunga, and belongs to a different order of plants, the *Scrophulariaceæ* (healers of scrofula).

It grows quite commonly in brooks and ditches, as a succulent plant with smooth leaves, and small flowers of bright blue, being found in situations favourable to the growth of the watercress. It is the *brok lempe* of old writers, *Veronica beccabunga*, the syllable *bec* signifying a beck or brook; or perhaps the whole title comes from the Flemish *beck pungen*, mouth-smart, in allusion to the pungent taste of the plant.

"It is eaten," says Gerard, "in salads, as watercresses are, and is good against that *malum* of such as dwell near the German seas, which we term the scurvie, or skirby, being used after the same manner that watercress and scurvy-grass is used, yet is it not of so great operation and virtue." The leaves and stem are slightly acid and astringent, with a somewhat bitter taste, and frequently the former are mixed by sellers of watercresses with their stock-in-trade.

A full dose of the juice of fresh Brooklime is an easy purge; and the plant has always been a popular Simple for scrofulous affections, especially of the skin. Chemically, this Water Pimpernel contains some tannin, and a special bitter principle; whilst, in common with most of the Cruciferous plants, it is endowed with a pungent volatile oil, and some sulphur. The bruised plant has been applied externally for healing ulcers, burns, whitlows, and for the mitigation of swollen piles.

The Bog Pimpernel (*Anagallis tenella*), is common in boggy ground, having erect rose-coloured leaves larger than those of the Poor Man's Weather Glass.

PINK.

THE Clove Pink, or Carnation of our gardens, though found apparently wild on old castle walls in England, is a naturalised flower in this country. It is, botanically, the *Dianthus Caryophyllus*, being so named as *anthos*, the flower, *dios*, of Jupiter: whilst redolent of *Caryophylli*, Cloves. The term Carnation has been assigned to the Pink, either because the blossom has the colour, *carnis*, of flesh: or, as more correctly spelt by our older writers, Coronation, from the flowers being employed in making chaplets, *coronæ*. Thus Spenser says:—

> "Bring Coronations, and Sops in Wine,
> Worn of paramours."—*Shepherd's Kalendar*.

This second title, Sops in Wine, was given to the plant because the flowers were infused in wine for the sake of their spicy flavour; especially in that presented to brides after the marriage ceremony. Further, this Pink is the Clove Gilly (or *July*) flower, and gives its specific name to the natural order *Caryophyllaceæ*. The word Pink is a corruption of the Greek Pentecost (fiftieth), which has now come to signify a festival of the Church. In former days the blossoms were commended as highly cordial: their odour is sweet and aromatic, so that an agreeable syrup may be made therefrom. The dried petals, if powdered, and kept in a stoppered bottle, are of service against heartburn and flatulence, being given in a dose of from twenty to sixty grains. Gerard says, "a conserve made of the flowers with sugar is exceeding cordiall, and wonderfully above measure doth comfort the heart, being eaten now and then. A water distilled from Pinks has been commended as excellent for curing epilepsy, and if a conserve be composed of them, this is the life and delight of the human race." The flower was at one time called *ocellus*, from the eye-shaped markings of its corolla. It is nervine and antispasmodic. By a mistake Turner designated the Pink Incarnation.

PLANTAIN.

THE Plantains (*Plantaginaceæ*), from *planta*, the sole of the foot, are humble plants, well known as weeds in fields and by roadsides, having ribbed leaves and spikes of flowers conspicuous by their long stamens. As Herbal Simples, the Greater Plantain, the Ribwort Plantain, and the Water Plantain, are to be specially considered.

The Greater Plantain of the waysides affords spikes of seeds which are a favourite food of Canaries, and which, in common with the seeds of other sorts, yield a tasteless mucilage, answering well as a substitute for linseed. The leaves of the Plantains have a bitter taste, and are somewhat astringent.

The generic name *Plantago* is probably derived from the Latin *planta*, the sole of the foot, in allusion to the broad, flat leaves lying close on the ground, and *ago*, the old synonym for *wort*, a cultivated plant.

This greater Plantain (*Plantago major*) is also termed Waybred, Waybread, or Waybroad, "spread on the way," and has followed our colonists to all parts of the globe, being therefore styled "The Englishman's Foot" and "Whiteman's Foot." The shape of the leaf in the larger species resembles a footprint. The root has a sweet taste, and gives the saliva a reddish tinge.

Dioscorides advised that it should be applied externally for sores of every kind, and taken internally against hæmorrhages. In the *Romeo and Juliet* of Shakespeare, Romeo says, "Your Plantain leaf is excellent for broken shin." Country persons apply these leaves to open sores and wounds, or make a poultice of them, or give fomentations with a hot decoction of the same, or prepare a gargle from the decoction when cold.

The expressed juice of the greater Plantain has proved of curative effect in tubercular consumption, with spitting of blood. This herb is said to furnish a cure for the venomous bite of the rattlesnake, as discovered by the negro Cæsar in South Carolina.

It is of excellent curative use against the intermittent fevers of Spring, but for counteracting autumnal (*septic*) fevers it is of no avail.

The virtues of the greater Plantain as an application to wounds and sores were known of old. It possesses a widespread repute in Switzerland as a local remedy for toothache, the root or leaves being applied against the ear of the affected side. Those persons who proved the plant by taking it experimentally in various doses, suffered much pain in the teeth and jaws. Accordingly, Dr. Hale found that, of all his remedies for the toothache, none could compare with the *Plantago major*.

It gives rise to an active flow of urine when taken in considerable doses, and when administered in small doses of the diluted tincture, it has proved curative of bed wetting in young children. Gerard tells that "Plantain leaves stuped stayeth the inordinate flux of the terms, though it hath continued many years." For inflamed protruding piles, a broad-leaved Plantain reduced to a pulp, and kept bound to the parts by a compress, will give sure and speedy relief. Highlanders call it *Slanlus*, the healing plant.

The Ribwort Plantain (*Plantago lanceolata*), Ribgrass, Soldiers, or Cocks and Hens, is named from the strong parallel veins in its leaves. The flower stalks are termed *Kemps*, from *campa*, a warrior. The leaves are astringent, and useful for healing sores when applied thereto, and for dressing wounds. This Plantain is also named Hardheads, Fighting Cocks, and in Germany, Devil's Head, being used in divination. Children challenge one another to a game of striking off the heads.

Toads are thought to cure themselves of their ailments by eating its leaves. In Sussex, it is known as Lamb's Tongue. The powdered root of the Ribwort Plantain is of use for curing vernal ague, a dessertspoonful being given for a dose, two or three times in a day.

The Water Plantain (*Alisma Plantago*), belonging to a different natural order, is common on the margins of our rivers and ditches, getting its name from the Celtic *alos*, water, and being called also the greater Thrumwort, from *thrum*, the warp end of a weaver's web. The root and leaves contain an acrid juice, dispersed by heat, which is of service for irritability of the bladder. After the root is boiled so as to dissipate this medicinal juice it makes an edible starchy vegetable.

This plant is commonly classed with the Plantains because its leaves resemble theirs; but in general characteristics and qualities it more properly belongs to the *Ranunculaceæ*.

Its fresh leaves applied to the skin will raise a blister, and may be used for such a purpose, especially to relieve the swollen legs of dropsical subjects when the vesicles should be punctured and the serum drawn off. They contain a pungent butyraceous volatile oil. The seeds dislodged from the dry, ripe plant, by striking it smartly on a table, are good in decoction against bleedings, and are employed by country people for curing piles. About the Russian Empire the Water Plantain is still regarded as efficacious against hydrophobia. Dr. George Johnston says: "In the Government of Isola it has never failed of a cure for the last twenty-five years." Reduced to powder it is spread over bread and butter, and is eaten. Likewise, cures of rabid dogs by this plant are reported; and in America it is renowned as a remedy against the bite of the rattlesnake. The tubers contain a nutritious substance, and are eaten by the Tartars.

Apropos of this "Water Plantain" a Teesdale proverb says: "He's nar a good weaver that leaves lang *thrums*."

The small seeds of a Plantain grass which grows commonly in Southern Europe, the Fleawort, or *Plantago Psyllium*, have been known from time immemorial as an easy and popular aperient. In France these Psyllium seeds, given in a dessertspoonful dose, are widely prescribed as a laxative in lieu of mineral aperient waters, or the morning Seidlitz. They act after being soaked for some hours in cold water, by their mucilage, and when swallowed, by virtue of a laxative oil set free within the intestines. The grass is well known in some parts as "Clammy Plantain," and it has leafless heads with toothed leaves. These seeds are dispensed by the London druggists who supply French medicines.

POPPY.

THE Scarlet Poppy of our cornfields (*Papaver Rhœas*) is one of the most brilliant and familiar of English wild flowers, being strikingly conspicuous as a weed by its blossoms rich in scarlet petals, which are black at the base. The title *Papaver* has been derived from *pap*, a soft food given to young infants, in which it was at one time customary to boil Poppy seeds for the purpose of inducing sleep. Provincially this plant bears the titles of "Cop Rose" (from its rose-like flowers, and the button-like form of its cop, or capsule) and "Canker Rose," from its detriment to wheat crops.

The generic term *Rhœas* comes from *reo*, to fall, because the scarlet petals have so fragile a hold on their receptacles; and the plant has been endowed with the sobriquet, "John Silver Pin, fair without and foul within." In the Eastern counties of England any article of finery brought out only occasionally, and worn with ostentation by a person otherwise a slattern, is called "Joan Silver Pin." After this sense the appellation has been applied to the Scarlet Poppy. Its showy flower is so attractive to the eye, whilst its inner juice is noxious, and stains the hands of those who thoughtlessly crush it with their fingers.

> "And Poppies a sanguine mantle spread,
> For the blood of the dragon St. Margaret shed."

Robert Turner naively says, "The Red Poppy Flower (*Papaver erraticum*) resembleth at its bottom the settling of the 'Blood in pleurisie'"; and, he adds, "how excellent is that flower in diseases of the pleurisie with similar surfeits hath been sufficiently experienced."

It is further called Blindy Buff, Blind Eyes, Headwarke, and Headache, from the stupefying effects of smelling it. Apothecaries make a syrup of a splendid deep colour from its vividly red petals; but this does not exercise any soporific action like that concocted from the white Poppy, which is a sort of modified opiate, suitable for infants under certain conditions, when sanctioned by a doctor. Otherwise, all sedatives of a narcotic sort are to be strongly condemned for use by mothers, or nurses:—

> "But a child that bids the world 'Good-night'
> In downright earnest, and cuts it quite,
> (A cherub no art can copy),
> 'Tis a perfect picture to see him lie,
> As if he had supped on dormouse pie,
> An ancient classical dish, by-the-bye,
> With a sauce of syrup of Poppy."

Petronius, in the time of Nero, A.D. 80, "delivered an odd receipt for dressing dormouse sausages, and serving them up with Poppies and honey, which must have been a very soporiferous dainty, and as good as owl pye to such as want a nap after dinner."

The white Poppy is specially cultivated in Britain for the sake of its seed capsules, which possess attributes similar to opium, but of a weaker strength. These capsules are commonly known as Poppyheads, obtained from the druggist for use in domestic fomentations to allay pain. Also from the capsules, without their seeds, is made the customary syrup of White Poppies, which is so familiar as a sedative for childhood; but it should be always remembered that infants of tender years are highly susceptible to the influence even of this mild form of opium. The true gum opium, and laudanum, which is its tincture, are derived from Eastern Poppies (*Papaver somniferum*) by incisions made in the capsules at a proper season of the year. The cultivated Poppy of the garden will afford English opium in a like manner, but it is seldom used for this purpose. A milky juice exudes when the capsules of these cultivated flowers are cut, or bruised. They are familiar to most children as drumsticks, plucked in the garden after the gaudy petals of the flowers have fallen off. The leaves and stems likewise afford some of the same juice, which, when inspissated, is known as English opium. The seeds of the white Poppy yield by expression a bland nutritive oil, which may be substituted for that of olives, or sweet almonds, in cooking, and for similar uses. Dried Poppy-heads, formerly in constant request for making hot soothing stupes, or for application directly to a part in pain, are now superseded for the most part by the many modern liquid preparations of opium handy for the purpose, to be mixed with hot water, or applied in poultices.

For outward use laudanum may be safely added to stupes, hot or cold, a teaspoonful being usually sufficient for the purpose, or perhaps two, if the pain is severe; and powdered opium may be incorporated with one or another ointment for a similar object. If a decoction of Poppy capsules is still preferred, it should be made by adding to a quarter-of-a-pound of white Poppy heads (free from seeds, and broken up in a mortar) three pints of boiling water; then boil for ten or fifteen minutes, and strain off the decoction, which should measure about two pints.

Dr. Herbert Snow, resident physician at the Brompton Cancer Hospital, says (1895) he has found: "after a long experience, Opium exhibits a strong inhibitive influence on the cancer elements, retarding and checking the cell growth, which is a main feature of the disease. Even when no surgical operation has been performed, Opium is the only drug which markedly checks cancer growth: and the early employment of this medicine will usually add years of comfortable life to the otherwise shortened space of the sufferer's existence." Opium gets its name from the Greek *apos*, juice.

The seeds of the white Poppy are known as mawseed, or balewort, and are given as food to singing birds. In old Egypt these seeds were mixed with flour and honey, and made into cakes.

Pliny says: "The rustical peasants of Greece glazed the upper crust of their loaves with yolks of eggs, and then bestrewed them with Poppy seeds," thus showing that the seeds were then considered free from narcotic properties. And in Queen Elizabeth's time these seeds were strewn over confectionery, whilst the oil expressed from them was "delightful to be eaten when taken with bread."

White Poppy capsules, when dried, furnish papaverine and narcotine, with some mucilage, and a little waxy matter. The seeds contained within the capsules yield Poppy seed oil, with a fixed oil, and a very small quantity of morphia—about five grains in a pound of white Poppy seeds. In some parts of Russia the seeds are put into soups.

The Poppy was cultivated by the Greeks before the time of Hippocrates. It has long been a symbol of death, because sending persons to sleep. Ovid says, concerning the Cave of Somnus:—

> "Around whose entry nodding Poppies grow,
> And all cool Simples that sweet rest bestow."

The common scarlet Poppy was called by the Anglo-Saxons "Chesebolle," "Chebole," or "Chybolle," from the ripe capsule resembling a round cheese.

There is a Welsh Poppy, with yellow flowers; and a horned Poppy, named after Glaucus, common on our sea coasts, with sea-green leaves, and large blossoms of golden yellow. Glaucus, a fisherman of Bœotia, observed that all the fishes which he caught received fresh vigour when laid on the ground, and were immediately able to leap back into the sea. He attributed these effects to some herb growing in the grass, and upon tasting the leaves of the Sea Poppy he found himself suddenly moved with an intense desire to live in the sea; wherefore he was made a sea-god by Oceanus and Tethys. Borlase says: "That in the Scilly Islands the root of the Sea Poppy is so much valued for removing all pains in the breast, stomach, and intestines, as well as so good for disordered lungs, whilst so much better there than in other places, that the apothecaries of Cornwall send thither for it; and some persons plant these roots in their gardens in Cornwall, and will not part with them under sixpence a root." The scarlet petals of the wild Poppy, very abundant in English cornfields, when treated with sulphuric acid make a splendid red dye. With gorgeous tapestry cut from these crimson petals, the clever "drapery bee" (*Apis papaveris*) upholsters the walls of her solitary cell. Bruised leaves of the wild, or the garden Poppy, if applied to a part which has been stung by a bee or a wasp, will give prompt relief.

POTATO.

Our invaluable Potato, which enters so largely into the dietary of all classes, belongs to the Nightshade tribe of dangerous plants, though termed "solanaceous" as a natural order because of the sedative properties which its several genera exercise to lull pain.

This Potato, the *Solanum tuberosum*, is so universally known as a plant that it needs no particular description. It is a native of Peru, and was imported in 1586 by Thomas Heriot, mathematician and colonist, being afterwards taken to Ireland from Virginia by Sir Walter Raleigh, and passing from thence over into Lancashire. He knew so little of its use that he tried to eat the fruit, or poisonous berries, of the plant. These of course proved noxious, and he ordered the new comers to be rooted out. The gardener obeyed, and in doing so first learnt the value of their underground wholesome tubers. But not until the middle of the eighteenth century, were they common in this country as an edible vegetable. "During 1629," says Parkinson, "the Potato from Virginia was roasted under the embers, peeled and sliced: the tubers were put into sack with a little sugar, or were baked with cream, marrow, sugar, spice, etc., in pies, or preserved and candied by the comfit makers." But he most probably refers here to the Batatas, or sweet Potato, a *Convolvulus*, which was a popular esculent vegetable at that date, of tropical origin, and to which our Potato has since been thought to bear a resemblance.

This Batatas, or sweet Potato, had the reputation, like Eringo root, of being able to restore decayed vigour, and so Falstaff is made by Shakespeare to say: "Let the sky rain potatoes, hail kissing comfits, and snow eringoes." For a considerable while after their introduction the Potato tubers were grown only by men of fortune as a delicacy; and the general cultivation of this vegetable was strongly opposed by the public, chiefly by the Puritans, because no mention of it could be found in the Bible.

Also in France great opposition was offered to the recognised use of Potatoes: and it is said that Louis the Fifteenth, in order to bring the plant into favour, wore a bunch of its flowers in the button hole of his coat on a high festival. Later on during the Revolution quite a mania prevailed for Potatoes. Crowds perambulated the streets of Paris shouting for "la liberté, et des Batatas"; and when Louis the Sixteenth had been dethroned the gardens of the Tuileries were planted with Potatoes. Cobbett, in this country, exclaimed virulently against the tuber as "hogs' food," and hated it as fiercely as he hated tea. The stalks, leaves, and green berries of the plant share the narcotic and poisonous attributes of the nightshades to which it belongs; and the part which we eat, though often thought to be a root, is really only an underground stem, which has not been acted on by light so as to develop any poisonous tendencies, and in which starch is stored up for the future use of the plant.

The stalks, leaves, and unripe fruit yield an active principle apparently very powerful, which has not yet been fully investigated. There are two sorts of tubers, the red and the white. A roasted Potato takes two hours to digest; a boiled one three hours and a half. "After the Potato," says an old proverb, "cheese."

Chemically the Potato contains citric acid, like that of the lemon, which is admirable against scurvy: also potash, which is equally antiscorbutic, and phosphoric acid, yielding phosphorus in a quantity less only than that afforded by the apple, and by wheat. It is of the first importance that the potash salts should be retained by the Potato during cooking: and the tubers should therefore be steamed with their coats on; else if peeled, and then steamed, they lose respectively seven and five per cent. of potash, and phosphoric acid. If boiled after peeling they lose as much as thirty-three per cent. of potash, and twenty-three per cent. of phosphoric acid.

"The roots" says Gerard, "were forbidden in Burgundy, for that they were persuaded the too frequent use of them causeth the leprosie." Nevertheless it is now believed that the Potato has had much to do with expelling leprosy from England. The affliction has become confined to countries where the Potato is not grown.

Boiled or steamed Potatoes should turn out floury, or mealy, by reason of the starch granules swelling up and filling the cellular tissue, whilst absorbing the albuminous contents of its cells. Then the albumen coagulates, and forms irregular fibres between the starch grains. The most active part of the tuber lies just beneath the skin, as may be shown by pouring some tincture of guaiacum over the cut surface of a Potato, when a ring of blue forms close to the skin, and is darkest there while extending over the whole cut surface. Abroad there is a belief the Potato thrives best if planted on Maundy Thursday. Rustic names for it are: Taiders, Taities, Leather Coats, Leather Jackets, Lapstones, Pinks, No Eyes, Flukes, Blue Eyes, Red Eyes, and Murphies; in Lancashire Potatoes are called Spruds, and small Potatoes, Sprots.

The peel or rind of the tuber contains a poisonous substance called "solanin," which is dissipated and rendered inert when the whole Potato is boiled, or steamed. Stupes of hot Potato water are very serviceable in some forms of rheumatism. To make the decoction for this purpose, boil one pound of Potatoes (not peeled, and divided into quarters,) in two pints of water slowly down to one pint; then foment the swollen and painful parts with this as hot as it can be borne. Similarly some of the fresh stalks of the plant, and its unripe berries, as well as the unpeeled tubers cut up as described, if infused for some hours in cold water, will make a liquor in which the folded linen of a compress may be loosely rung out, and applied most serviceably under waterproof tissue, or a double layer of dry flannel. The carriage of a small raw Potato in the trousers' pocket has been often found preventive of rheumatism in a person predisposed thereto, probably by reason of the sulphur, and the narcotic principles contained in the peel. Ladies in former times had their dresses supplied with special bags, or pockets, in which to carry one or more small raw Potatoes about their person for avoiding rheumatism.

If peeled and pounded in a mortar, uncooked Potatoes applied cold make a very soothing cataplasm to parts that have been scalded, or burnt. In Derbyshire a hot boiled Potato is used against corns; and for frost-bites the mealy flour of baked potatoes, when mixed with sweet oil and applied, is very healing.

The skin of the tuber contains *corky* wood which swells in boiling with the jackets on, and which thus serves to keep in all the juices so that the digestibility of the Potato is increased; at the same time water is prevented from entering and spoiling the flavour of the vegetable. The proportion of muscle-forming food (nitrogen) in the Potato is very small, and it takes ten and a half pounds of the tubers to equal one pound of butcher's meat in nutritive value.

The Potato is composed mainly of starch, which

affords animal heat and promotes fatness. The Irish think that these tubers foster fertility; they prefer them with the jackets on, and somewhat hard in the middle—"with the bones in." A potato pie is believed to invigorate the sexual functions.

New Potatoes contain as yet no citric acid, and are hard of digestion, like sour crude apples; their nutriment, as Gerard says, "is sadly windy," the starch being immature, and not readily acted on by the saliva during mastication. "The longer I live," said shrewd Sidney Smith, "the more I am convinced that half the unhappiness in the world proceeds from a vexed stomach, or vicious bile: from small stoppages, or from food pressing in the wrong place. Old friendships may be destroyed by toasted cheese; and tough salted meat has led a man not infrequently to suicide."

A mature Potato yields enough citric acid even for commercial purposes; and there is no better cleaner of silks, cottons, and woollens, than ripe Potato juice. But even of ripe Potatoes those that break into a watery meal in the boiling are always found to prove greatly diuretic, and to much increase the quantity of urine.

By fermentation mature Potatoes, through their starch and sugar, yield a wine from which may be distilled a Potato spirit, and from it a volatile oil can be extracted, called by the Germans, *Fuselöl.* This is nauseous, and causes a heavy headache, with indigestion, and biliary disorders together with nervous tremors. Chemically it is amylic ether.

Also when boiled with weak sulphuric acid, the Potato starch is changed into glucose, or grape sugar, which by fermentation yields alcohol: and this spirit is often sold under the name of British brandy.

A luminosity strong enough to enable a bystander to

read by its light issues from the common Potato when in a state of putrefaction. In Cumberland, to have "taities and point to dinner," is a figurative expression which implies scanty fare. At a time when the duty on salt made the condiment so dear that it was scarce in a household, the persons at table were fain to point their Potatoes at the salt cellar, and thus to cheat their imaginations. Carlyle asks in *Sartor Resartus* about "an unknown condiment named 'point,' into the meaning of which I have vainly enquired; the victuals *potato and point* not appearing in any European cookery book whatever."

German ladies, at their five o'clock tea, indulge in Potato talk (*Kartoffel gesprach*) about table dainties, and the methods of cooking them. Men likewise, from the four quarters of the globe, in the days of our childhood, were given to hold similar domestic conclaves, when :—

"Mr. East made a feast,
Mr. North laid the cloth,
Mr. West brought his best,
Mr. South burnt his mouth
Eating a cold Potato."

With pleasant skill of poetic alliteration, Sidney Smith wrote in ordering how to mix a sallet :—

"Two large Potatoes passed through kitchen sieve,
Unwonted softness to a salad give."

And Sir Thomas Overbury wittily said about a dolt who took credit for the merits of his ancestors: "Like the Potato, all that was good about him was underground."

PRIMROSE.

THE Common Primrose (*Primula veris*) is the most widely known of our English wild flowers, and appears in the Spring as its earliest herald.

It gets its name from the Latin *primus*, first, being named in old books and M.S. *Pryme rolles*, and in the *Grete Herball*, Primet, as shortened from Primprint.

In North Devon it is styled the Butter Rose, and in the Eastern counties it is named (in common with the Cowslip) Paigle, Peagle, Pegyll, and Palsy plant.

Medicinally also it possesses similar curative attributes, though in a lesser degree, to those of the Cowslip. Both the root and the flowers contain a volatile oil, and "primulin" which is identical with mannite: whilst the acrid principle is "saponin." Alfred Austin, Poet Laureate, teaches to "make healing salve with early Primroses."

Pliny speaks of the Primrose as almost a panacea: *In aquâ potam omnibus morbis mederi tradunt.* An infusion of the flowers has been always thought excellent against nervous disorders of the hysterical sort. It should be made with from five to ten parts of the petals to one hundred of water. "Primrose tea" says Gerard, "drunk in the month of May, is famous for curing the phrensie."

The whole plant is sedative and antispasmodic, being of service by its preparations to relieve sleeplessness, nervous headache, and muscular rheumatism. The juice if sniffed up into the nostrils will provoke violent sneezing, and will induce a free flow of water from the lining membranes of the nostrils for the mitigation of passive headaches: though this should not be tried by a person of full habit with a determination of blood to the head. A teaspoonful of powdered dry Primrose root will act as an emetic. The whole herb is somewhat expectorant.

When the petals are collected and dried they become of a greenish colour: whilst fresh they have a honey-like odour, and a sweetish taste.

Within the last few years a political significance and popularity have attached themselves to the Primrose beyond every other British wild flower. It arouses the patriotism of the large Conservative party, and enlists the favour of many others who thoughtlessly follow an attractive fashion, and who love the first fruits of early Spring. Botanically the Primrose has two varieties of floral structure: one "pin-eyed," with a tall pistil, and short stamens; the other "thrum-eyed," showing a rosette of tall stamens, whilst the short pistil must be looked for, like the great Panjandrum himself, "with a little round button at the top," half way down the tube. Darwin was the first to explain that this diversity of structure ensures cross fertilisation by bees and allied insects. Through advanced cultivation at the hands of the horticulturist the Primula acquires in some instances a noxious character. For instance, the *Primula biconica*, which is often grown in dwelling rooms as a window plant, and commonly sold as such, will provoke an erysipelatous vesicular eruption of a very troublesome and inflamed character on the hands and face of some persons who come in contact with the plant by manipulating it to take cuttings, or in other ways. A knowledge of this fact should suggest the probable usefulness of the said Primula, when made into a tincture, and given in small diluted doses thereof, to act curatively for such an eruption if attacking the sufferer from idiopathic causes.

The Latins named the Ligustrum (our Privet) Primrose. Coles says concerning it (17th century): "This herbe is called Primrose; it is good to 'Potage.'" They also applied the epithet, "Prime rose" to a lady.

The Evening Primrose (*Œnothera biennis,* or *odorata*) is found in this country on sand banks in the West of England and Cornwall; but it is then most probably a garden scape, and an alien, its native habitat being in Canada and the United States of America. We cultivate it freely in our parterres as a brilliant, yellow, showy flower. It belongs to the natural order, *Onagraceæ*, so called because the food of wild asses; and was the "vini venator" of Theophrastus, 350 B.C. The name signifies having the odour of wine, *oinos* and *theera*. Pliny said: "It is an herbe good as wine to make the heart merrie. It groweth with leaves resembling those of the almond tree, and beareth flowers like unto roses. Of such virtue is this herbe that if it be given to drink to the wildest beast that is, it will tame the same and make it gentle." The best variety of this plant is the *Œnothera macrocarpa*.

The bark of the Evening Primrose is mucilaginous, and a decoction made therefrom is of service for bathing the skin eruptions of infants and young children. To answer such purpose a decoction should be made from the small twigs, and from the bark of the larger branches, retaining the leaves. This has been found further of use for diarrhœa associated with an irritable stomach, and asthma. The infusion, or the liquid extract, acts as a mild but efficient sedative in nervous indigestion, from twenty to thirty drops of the latter being given for a dose. The ascertained chemical principle of the plant, *Œnotherin*, is a compound body. Its flowers open in the evening, and last only until the next noon; therefore this plant is called the "Evening Primrose," or "Evening Star."

Another of the Primrose tribe, the Cyclamen, or Sowbread (*Panis porcinus*), is often grown in our gardens, and for ornamenting our rooms as a pot plant. Its name means (Greek) "a circle," and refers to the reflected corolla, or to the spiral fruit-stalks; and again, from the tuber being the food of wild swine. Gerard said it was reported in his day to grow wild on the Welsh mountains, and on the Lincolnshire hills: but he failed to find it. Nevertheless it is now almost naturalised in some parts of the South, and East of England. As the petals die, the stalks roll up and carry the capsular berries down to the surface of the ground. A medicinal tincture is made (H.) from the fresh root when flowering. The ivy-leaved variety is found in England, with nodding fresh-coloured blossoms, and a brown intensely acrid root. Besides starch, gum, and pectin, it yields chemically, "cyclamin," or "arthanatin," with an action like "saponin," whilst the juice is poisonous to fish. When applied externally as a liniment over the bowels, it causes them to be purged. Gerard quaintly and suggestively declares "It is not good for women with childe to touch, or take this herbe, or to come neere unto it, or to stride over the same where it groweth: for the natural attractive vertue therein contained is such that, without controversie, they that attempt it in manner above said, shall be delivered before their time; which danger and inconvenience to avoid, I have fastened sticks in the ground about the place in my garden where it groweth, and some other sticks also crosswaies over them, lest any woman should by lamentable experiment find my words to be true by stepping over the same. Again, the root hanged about women in their extreme travail with childe, causeth them to be delivered incontinent: and the leaves put into the place hath the like effect." Inferentially a tincture of the plant should be good for falling and displacement of the womb. "Furthermore, Sowbread, being beaten, and made into little flat cakes, is reputed to be a good amorous medicine, to make one in love."

In France, another Primula, the wild Pimpernel, occurs as a noxious herb, and is therefore named *Mouron.*

QUINCE.

THE Quince (*Cydonia*) is cultivated sparingly in our orchards for the sake of its highly fragrant, and strong-smelling fruit, which as an adjunct to apples is much esteemed for table uses.

It may well be included among remedial Herbal Simples because of the virtues possessed by the seeds within the fruit. The tree is a native of Persia and Crete; bearing a pear-shaped fruit, golden yellow when gathered, and with five cells in it, each containing twelve closely packed seeds. These are mucilaginous when unbroken, and afford the taste of bitter almonds.

When immersed in water they swell up considerably, and the mucilage will yield salts of lime with albumen.

Bandoline is the mucilage of Quince seeds to which some Eau de Cologne is added: and this mixture is employed for keeping the hair fixed when dressed by the *Coiffeur.*

The mucilage of Quince seeds is soothing and protective to an irritated or inflamed skin; it may also be given internally for soreness of the lining mucous membranes of the stomach and bowels, as in gastric catarrh, and for cough with a dry sore throat. One dram of the seeds boiled slowly in half-a-pint of fresh water until the liquor becomes thick, makes an excellent mucilage as a basis for gargles and injections; or, one part of the seeds to fifty parts of rosewater, shaken together for half-an-hour.

From growing at first in Cydon, now Candia, the tree got its name *Cydonia*: its old English title was Melicotone; and in ancient Rome it was regarded as a sacred fruit, being hung upon statues in the houses of the great. Now we banish the tree, because of its strong pene trating odour, to a corner of the garden.

Lord Bacon commended "quiddemy," a preserve of Quinces, for strengthening the stomach; and old Fuller said of this fruit, "being not more pleasant to the palate than restorative to the health, they are accounted a great cordiall." Jam made from the Quince (*Marmelo*) first took the name of Marmalade, which has since passed on to other fruit conserves, particularly to that of the Seville Orange. In France the Quince is made into a *compôte* which is highly praised for increasing the digestive powers of weakly persons. According to Plutarch Solon made a law that the Quince should form the invariable feast of the bridegroom (and some add likewise of the bride) before retiring to the nuptial couch. Columella said: "Quinces yield not only pleasure but health." The Greeks named the Quince "Chrysomelon," or the Golden Apple; so it is asserted that the golden fruit of the Hesperides were Quinces, and that these tempted Hercules to attack their guardian dragon. Shakespeare makes Lady Capulet when ordering the wedding feast,

"Call for dates, and Quinces in the pastry."

In Persia the fruit ripens, and is eaten there as a dessert delicacy which is much prized. If there be but a single Quince in a caravan, no one who accompanies it can remain unconscious of its presence.

In Sussex at one time a popular wine was made of Quinces. They are astringent to stay diarrhœa; and a syrup may be concocted from their juice to answer this purpose. For thrush and for excoriations within the mouth and upper throat, one drachm of the seeds should be boiled in eight fluid ounces of water until it acquires a proper demulcent mucilaginous consistence. "Simon Sethi writeth," says Gerard: "that the woman with child that eateth many Quinces during the time of her breeding, shall bring forth wise children, and of good understanding." Gerard says again: "The marmalad, or Cotiniat made of Quinces and sugar is good and profitable to strengthen the stomach that it may retain and keep the meat therein until it be perfectly digested. It also stayeth all kinds of fluxes both of the belly, and of other parts, and also of blood. Which cotiniat is made in this manner. Take four Quinces, pare them, cut them in pieces, and cast away the core: then put into every pound of Quinces a pound of sugar, and to every pound of sugar a pint of water. These must be boiled together over a still fire till they be very soft: next let it be strained, or rather rubbed through a strainer, or a hairy sieve, which is better. And then set it over the fire to boil again until it be stiff: and so box it up: and as it cooleth, put thereto a little rose water, and a few grains of musk mingled together, which will give a goodly taste to the cotiniat. This is the way to make marmalad." "The seed of Quinces tempered with water doth make a mucilage, or a thing like jelly which, being held in the mouth is marvellous good to take away the roughness of the tongue in hot burning fevers." Lady Lisle sent some cotiniat of Quinces to Henry the Eighth by her daughter Katharine. They were reputed a sexual stimulant. After being boiled and preserved in syrup, Quinces give a well known pleasant flavour to apple pie. As the fruit is free from acid, or almost so, its marmalade may be eaten by the goutily disposed with more impunity than that made with the Seville orange. An after taste suggestive of garlic is left on the palate by masticating Quince marmalade.

In the modern treatment of chronic dysentery the value of certain kinds of fresh fruit has come to be medically recognised. Of these may be specified strawberries, grapes, fresh figs, and tomatoes, all of which are seed fruits as distinguished from stone fruit. It is essential that they shall be absolutely sound, and in good condition. Dr. Saumaurez Lacy, of Guernsey, has successfully practised this treatment for many years, and it has been recently employed by others for chronic dysentery, and diarrhœa, with most happy results.

RADISH.

THE common garden Radish (*Raphanus sativus*) is a Cruciferous plant, and a cultivated variety of the Horse Radish. It came originally from China, but has been grown all over Europe from time immemorial. Radishes were celebrated by Dioscorides and Pliny as above all roots whatsoever, insomuch, that in the Delphic temple there was a Radish of solid gold, *raphanus ex auro dicatus*: and Moschinus wrote a whole volume in their praise; but Hippocrates condemned them as *vitiosas, innatantes, ac œgre concoctiles.*

Among the oblations offered to Apollo in his temple at Delphi, turnips were dedicated in lead, beet in silver, and radishes in wrought gold. The wild Radish is *Raphanus raphanistrum.* The garden Radish was not grown in England before 1548.

Later on John Evelyn wrote in his *Acetaria*: "And indeed (besides that they decay the teeth) experience tells us that, as the Prince of Physicians writes, it is hard of digestion, inimicous to the stomach, causing nauseous eructations, and sometimes vomiting, though otherwise diuretic, and thought to repel the vapours of wine when the wits were at their genial club." "The Radish" says Gerard, "provoketh urine, and dissolveth cluttered sand."

The roots, which are the edible part, consist of a watery fibrous pulp, which is comparatively bland, and of an external skin furnished with a pungent volatile aromatic oil which acts as a condiment to the phlegmatic pulp. "Radishes are eaten with salt alone as carrying their pepper in them." The oil contained in the roots, and likewise in the seeds, is sulphuretted, and disagrees with persons of weak digestion. A young Radish, which is quickly grown and tender, will suit most stomachs, especially if some of the leaves are masticated together with the root; but a Radish which is tough, strong, and hollow, "*fait penser à l'ile d'Elbe: il revient.*"

The pulp is chemically composed chiefly of nitrogenous substance, being fibrous and tough unless when the roots are young and quickly grown. On this account they should not be eaten when at all old and hard by persons of slow digestion, because apt to lodge in the intestines, and to become entangled in their cæcal pouch, or in its appendix. But boiled Radishes are almost equal to asparagus when served at table, provided they have been cooked long enough to become tender, that is, for almost an hour. The syrup of Radishes is excellent for hoarseness, bronchial difficulty of breathing, whooping cough, and other complaints of the chest.

For the cure of corns, if after the feet have been bathed, and the corns cut, a drop or two of juice be squeezed over the corn from the fresh pulp of a Radish on several consecutive days, this will wither and disappear. Also Radish roots sliced when fresh, and applied to a carbuncle will promote its healing. An old Saxon remedy against a woman's chatter was to "taste at night a root of Radish when fasting, and the chatter will not be able to harm him." In some places the Radish is called Rabone.

From the fresh plant, choosing a large Spanish Radish, with a turnip-shaped root, and a black outer skin, and collected in the autumn, a medicinal tincture (H.) is made with spirit of wine. This tincture has proved beneficial in cases of bilious diarrhœa, with eructations, and mental depression, when a chronic cough is also liable to be present. Four or five drops should be given with a tablespoonful of cold water, twice or three times in the day. The Black Radish is found useful against whooping cough, and is employed for this purpose in Germany, by cutting off the top, and then making a hole in the root. This is filled with treacle, or honey, and allowed to stand for a day or two; then a teaspoonful of the medicinal liquid is given two or three times in the day. Roman physicians advised that Radishes should be eaten raw, with bread and salt in the morning before any other food. And our poet Thomson describes as an evening repast:—

"A Roman meal
Such as the mistress of the world once found
Delicious, when her patriots of high note,
Perhaps by moonlight at their humble doors,
Under an ancient Oak's domestic shade,
Enjoy'd spare feast, a RADISH AND AN EGG."

RAGWORT.

THE Ragwort (*Senecio Jacobæa*) is a very common plant in our meadows, and moist places, closely allied to the

Groundsel, and well known by its daisy-like flowers, but of a golden yellow colour, with rays in a circle surrounding the central receptacle, and with a strong smell of honey.

This plant goes popularly by the name of St. James's wort, or Canker wort, or (near Liverpool) Fleawort, and in Yorkshire, Seggrum; also Jacoby and Yellow Top. The term Ragwort, or Ragweed, is a corruption of Ragewort, as expressing its supposed stimulating effects on the sexual organs. For the same reason the *pommes d'amour* (Love Apples, or Tomatoes) are sometimes called Rage apples. The Ragwort was formerly thought to cure the staggers in horses, and was hence named Stagger wort, or because, says Dr. Prior, it was applied to heal freshly cut young bulls, known as Seggs, or Staggs. So also it was called St. James's wort, either because that great warrior and saint was the patron of horses, or because it blossoms on his day, July 25th: sometimes also the plant has been styled Stammer wort. Furthermore it possesses a distinct reputation for the cure of cancer, and is known as Cankerwort, being applied when bruised, either by itself, or combined with Goosegrass.

Probably the lime which the whole plant contains in a highly elaborated state of subdivision has fairly credited it with anti-cancerous powers. For just such a reason Sir Spencer Wells commended powdered egg shells and powdered oyster shells as efficacious in curing certain cases under his immediate observation of long-standing cancer, when steadily given for some considerable time.

A poultice made of the fresh leaves, and applied externally two or three times in succession "will cure, if ever so violent, the old ache in the hucklebone known as sciatica." Chemically the active principle of the

Ragwort is "senecin," a dark resinous substance, of which two grains may be given twice or three times in the day.

Also the tincture, made with one part of the plant to ten parts of spirit of wine (tenuior), may be taken in doses of from five to fifteen drops, with a spoonful of water three times in the day.

Either form of medicine will correct monthly irregularities of women where the period is delayed, or difficult, or arrested by cold. It must be given steadily three times a day for ten days or a fortnight before the period becomes re-established. In suitable cases the Senecio not only anticipates the period, but also increases the quantity: and where the monthly time has never been established the Ragwort is generally found useful.

This herb—like its congener, the common Groundsel—has lancinated, juicy leaves, which possess a bitter saline taste, and yield earthy potash salts abundantly. Each plant is named "Senecio" because of the grey woolly pappus of its seeds, which resemble the silvered hair of old age. In Ireland the Ragwort is dedicated to the fairies, and is known as the Fairies' Horse, on the golden blossoms of which the good little people are thought to gallop about at midnight.

RASPBERRY.

THE Raspberry (*Rubus Idæus*) occurs wild plentifully in the woods of Scotland, where children gather the fruit early in summer. It is also found growing freely in some parts of England—as in the Sussex woods—and bearing berries of as good a quality as that of the cultivated Raspberry, though not so large in size.

Another name for the fruit is *Framboise*, which is

a French corruption of the Dutch word *brambezie*, or brambleberry.

Again, the Respis, or Raspberry, was at one time commonly known in this country as Hindberry, or the gentler berry, as distinguished from one of a harsher and coarser sort, the Hartberry. "Respberry" signifies in the Eastern Counties of England a shoot, or sucker, this name being probably applied because the fruit grows on the young shoots of the previous year.

Raspberry fruit is fragrant and cooling, but sugar improves its flavour. Like the strawberry, if eaten without sugar and cream, it does not undergo any acetous fermentation in the stomach, even with gouty or strumous persons. When combined with vinegar and sugar it makes a liqueur which, if diluted with water, is most useful in febrile disorders, and which is an excellent addition to sea stores as preventive of scurvy.

The Latins named this shrub "the bramble of Ida," because it grew in abundance on that classic mountain where the shepherd Paris adjudged to Venus the prize for beauty—a golden apple—on which was divinely inscribed the words, *Detur pulchriori*—"Let this be awarded to the fairest of womankind."

The fresh leaves of the Raspberry are the favourite food of kids. There are red, white, yellow, and purple varieties of this fruit. Heat develops the richness of its flavour; and Raspberry jam is the prince of preserves.

Again, a wine can be brewed from the fermented juice, which is excellent against scurvy because of its salts of potash—the citrate and malate.

Raspberry vinegar, made by pouring vinegar repeatedly over successive quantities of the fresh fruit, is a capital remedy for sore throat from cold, or of the relaxed kind; and when mixed with water it furnishes a most refreshing drink in fevers. But the berries should be used immediately after being gathered, as they quickly spoil, and their fine flavour is very evanescent. The vinegar can be extemporised by diluting Raspberry jelly with hot vinegar, or by mixing syrup of the fruit with vinegar.

In Germany a conserve of Raspberries which has astringent effects is concocted with two parts of sugar to one of juice expressed from the fruit. Besides containing citric and malic acids, the Raspberry affords a volatile oil of aromatic flavour, with crystallisable sugar, pectin, colouring matter, mucus, some mineral salts, and water.

Gerard says: "The fruit is good to be given to them that have weake, and queasie stomackes."

A playful example of the declension of a Latin substantive is given thus:—

"*Musa, Musa,*
The Gods were at tea:
Musæ, Musam,
Eating Raspberry jam:
Musa, Musāh,
Made by Cupid's mamma."

RHUBARB (Garden), *see* **Dock,** *page* 159.

RICE.

RICE, or Ryse, the grain of *Oryza sativa*, a native cereal of India, is considered here scarcely as a Herbal Simple, but rather as a common article of some medicinal resource in the store cupboard of every English household, and therefore always at hand as a vegetable remedy.

Among the Arabs Rice is considered a sacred food:

and their tradition runs that it first sprang from a drop of Mahomet's perspiration in Paradise.

Being composed almost exclusively of starch, and poorer in nitrogen, as well as in phosphoric acid, than other cereals, it is less laxative, and is of value as a demulcent to palliate irritative diarrhœa, and to allay intestinal distress.

A mucilage of Rice made by boiling the well-washed grain for some time in water, and straining, contains starch and phosphate of lime in solution, and is therefore a serviceable emollient. But when needed for food the grain should be steamed, because in boiling it loses the little nitrogen, and the greater part of the lime phosphate which it has scantily contained.

Rice bread and Rice cakes, simply made, are very light and easy of digestion. The gluten confers the property of rising on dough or paste made of Rice flour. But as an article of sustenance Rice is not well suited for persons of fermentative tendencies during the digestion of their food, because its starch is liable to undergo this chemical change in the stomach.

Dr. Tytler reported in the *Lancet* (1833), cases resembling malignant cholera from what he termed the *morbus oryzœus*, as provoked by the free and continued use of Rice as food. And Boutins, in 1769, published an account of the diseases common to the East Indies, in which he stated that when Rice is eaten more or less exclusively, the vision becomes impaired. But neither of these allegations seems to have been afterwards authoritatively confirmed.

Chemically, Rice consists of starch, fat, fibrin, mineral matter such as phosphate of lime, cellulose, and water.

A spirituous liquor is made in China from the grain of Rice, and bears the name "arrack."

Rice cannot be properly substituted in place of succulent green vegetables dietetically for any length of time, or it would induce scurvy. The Indians take stewed Rice to cure dysentery, and a decoction of the grain for the purpose of subduing inflammatory disorders.

Paddy, or Paddee, is Rice from which the husk has not been removed before crushing. It has been said by some that the cultivation of Rice lowers vitality, and shortens life.

In Java a special Rice-pudding is made by first putting some raw Rice in a conical earthen pot wide at the top, and perforated in its body with holes. This is placed inside another earthen pot of a similar shape but not perforated, and containing boiling water. The swollen Rice soon stops up the holes of the inner pot, and the Rice within becomes of a firm consistence, like pudding, and is eaten with butter, sugar, and spices.

An ordinary Rice-pudding is much improved by adding some rosewater to it before it is baked.

This grain has been long considered of a pectoral nature, and useful for persons troubled with lung disease, and spitting of blood, as in pulmonary consumption. The custom of throwing a shower of Rice after and over a newly married couple is very old, though wheat was at first the chosen grain as an augury of plenty. The bride wore a garland of ears of corn in the time of Henry the Eighth.

ROSES.

CERTAIN curative properties are possessed both by the Briar, or wild Dog Rose of our country hedges, and by the cultivated varieties of this queen of flowers in our Roseries. The word Rose means red, from the Greek *rodon*, connected also with *rota*, a wheel, which resembles the outline of a Rose. The name Briar is from the Latin *bruarium*, the waste land on which it grows. The first Rose, of a dark red colour, is held to have sprung from the blood of Adonis. The fruit of the wild Rose, which is so familiar to every admirer of our hedgerows in the summer, and which is the common progenitor of all Roses, is named Hips. "Heps maketh," says Gerard, "most pleasant meats or banquetting dishes, as tarts and suchlike, the concoction whereof I commit to the cunning cook, and teeth to eat them in the rich man's mouth."

Hips, derived from the old Saxon, *hiupa*, *jupe*, signifies the Briar rather than its fruit. They are called in some parts, "choops," or "hoops." The woolly down which surrounds the seeds within the Hips serves admirably for dispelling round worms, on which it acts mechanically without irritating the mucous membrane which lines the bowels.

When fully ripe and softened by frost, the Hips, after removal of their hard seeds, and when plenty of sugar is added, make a very nice confection, which the Swiss and Germans eat at dessert, and which forms an agreeable substitute for tomato sauce. Apothecaries employ this conserve in the preparing of electuaries, and as a basis for pills. They also officinally use the petals of the Cabbage Rose (*Centifolia*) for making Rose water, and the petals of the Red Rose (*Gallica*) for a cooling infusion, the brilliant colour of which is much improved by adding some diluted sulphuric acid; and of these petals they further direct a syrup to be concocted.

Next in development to the Dog Rose, or Hound's Rose, comes the Sweetbriar (Eglantine), with a delicate perfume contained under its glandular leaves. "*Frag-*

rantia ejus olei omnia alia odoramenta superest." This (*Rosa rubiginosa*) grows chiefly on chalk as a bushy shrub. Its poetic title, Eglantine, is a corruption of the Latin *aculeius*, prickly. A legend tells that Christ's crown of thorns was made from the Rose-briar, about which it has been beautifully said :—

> " Men saw the thorns on Jesus' brow,
> But Angels saw the Roses."

Pliny tells a remarkable story of a soldier of the Prætorian guard, who was cured of hydrophobia, against all hope, by taking an extract of the root of the *Kunoroddon*, Dog Rose, in obedience to the prayer of his mother, to whom the remedy was revealed in a dream ; and he says further, that it likewise restored whoever tried it afterwards. Hence came the title *Canina*. '*Parceque elle a longtemps été en vogue pour guerir de la rage.*"

But the term, Dog Rose, is generally thought to merely signify a flower of lower quality than the nobler Roses of garden culture.

The five graceful fringed leaflets which form the special beauty of the Eglantine flower and bud, have given rise to the following Latin enigma (translated):—

> " Of us five brothers at the same time born,
> Two from our birthday always beards have worn :
> On other two none ever have appeared,
> While our fifth brother wears but half a beard."

From Roses the Romans prepared wine and confections, also subtle scents, sweet-smelling oil, and medicines. The petals of the crimson French Rose, which is grown freely in our gardens, have been esteemed of signal efficacy in consumption of the lungs since the time of Avicenna, A.D. 1020, who states that he cured many patients by prescribing as much of the conserve as they could manage to swallow daily. It was combined with milk, or with some other light nutriment; and generally from thirty to forty pounds of this medicine had to be consumed before the cure was complete. Julius Cæsar hid his baldness at the age of thirty with Roman Roses.

"Take," says an old MS. recipe of Lady Somerset's, "Red Rose buds, and clyp of the tops, and put them in a mortar with ye waight of double refined sugar; beat them very small together, then put it up; must rest three full months, stirring onces a day. This is good against the falling sickness."

It is remarkable that while the blossoms of the Rose Order present various shades of yellow, white, and red, *blue* is altogether foreign to them, and unknown among them.

As the Thistle is symbolical of Scotland, the Leek of Wales, and the Shamrock of Ireland: so the sweet, pure, simple, honest Rose of our woods is the apt-chosen emblem of Saint George, and the frank, bonny, blushing badge of Merrie England.

The petals of the Cabbage Rose (*Centifolia*), which are closely folded over each other like the leaves of a cabbage, have a slight laxative action, and are used for making Rose-water by distillation, whether when fresh, or after being preserved by admixture with common salt. This perfumed water has long enjoyed a reputation for the cure of inflamed eyes, more commonly when combined with zinc, or with sugar of lead. Hahnemann quotes the same established practice as a tacit avowal that there exists in the leaves of the Rose some healing power for certain diseased conditions of the eyes, which virtue is really founded on the homœopathic property possessed by the Rose, of exciting a species of ophthalmia in healthy persons; as was observed by Echtius, Ledelius, and Rau.

It is recorded also in his *Organon of Medicine*, that persons are sometimes found to faint at the smell of Roses (or, as Pope puts it, to "die of a rose in aromatic pain"); whereas the Princess Maria cured her brother, the Emperor Alexius, who suffered from faintings, by sprinkling him with Rose-water, in the presence of his aunt Eudoxia.

The wealthy Greeks and Romans strewed Roses on the tombs of departed friends, whilst poorer persons could only afford a tablet at the grave bearing the prayer:

> "Sparge, precor, rosas super mea busta, viator."

> "Scatter Roses, I beseech you, over my ashes, O pitiful passer-by."

But nowadays many persons have an aversion to throwing a Rose into a grave, or even letting one fall in.

Roses and reticence of speech have been linked together since the time of Harpocrates, whom Cupid bribed to silence by the gift of a golden Rose-bud; and therefore it became customary at Roman feasts to suspend over the table a flower of this kind as a hint that the convivial sayings which were then interchanged were not to be talked of outside. What was spoken "sub vino" was not to be published "sub divo":

> "Est rosa flos veneris, cujus quo facta laterent
> Harpocrati, matris dona, dicavit amor;
> Inde rosam mensis hospes suspendit amicis,
> Conviva ut sub eâ dicta tacenda sciat."

For the same reason the Rose is found sculptured on the ceilings of banqueting rooms ; and in 1526 it began to be placed over Confessionals. Thus it has come about that the Rose is held to be the symbol of secrecy, as well as the flower of love, and the emblem of beauty: so that the significant phrase "sub rosa,"—under the Rose,—conveys a recognised meaning, understood, and respected by everyone. The bed of Roses is not altogether a poetic fiction. In old days the Sybarites slept upon mattresses which were stuffed with Rose petals: and the like are now made for persons of rank on the Nile.

A memorial brass over the tomb of Abbot Kirton, in Westminster Abbey, bears testimony to the high value he attached during life to Roses curatively :—

"Sis, Rosa, flos florum, morbis medicina meorum."

Many country persons believe, that if Roses and Violets are plentiful in the autumn, some epidemic may be expected presently. But this conclusion must be founded like that which says, "a green winter makes a fat churchyard," on the fact that humid warmth continued on late in the year tends to engender putrid ferments, and to weaken the bodily vigour.

Attar of Roses is a costly product, because consisting of the comparatively few oil globules found floating on the surface of a considerable volume of Rose-water thrice distilled. It takes five hundredweight of Rose petals to produce one drachm by weight of the finest Attar, which is preserved in small bottles made of rock crystal. The scent of the minutest particle of the genuine essence is very powerful and enduring :—

"You may break, you may ruin, the vase if you will,
But the scent of the Roses will hang round it still."

The inscription, *Rosamundi, non Rosa munda,* was graven on the tomb of fair Rosamund, the inamorata of Henry the Seventh :—

> " Hic jacet in tombâ Rosa Mundi, non Rosa munda ;
> Non redolet, sed olet quæ redolere solet."

> " Here Rose the graced, not Rose the chaste, reposes ;
> The smell that rises is no smell of Roses."

In Sussex, the peculiar excrescence which is often found on the Briar, as caused by the puncture of an insect, and which is known as the canker, or " robin redbreast's cushion," is frequently worn round the neck as a protective amulet against whooping cough. This was called in the old Pharmacopeias " Bedeguar," and was famous for its astringent properties. Hans Andersen names it the " Rose King's beard."

The Rosary was introduced by St. Dominick to commemorate his having been shown a chaplet of Roses by the Blessed Virgin. It consisted formerly of a string of beads made of Rose leaves tightly pressed into round moulds and strung together, when real Roses could not be had. The use of a chaplet of beads for recording the number of prayers recited is of Eastern origin from the time of the Egyptian Anchorites.

The Rock Rose (a *Cistus*), grows commonly in our hilly pastures on a soil of chalk, or gravel, bearing clusters of large, bright, yellow flowers, from a small branching shrub. These flowers expand only in the sunshine, and have stamens which, if lightly touched, spread out, and lie down on the petals. The plant proves medicinally useful, particularly if grown in a soil containing magnesia. A tincture is prepared (H.) from the whole plant, English or Canadian, which is useful for curing shingles, on the principle of its producing, when taken by healthy provers in doses of various potencies, a cutaneous outbreak on the trunk of the body closely resembling the characteristic symptoms of shingles, whilst attended with nervous distress, and with much burning of the affected skin. The plant has likewise a popular reputation for healing scrofula, and its tincture is beneficial for reducing enlarged glands, as of the neck and throat; also for strumous swelling of the knee joint, as well as of other joints. It is a "helianthemum" of the Sunflower tribe.

The Canadian Rock Rose is called Frostwort and Frostweed, because crystals of ice shoot from the cracked bark below the stem during freezing weather in the autumn.

A decoction of our plant has proved useful in prurigo (itching), and as a gargle for the sore throat of scarlet fever. For shingles, from five to ten drops of the tincture, third decimal strength, should be given with a spoonful of water three times a day.

ROSEMARY.

THE Rosemary is a well-known, sweet-scented shrub, cultivated in our gardens, and herb beds on account of its fragrancy and its aromatic virtues. It came originally from the South of Europe and the Levant, and was introduced into England before the Norman Conquest. The shrub (*Rosmarinus*) takes its compound name from *ros*, dew, *marinus*, belonging to the sea; in allusion to the grey, glistening appearance of the plant, and its natural locality, as well as its odour, like that of the sea. It is ever green, and bears small, pale, blue flowers.

Rosemary was thought by the ancients to refresh the memory and comfort the brain. Being a cordial herb it was often mentioned in the lays, or amorous ballads, of the Troubadours; and was called "Coronaria" because women were accustomed to make crowns and garlands thereof.

> "What flower is that which regal honour craves?
> Adjoin the Virgin: and 'tis strewn o'er graves."

In some parts of England Rosemary is put with the corpse into the coffin, and sprigs of it are distributed among the mourners at a funeral, to be thrown into the grave. Gay alludes to this practice when describing the burial of a country lass who had met with an untimely death :—

> "To show their love, the neighbours far and near
> Followed, with wistful looks, the damsel's bier;
> Sprigged Rosemary the lads and lasses bore,
> While dismally the Parson walked before;
> Upon her grave the Rosemary they threw,
> The Daisy, Butter flower, and Endive blue."

In *Romeo and Juliet*, Father Lawrence says :—

> "Dry up your tears, and stick your Rosemary
> On this fair corse."

The herb has a pleasant scent and a bitter, pungent taste, whilst much of its volatile, active principle resides in the calices of the flowers; therefore, in storing or using the plant these parts must be retained. It yields its virtues partially to water, and entirely to rectified spirit of wine.

In early times Rosemary was grown largely in kitchen gardens, and it came to signify the strong influence of the matron who dwelt there :—

> "Where Rosemary flourishes the woman rules."

The leaves and tops afford an essential volatile oil, but not so much as the flowers.

A spirit made from this essential oil with spirit of wine will help to renovate the vitality of paralyzed limbs, if rubbed in with brisk friction. The volatile oil includes a special camphor similar to that possessed by the myrtle. The plant also contains some tannin, with a resin and a bitter principle. By old writers it was said to increase the flow of milk.

The oil is used officinally for making a spirit of Rosemary, and is added to the compound tincture of Lavender, as well as to Soap liniment. By common consent it is agreed that the volatile oil (or the spirit) when mixed in washes will specially stimulate growth of the hair. The famous Hungary water, first concocted for a Queen of Hungary who, by its continual use, became effectually cured of paralysis, was prepared by putting a pound and a half of the fresh tops of Rosemary, when in full flower, into a gallon of proof spirit, which had to stand for four days, and was then distilled.

Hungary water (*l'eau de la reine d'Hongrie*) was formerly very famous for gout in the hands and feet. Hoyes says, the formula for composing this water, written by Queen Elizabeth's own hand in golden characters, is still preserved in the Imperial Library at Vienna.

An ounce of the dried leaves and flowers treated with a pint of boiling water, and allowed to stand until cold, makes one of the best hair washes known. It has the singular power of preventing the hair from uncurling when exposed to a damp atmosphere. The herb is used in the preparation of *Eau de Cologne*.

Rosemary wine, taken in small quantities, acts as a quieting cordial to a heart of which the action is excitable or palpitating, and it relieves any accompanying dropsy by stimulating the kidneys. This wine may be made by chopping up sprigs of Rosemary, and pouring on them some sound white wine, which after two or three days, may be strained off and used. By stimulating the nervous system it proves useful against the headaches of weak circulation and of languid health. "If a garlande of the tree be put around the heade it is a remedy for the stuffing of the head that cometh from coldness."

The green-leaved variety of Rosemary is the sort to be used medicinally. There are also silver and gold-leaved diversities. Sprigs of the herb were formerly stuck into beef whilst roasting as an excellent relish. A writer of 1707 tells of "Rosemary-preserve to dress your beef."

The toilet of the Ancients was never considered complete without an infusion, or spirit of Rosemary; and in olden times Rosemary was entwined in the wreath worn by the bride at the altar, being first dipped in scented water. Anne of Cleves, one of Henry the Eighth's wives, wore such a wreath at her wedding; and when people could afford it, the Rosemary branch presented to each guest was richly gilded.

The custom which prevailed in olden times of carrying a sprig of Rosemary in the hand at a funeral, took its rise from the notion of an alexipharmick or preservative powder in this herb against pestilential disorders; and hence it was thought that the smelling thereof was a powerful defence against any morbid effluvia from the corpse.

For the same reason it was usual to burn Rosemary in the chambers of the sick, just as was formerly done with frankincense, which gave the Greeks occasion to call the Rosemary *Libanotis.* In the French language of flowers this herb represents the power of rekindling lost energy. "The flowers of Rosemary," says an old author, "made up into plates (lozenges), with sugar, and eaten, comfort the heart, and make it merry, quicken the spirits, and make them more lively." "There's Rosemary for you—that's for remembrance! Pray you, love, remember!" says Ophelia in *Hamlet*. The spirit of Rosemary is kept by all druggists, and may be safely taken in doses of from twenty to thirty drops with a spoonful or two of water. Rosemary tea will soon relieve hysterical depression. Some persons drink it as a restorative at breakfast. It will help to regulate the monthly flow of women. An infusion of the herb mixed with poplar bark, and used every night, will make the hair soft, glossy, and strong.

In Northern Ireland is found the Wild Rosemary, or Marsh Tea (*Ledum palustre*), which has admirable curative uses, and from which, therefore, though it is not a common plant in England, a medicinal tincture (H.) is made with spirit of wine.

The herb belongs to the Rock Rose tribe, and contains citric acid, leditannic acid, resin, wax, and a volatile principle called "ericinol."

This plant is of singular use as a remedy for chilblains, as well as to subdue the painful effects of a sting from a wasp or bee; also to relieve gouty pains, which attack severely, but do not cause swelling of the part, especially as regards the fingers and toes. Four or five drops of the tincture should be taken for a dose with a tablespoonful of cold water, three or four times in the day; and linen rags soaked in a lotion made with a teaspoonful of the tincture added to half a tumblerful of cold water, should be kept applied over the affected part.

It equally relieves whitlows; and will heal punctured wounds, if arnica, or the Marigold, or St. John's Wort is not indicated, or of use. When tested by provers in large doses, it has caused a widespread eruption of eczema, with itching and tingling of the whole skin, extending into the mouth and air passages, and occasioning a violent spasmodic cough. Hence, one may fairly assume (and this has been found to hold good), that a gouty, spasmodic cough of the bronchial tubes, attended with gouty eczema, and with pains in the smaller joints, will be generally cured by tincture or infusion of the Wild Rosemary in small doses of a diluted strength, given several times a day, the diet at the same time being properly regulated. Formerly this herb was used in Germany for making beer heady; but it is now forbidden by law.

RUE.

THE wild Rue is found on the hills of Lancashire and Yorkshire, being more vehement in smell and in operation than the garden Rue. This latter, *Ruta graveolens*, (powerfully redolent), the common cultivated Rue of our kitchen gardens, is a shrub with a pungent aromatic odour, and a bitter, hot, penetrating taste, having leaves of a bluish-green colour, and remaining verdant all the year round. It is first mentioned as cultivated in England by Turner, in his *Herbal*, 1562, and has since become one of the best known and most widely grown Simples for medicinal and homely uses. The name *Ruta* is from the Greek *reuo*, to set free, because this herb is so efficacious in various diseases. The Greeks regarded Rue as an anti-magical herb, since it served to remedy the nervous indigestion and flatulence from which they suffered when eating before strangers: which infirmity they attributed to witchcraft. This herb was further termed of old "Serving men's joy," because of the multiplicity of common ailments which it was warranted to cure. It constituted a chief ingredient of the famous antidote of Mithridates to poisons, the formula of which was found by Pompey in the satchel of the conquered King. The leaves are so acrid, that if they be much handled they inflame the skin; and the wild plant possesses this acridity still more strongly.

Water serves to extract the virtues of the cultivated shrub better than spirit of wine is able to do. The juice of Rue is of great efficacy in some forms of epilepsy, operating for the most part insensibly, though sometimes causing vomiting or purging.

Piperno, a Neapolitan physician, in 1625, commended Rue as a specific against epilepsy and vertigo. For the former malady at one time some of this herb was suspended round the neck of the sufferer, whilst "forsaking the devil with all his works, and invoking the Lord Jesus." Goat's Rue, *Galega*, is likewise of service in epilepsy and convulsions.

If a leaf or two of Rue be chewed, a refreshing aromatic flavour will pervade the mouth, and any nervous headache, giddiness, hysterical spasm, or palpitation, will be quickly relieved. Two drachms of powdered Rue, if taken every day regularly as a dose for a long while together, will often do wonders. It was much used by the ancients, and Hippocrates commended it. The herb is strongly stimulating and anti-spasmodic; its most important constituent being the volatile oil, which contains caprinic, pelargonic, caprylic, and œnanthylic acids. The oxygenated portion is caprinic aldehyde. In too full doses the oil causes aching of the loins, frequent urination, dulness and weight of mind, flushes of heat, unsteadiness of gait, and increased frequency of the pulse, but with diminished force. Similar symptoms are produced during an attack of the modern epidemical influenza; as like-wise by oil of wormwood, and some other essential oils.

Externally, Rue is an active irritant to the skin, the bruised leaves blistering the hands, and causing a pustular eruption. Gerard says, "The wild Rue venometh the hands that touch it, and will also infect the face; therefore it is not to be admitted to meat, or medicine." It stimulates the monthly function in women, but must be used with caution.

The decoction and infusion are to be made from the fresh plant, or (when this plant cannot be got), the oil may be given in a dose of from one to five drops. Externally, compresses saturated with a strong decoction of the plant when applied to the chest, have been used beneficially for chronic bronchitis.

Rue is best adapted to those of phlegmatic habit, and of languid constitutional energies. It is often employed in the form of tea. The *Schola Salernitana* says about this plant:—

> "Ruta viris minuit venerem, mulieribus addit
> Ruta facit castum, dat lumen, et ingerit astum
> Coctaque ruta facit de pulicibus loca tuta."
>
> "Rue maketh chaste: and eke preserveth sight;
> Infuseth wit, and putteth fleas to flight."

The leaves promote the menses, being given in doses of from fifteen to twenty grains. "Pliny," says John Evelyn, "reports Rue to be of such effect for the preservation of sight that the painters of his time used to devour a great quantity of it; and the herb is still eaten by the Italians frequently mingled amongst their salads." With respect to its use in epilepsy, Julius Cæsar Baricellus said: "I gave to my own children two scruples of the juice of Rue, and a small matter of gold; and, by the blessing of God, they were freed from their fits." The essential oil of Rue may be used for the same purpose, and in like manner.

Formerly this plant was thought to bestow second sight; and so sacred a regard was at one time felt for it in our islands, that the missionaries sprinkled their holy water from brushes made of the Rue; for which cause it was named "Herb of Grace."

Gerard tells us: "The garden Rue, which is better than the wild Rue for physic's use, grows most profitably (as Dioscorides said) under a fig tree." Country people boil its leaves with treacle, thus making a conserve of them. These leaves are curative of croup in poultry.

In the early part of the present century it was customary for judges, sitting at Assize, to have sprigs of Rue placed on the bench of the dock, as defensive against the pestilential infection brought into court from gaol by the prisoners. The herb was supposed to afford powerful protection from contagion.

At the present time the medicinal tincture (H.) is used for the treatment of rheumatism when developed in the membranes which invest the bones.

If bruised and applied, the leaves will ease the severe pain of sciatica. The expressed juice taken in small quantities is a noted remedy for nervous nightmare. A quaint old rhyme says of the plant:—

"Nobilis est ruta quia lumina reddit acuta."

"Noble is Rue! it makes the sight of eyes both sharp and clear;
With help of Rue, oh! blear-eyed man! thou shalt see far and near."

This is essentially the case when the vision has become dim through over exertion of the eyes. It was with "Euphrasy and Rue" the visual nerve of Adam was purged by Milton's Angel.

As a preserver of chastity Ophelia was made by Shakespeare to give Rue to Hamlet's mother, the Queen of Denmark.

RUSHES.

THE true Rushes (*Juncaceæ*) include the Soft Rush (*effusus*); the Hard Rush (*glaucus*); and the Common Rush (*conglomeratus*). The Bulrush (Pool Rush) is a Sedge; the Club Rush is a Typha; and the flowering Rush, a Butomus. "Rish" was the old method of spelling the name.

A medicinal tincture is made (H.) from the fresh root of the *juncus effusus*. It will be found helpful against spinal irritability, with some crampy tightness felt in the arms and legs, together with headache and flatulent indigestion. Four or five drops should be given for a dose, with a spoonful of water, three or four times in the day.

This, the Soft Rush, is commonly used for tying the bines of hops to the poles; and, as these bines grow larger in size, the rushes wither, setting the bines free in a timely fashion. To find a green-topped Seave, or Rush, and a four-leaved Clover, is, in rural estimation, equally lucky.

The generic title, *Juncus*, has been applied because Rushes are *in conjunction* when plaited together for making cordage.

The common Rush is found by roadsides in damp pastures, and is readily known by its long, slender, round, naked stem, containing pith, and showing about the middle of July a dense globular head of brown flowers. Rushes of this sort were employed by our remote ancestors for strewing, when fresh and green, about the floor of the hall after discontinuing its big fire at Eastertide. Shakespeare says in *Romeo and Juliet*:—

> "Wantons, light of heart,
> Tickle the senseless rushes with their heels."

In obedience to a bequest (1494), Rushes are still strewn about the pavement of Redcliff Church at Bristol every Whit-Sunday. The common phrase, "not worth a Rush," took its origin from this general practice. Distinguished guests were honoured in mediæval times with clean fresh Rushes; but those of inferior rank had either the Rushes left by their superiors, or none at all.

The sweet-scented "Flag," or Rush (*Acorus calamus*), was always used by preference when it could be procured. It is a native of this country, growing on watery banks, and very plentiful in the rivers of Norfolk, from whence the London market is supplied. The roots have a warm, bitter taste, and the essential oil is highly aromatic, this being used for preparing aromatic vinegar. In Norfolk the powdered dry rhizome is given for ague. With sugar it makes an agreeable cordial conserve. (*See Flag (Sweet), page* 201). For preserving the aromatic qualities within the dried rhizome, or root, it should be kept in stock unpeeled. This contains "oleum calami," and the bitter principle "acorin." Some of the root may be habitually chewed for the relief of chronic indigestion. The odorous delights of a pastoral time passed near these sweetly-fragrant plants have been happily alluded to in the well-known lines of idyllic verse :—

> "Green grow the Rushes, oh!
> Green grow the Rushes, oh!
> The sweetest hours that e'er I spent
> Were spent among the lasses, oh!"

> "Virent junci fluviales,
> Junci prope lymphas:
> Ah! quam ridet quœ me vīdet
> Hora inter Nymphas!"

The old saying, "As fit as Tib's Rush for Tom's forefinger," alludes to an ancient custom of making spurious marriages with a ring constructed from a Rush. Tom and Tib were vulgar epithets applied in Shakespeare's time to the rogue, and the wanton.

The Bulrush (*Scirpus lacustris*) is a tall, aquatic plant, which belongs to the Sedge tribe. It name was formerly spelt "Pole Rush," and was given because this grows in pools of water, and not like other Rushes, in mire. Bottoms of chairs are frequently made with its stems. Its seed is prepared medicinally, being astringent and somewhat sedative; "So soporiferous," says Gerard, "that care must be had in the administration thereof, lest in provoking sleep you induce a drowsiness, or dead sleep." Street hawkers, in Autumn, offer as Bulrushes the tall, round spikes of the Great Reed Mace, which is not a true Rush. Artists are responsible in the first instance for the mistake—notably Paul De la Roche, in his famous picture of "The Finding of Moses." The future great leader of the Israelites is there depicted in an ark amid a forest of Great Cat's-tail Reeds.

The flowering Rush, or water gladiole, which grows by the banks of rivers is called botanically "butomus," from the Greek, *bous*, an ox, and *temno*, to cut, because the sharp edges of the erect three-cornered leaf-blades wound the cattle which come in contact with them, or try to eat them. Its root is highly esteemed in Russia for the cure of hydrophobia, being regarded by the doctors as a specific for that disease. Its flowers are large, and of a splendid rose colour. The seeds promote the monthly flow in women, act on disordered kidneys, prove astringent against fluxes, and serve to woo sleep in nervous wakefulness. Gerard tells that "the seed of Rushes drieth the overmuch flowing of women's termes."

The Reed Mace, or Cat's-tail, is often incorrectly called Bulrush, though it is a typha (*tuphos*, marsh) plant.

The Bog Asphodel (*Narthecium ossifragum*) grows in bogs, and bears a spike of yellow, star-like flowers. Its second nominative was given to signify its causing the bones of cattle which feed thereon to become soft; but probably this morbid state is incurred rather through the exhalations arising from the bogs where the cattle are pastured. To the same plant has been given also the name "Mayden heere," because young damsels formerly used it for making their hair yellow.

The Great Cat's-tail (*Typha palustris*), or Great Reed Mace, a perennial reed common in Great Britain, affords by the tender white part of its stalks when peeled near the root, a crisp, cooling, pleasant article of food. This is eaten raw with avidity by the Cossacks. Aristophanes makes mention of the Mace in his comedy of frogs who were glad to have spent their day skipping about *inter Cyperum et Phleum*, among Galingale and Cat's-tail. Sacred pictures which represent our Saviour wearing the crown of thorns, place this reed in His hands as given Him in mockery for a kingly Mace. The same *Typha* has been further called "Dunse-down," from making persons "dunch," or deaf, if its soft spikes accidentally run into the ears. "*Ejus enim paniculæ flos si aures intraverit, exsurdat.*" It is reasonable to suppose that, on the principle of similars, a preparation of this plant, if applied topically within the ear, as well as taken medicinally, will be curative of a like deafness. Most probably the injury to the hearing caused by the spikes at first is toxic as well as of the nature of an injury. The Poet Laureate sings of "Sleepy breath made sweet with Galingale" (*Cyperus longus*). Other names again are, "Chimney-sweeper's brush"; "Blackheads" until ripe, then "Whiteheads"; and "Water torch," because its panicles, if soaked in oil, will burn like a torch.

SAFFRON (Meadow and Cultivated).

THE Meadow Saffron (*Colchicum autumnale*) is a common wild Crocus found in English meadows, especially about the Midland districts. The flower appears in the autumn before the leaves and fruit, which are not produced until the following spring. Its corollæ resemble those of the true Saffron, a native of the East, but long cultivated in Great Britain, where it is sometimes found apparently wild. They are plants of the Iris order.

From the Meadow Saffron is obtained a corm or bulb, dug up in the spring, of which the well-known tincture of colchicum, a specific for rheumatism, is made; and from the true Saffron flowers are taken the familiar orange red stigmata, which furnish the fragrant colouring matter used by confectioners in cakes, and by the apothecary for his syrup of Saffron, etc.

The flower of the Meadow Saffron rises bare from the earth, and is, therefore, called "Upstart" and "Naked Lady." This plant owes its botanical name *Colchicum*, to Colchis, in Natalia, which abounded in poisonous vegetables, and gave rise to the fiction about the enchantress Medea. She renewed the vitality of her aged father, Æneas, by drawing blood out of his veins and refilling them with the juices of certain herbs. The fabled origin of the Saffron plant ran thus. A certain young man named Crocus went to play at quoits in a field with Mercurie, when the quoit of his companion happened by misfortune to hit him on the head, whereby, before long, he died, to the great sorrow of his friends. Finally, in the place where he had bled, Saffron was found to be growing: whereupon, the people, seeing the colour of the chine as it stood, adjusted it to come of the blood of Crocus, and therefore they gave it his name. The medicinal properties of Colchicum have been known from a very early period. In the reign of James the First (1615), Sir Theodore Mayerne administered the bulb to his majesty together with the powder of unburied skulls. In France, it has always been a favourite specific for gout; and during the reign of Louis the Fifteenth, it became very fashionable under the name of *Eau Médicinale;* but the remedy is somewhat dangerous, and should never be incautiously used. Instances are on record where fatal results have followed too large a medicinal dose, even on the following day, after taking sixty drops of the wine of Colchicum overnight; and when given in much smaller doses it sometimes acts as a powerfully irritating purgative, or as an emetic. The medicine should not be employed except by a doctor; its habitual use is very harmful.

The acrimony of the bulb may be modified in a measure if it, or its seeds, are steeped in vinegar before being taken as a medicine.

The French designate the roots of the Meadow Saffron (*Colchicum*) as "*Tue-chien*"; "*morte aux chiens,*" "death to dogs."

Alexander of Tralles, a Greek physician of the sixth century, was the first to advise Colchicum (*Hermodactylon*) for gout, with the effect that patients, immediately after its exhibition, found themselves able to walk. "But," said he, and with shrewd truth, "it has this bad property, that it disposes those who take it curatively for gout or rheumatism, to be afterwards more frequently attacked with the disease than before."

Our druggists supply an officinal tincture of Colchicum (Meadow Saffron) made from the seeds, the dose of which is from ten to thirty drops, with a spoonful of water; also a wine infused from the bulb, of which the dose is the same as that of the tincture, twice or three times a day; and an acetous extract prepared from the thickened juice of the crushed bulbs, of which from half to two grains may be given in a pilule, or dissolved in water, twice or three times a day, until the active symptoms are subdued, and then less often for another day or two afterwards. The most important chemical constituent of the bulb, flowers, and seeds, is "Colchicin." Besides this there are contained starch, gum, sugar, tannin, and some fatty resinous matter. There is also a fixed oil in the seeds.

Crocus vernus, the True Saffron, grows wild about Halifax, and in the neighbourhood of Derby; but for commercial uses the supply of stigmata is had from Greece, and Asia Minor. This plant was cultivated in England as far back as during the reign of Edward the Third. It is said that a pilgrim then brought from the Levant to England the first root of Saffron, concealed in a hollow staff, doing the same thing at the peril of his life, and planting such root at Saffron Walden, in Essex, whence the place has derived its name.

The stigmata are picked out, then dried in a kiln, over a hair cloth, and pressed afterwards into cakes, of which the aromatic quality is very volatile. The plant was formerly cultivated at Saffron Walden, where it was presented in silver cups by the Corporation to some of our Sovereigns, who visited Walden for the ceremony. Five guineas were paid by the Corporation for the pound of Saffron which they purchased for Queen Elizabeth; and to constitute this quantity forty thousand flowers were required. The City Arms of Walden bears three Saffron plants, as given by a Charter of Edward the Sixth. Saffron Hill, in Holborn, London, belonged formerly to Ely House, and got its name from the crops of Saffron which were grown there: "*Occultā Spolia hi Croceo de colle ferebant*" (*Comic Latin Grammar*).

In our rural districts there is a popular custom of giving Saffron tea in measles, on the doctrine of colour analogy; to which notion may likewise be referred the practice of adding Saffron to the drinking water of canaries when they are moulting.

In England, it was fashionable during the seventh century to make use of starch stained yellow with Saffron; and in an old cookery book of that period, it is directed that "Saffron must be put into all Lenten soups, sauces, and dishes; also that without Saffron we cannot have well-cooked peas." Confectioners were wont to make their pastry attractive with Saffron. So the Clown says in Shakespeare's *Winter's Tale*, "I must have Saffron to colour the warden pies." We read of a Saffron-tub in the kitchen of Bishop Swinfield, 1296. During the fourteenth century Saffron was cultivated in the herbarium of the manor-house, and the castle. Throughout Devonshire this product is quoted to signify anything costly.

Henry the Eighth forbade persons to colour with Saffron the long locks of hair worn then, and called Glibbes. Lord Bacon said, "the English are rendered sprightly by a liberal use of Saffron in sweetmeats and broth": also, "Saffron conveys medicine to the heart, cures its palpitation, removes melancholy and uneasiness, revives the brain, renders the mind cheerful, and generates boldness." The restorative plant has been termed "*Cor hominis;*" "*Anima pulmonum,*" "the Heart of Man"; and there is an old saying alluding to one of a merry temper, "*Dormivit in sacco Croci,*" "he has slept in a sack of Saffron." It was called by the ancients "*Aurum philosophorum,*" contracted to "*Aroph.*" Also, *Sanguis Herculis*, and *Rex Vegetabilium*, "being given with good success to procure bodily lust." The English word Saffron comes from the Arabian—*Zahafram*—whilst the name Crocus of this golden plant is taken from the Greek *krokee*—a thread—signifying the dry thin stigmata of the flower. Old Fuller wrote "the Crocodile's tears are never true save when he is forced where Saffron groweth (whence he hath his name of *Croco-deilos*, or the Saffron-fearer), knowing himself to be all poison, and it all antidote." Frequently Marigold stigmata are cheaply used for adulterating the true Saffron.

Homer introduces Saffron as one of the flowers which formed the nuptial couch of Jupiter: and Solomon mentioned it as growing in his garden: "Spikenard and saffron: calamus, and cinnamon" (*Canticles* iv., 14). Pliny states that wine in which Saffron was macerated gave a fragrant odour to theatres about which it was sprinkled. The Cilician doctors advised Cleopatra to take Saffron for clearing her complexion.

The medicinal use of Saffron has always obtained amongst the Orientals. According to a treatise, *Crocologia* (1670), by Hartodt, it was then employed as a medicine, as a pigment, and for seasoning various kinds of food. The colouring matter of Saffron is a substance called polychroite, or crocin; and its slightly stimulating properties depend upon a volatile oil.

Boerhaave said that Saffron possesses the power of liquefying the blood; hence, "Women who use it too freely suffer from immoderate menses." A tincture is made (H.) from the Saffron of commerce, which is of essential use for controlling female hæmorrhages. Four or five drops of the tincture may be given with a spoonful of water every three or four hours for this purpose. The same tincture is good for impaired vision, when there is a sense of gauze before the eyes, which the person tries to wink, or wipe away. Smelling strongly and frequently at the Hay Saffron of commerce (obtained from Spain and France), will cause headache, stupor, and heavy sleep; whilst, during its internal use, the urine becomes of a deep yellow colour.

Of the syrup of Saffron, which is a slightly stimulating exhilarant, and which possesses a rich colour, from one to two teaspoonfuls may be given for a dose, with two tablespoonfuls of cold water. It serves to energise the organs within the middle trunk of both males and females; also to recruit an exhausted brain.

In Devonshire, Saffron used to be regarded as a most valuable remedy to restore consumptive patients, even when far advanced in the disease, and it was, therefore, esteemed of great worth :—

"Nec poteris croci dotes numerare, nec usus."

"Saffron is such a special remedy for those that have consumption of the lungs, and are—as we term it—at death's door, and almost past breathing, that it bringeth breath again, and prolongeth life for certain days, if ten, or twenty grains at most, be given in new, or sweet wine. It presently, and in a moment, removeth away difficulty of breathing, which most dangerously and suddenly happeneth."

In Westphalia, an apple mixed with Saffron, on the doctrine of signatures, is given on Easter Monday, against jaundice. Evelyn tells us: "The German housewives have a way of forming Saffron into balls, by mingling it with a little honey, which, when thoroughly dried, they reduce to powder, and sprinkle it over their sallets for a noble cordial." Those of Spain and Italy, we know, generally make use of this flower, mingling its golden tincture with almost everything they eat. But, an excessive use of Saffron proves harmful. It will produce an intense pain in the head, and imperil the reason. Half-a-scruple, *i.e.*, ten grains, should be the largest dose. In fuller doses this tincture will provoke a determination of blood to the head, with bleeding from the nose, and sometimes with a disposition to immoderate laughter. Small doses, therefore, of the diluted tincture, ought to relieve these symptoms when they occur as spontaneous illness. The inhabitants of Eastern countries regard Saffron as a fine restorative, and nuptial invitations are often powdered by them with this medicament.

In Ireland women dye their sheets with Saffron to preserve them from vermin, and to strengthen their own limbs.

> "Green herbs, red pepper, mussels, *Saffron*,
> Soles, onions, garlic, roach and dace;
> All these you eat at Ferre's tavern
> In that one dish of bouillabaisse."
>
> —*Thackeray*.

SAGE.

OUR garden Sage, a familiar occupant of the English herb bed, was formerly celebrated as a medicine of great virtue. This was the *Elalisphakos* of the Greeks, so called from its dry and withered looking leaves. It grows wild in the South of Europe, but is a cultivated Simple in England, France, and Germany. Like other labiate herbs it is aromatic and fragrant, because containing a volatile, camphoraceous, essential oil.

All parts of the plant have a strong-scented odour, and a warm, bitter, astringent taste. The Latin name, *Salvia*, has become corrupted through *Sauja*, *sauge*, to Sage, and is derived from *salvere*, "to be sound," in reference to the medicinally curative properties of the plant.

A well-known monkish line about it ran to this effect: *Cur moriatur homo cui Salvia crescit in horto?* "Why should a man die whilst Sage grows in his garden?" And even at this time, in many parts of England, the following piece of advice is carefully adopted every year:—

"He that would live for aye
Must eat Sage in May."

During the time of Charlemagne, the school of Salerno thought so highly of Sage that they originated the dictum quoted above of Saracenic old pharmacy, but they wisely added a second line:—

"Contra vim mortis non est medicamen in hortis."

The essential oil of the herb may be more readily dissolved in a spirituous than in a watery vehicle. Of this, the active principle is "salviol," which confers the power of resisting putrefaction on animal substances; whilst the bitterness and condimentary pungency of the herb enable the stomach to digest rich, luscious meats and gravies, if it be eaten therewith.

Hence has arisen the custom of stuffing ducks for the table, and geese, with the conventional Sage and onions. Or there is no better way of taking Sage as a stomachic wholesome herb than by eating it with bread and butter. In Buckinghamshire a tradition maintains that the wife rules where Sage grows vigorously in the garden: and it is believed that this plant will thrive or wither, just as the owner's business prospers or fails. George Whitfield, when at Oxford (1733), took only Sage-tea, with sugar, and coarse bread.

Old sayings tell of the herb, as *Salvia salvatrix; naturæ conciliatrix;* and the line runs:—

> "Salvia cum rutâ faciunt tibi pocula tuta,"

recommending to plant Rue among the Sage so as to keep away noxious toads.

The Chinese are as fond of Sage as we are of their fragrant teas; and the Dutch once carried on a profitable trade with them, by exchanging a pound of Sage leaves for each three-pound parcel of tea.

It was formerly thought that Sage, if used in the making of cheese, improved its flavour.

> "Marbled with Sage the hardening cheese she pressed."
>
> —*Gay.*

"Sage," says Gerard, "is singular good for the head and brain; it quickeneth the senses and memory; strengtheneth the sinews; restoreth health to those that hath the palsy; and takes away shaky trembling of the members." Agrippa called it "the holy herb," because women with child, if they be likely to come before their time, "do eat thereof to their great good."

Pepys, in his well-known Diary says, "between Gosport and Southampton we observed a little churchyard where it is customary to sow all the graves with Sage." In *Franche Comte* the herb is supposed to mitigate grief, mental and bodily.

> "Salvia comfortat nervos, manuumque tremorem
> Tollit; et ejus ope febris acuta fugit."

> "Sage helps the nerves, and by its powerful might
> Palsy is cured, and fever put to flight."

But if Sage be smelt for some time it will cause a sort of intoxication, and giddiness. The leaves, when dried and smoked in a pipe as tobacco, will lighten the brain.

In Sussex, a peasant will munch Sage leaves on nine consecutive mornings, whilst fasting, to cure ague.

A strong infusion of the herb has been used with success to dry up the breast milk for weaning; and as a gargle Sage leaf tea, when sweetened with honey, serves admirably. This decoction, when made strong, is an excellent lotion for ulcers, and to heal raw abrasions of the skin. The herb may be applied externally in bags as a hot fomentation. Some persons value the Wormwood Sage more highly than either of the other varieties.

In the Sage flower the stamens swing round their loosely-connected anther cells against the back of any blundering bee who is in search of honey, just as in olden days the bag of sand caught the shoulders of a clumsy youth when tilting at the Quintin.

Wild Meadow Sage (*Salvia verbenaca*), or Meadow Clary, grows in our dry pastures, but somewhat rarely, though it is better known as a cultivated herb in our kitchen gardens. The leaves and flowers afford a volatile oil, which is fragrant and aromatic.

Some have attributed the name *Salvia sclarea*, Clary (Clear eye) to the fact of the seeds being so mucilaginous, that when the eye is invaded by any small foreign body, their decoction will remove the same by acting as an emulsion to lubricate it away. The leaves and flowers may be usefully given in an infusion for hysterical colic and similar troubles connected with nervous weakness. Also they make a pleasant fermented wine. The Wood Sage is the Wood Germander,

Teucrium scorodinia, a woodland plant with sage-like leaves, containing a volatile oil, some tannin, and a bitter principle. This plant has been used as a substitute for hops. It was called "hind heal" from curing the hind when sick, or wounded, and was probably the same herb as *Elaphoboscum*, the Dittany, taken by harts in Crete. A snuff has been made from its powder to cure nasal polypi: also the infusion (freshly prepared), should be given medicinally, two tablespoonfuls for a dose: or, of the powder, from thirty to forty grains. The name "Germander" is a corruption from Chamœdrys, *chamai*, ground, and *drus*, oak, because the leaves are like those of the oak.

SAINT JOHN'S WORT (*see page* 287).

SAVIN.

SAVIN, the Juniper Savin (*Sabina*), or Saffern, is a herb which grows freely in our bed of garden Simples, if properly cared for, and which possesses medicinal virtues of a potential nature. The shrub is a native of southern Europe, being a small evergreen plant, the twigs of which are densely covered with little leaves in four rows, having a strong, peculiar, unpleasant odour of turpentine, with a bitter, acrid, resinous taste. The young branchlets are collected for medicinal use. They contain tannin, resin, a special volatile oil, and extractive matters.

A medicinal tincture (H.) is made from the fresh leaves, and the points of the shoots of the cultivated Savin. But this is a powerful medicine, and must be used with caution. In small doses of two or three drops with a tablespoonful of cold water it is of singular efficacy for arresting an active florid flux from the womb at the monthly times of women when occurring too profusely, the remedy being given every two, three, or four hours. Or from one to four grains of powdered Savin may be taken instead of each dose of the tincture.

The stimulating virtues of Savin befit it for cleansing carbuncles, and for benefiting baldness. When mixed with honey it has removed freckles with success; the leaves, dried and powdered, serve, when applied, to dispel obstinate warty excrescences about the genitals.

Rubbed together with cerate, or lard, powdered Savin is used for maintaining the sores of blisters, and of issues, open when it is desired to keep up their derivative action.

The essential oil will stimulate the womb to functional activity when it is passively congested and torpid. As to its elementary composition this oil closely resembles the spirit of turpentine; and when given in small well diluted doses as a tincture (made of the oil mixed with spirit of wine), such medicine does good service in relieving rheumatic pains and swellings connected with impaired health of the womb. For these purposes the ordinary tincture (H.) of Savin should be mixed, one part thereof with nine parts of spirit of wine, and given in doses of from six to ten drops with a tablespoonful of water. Dr. Pereira says about the herb: "According to my own observation, Savin is the most certain and powerful stimulator of the monthly courses in the whole of our *Materia Medica*; and I never saw any ill effects result from its administration." The essential oil may be preferred in a dose of from one to four drops on sugar, or in milk, when this functional activity is sought.

Savin was known of old as the "Devil's Tree," and the "Magician's Cypress," because much affected by witches and sorcerers when working their spells.

SCURVY GRASS.

ONE of the most useful, but not best known, of the Cruciferous wild plants which are specifics against Scrofula is our English Scurvy Grass.

It grows by choice near the sea shore, or in mountainous places; and even when found many miles from the sea its taste is salt. It occurs along the muddy banks of the Avon; also in Wales, and in Cumberland, more commonly near the coast, and likewise on the mountains of Scotland; again it may be readily cultivated in the garden for medicinal uses. If eaten as a salad in its fresh state it is the most effectual of all the antiscorbutic plants.

The herb is produced with an angular smooth shining stem, twelve or fourteen inches high, having narrow green leaves, and terminating in thick clusters of white flowers. Its leaves are good and wholesome when eaten in spring with bread and butter. The juice, when diluted with water, makes a good mouth-wash for spongy gums.

The whole plant contains tannin, and a bitter principle, which is butyl-mustard oil, and on which the medicinal properties depend. This oil is of great volatility and penetrating power; one drop instilled on sugar, or dissolved in spirit, communicates to a quart of wine the taste and smell of Scurvy Grass.

The fresh plant taken as such, or the expressed fresh juice, confers the benefits of the herb in by far the most effectual way. A distilled water, and a conserve prepared with the leaves, were formerly dispensed by druggists; and the fresh juice mixed with that of Seville oranges went by the name of "spring drinks," or "juices."

The plant is found in large quantities at Lymington

(Hants), on low banks almost dipping into the sea. Its expressed juice was formerly taken in beer, or boiled in milk as a decoction, flavoured with pepper, aniseed, etc.

This Scurvy Grass has the botanical name *Cochlearia*, or, in English, Spoonwort, so named from its leaves resembling in shape the bowl of an old-fashioned spoon. It is supposed to be the famous *Herba Britannica* of the ancients. Our great navigators have borne unanimous testimony to its never-failing value in scurvy; and it has been justly noticed that the plant grows most plentifully in altitudes where scurvy is specially troublesome and frequent. The green herb bruised may be applied as a poultice.

For making a decoction of the plant as a blood purifier, and against scurvy, put two ounces of the whole plant and its roots into a quart jug, and fill up with boiling water, taking care to keep this well covered. When it is cold take a wineglassful thereof three, or four times in the day.

Another name for the plant is Scruby grass. The fresh herb has a strong pungent odour when bruised, and a warm bitter taste. Its beneficial uses in scurvy, are due to the potash salts which it contains. Externally, the juice will cleanse and heal foul ulcers, and ill-favoured eruptions.

SEA PLANTS and SEA WEEDS.

OF marine plants commonly found, the Samphire and the Sea Holly have certain domestic and medicinal uses which give them a position as Simples; and of the more ordinary Sea Weeds (cryptogamous, or flowerless plants) some few are edible, though sparingly nutritious, whilst curative and medicinal virtues are attributed to several others, as Irish Moss, Scotch Dulse, Sea Tang, and the

Bladderwrack. It may be stated broadly that the Sea Weeds employed as remedial Simples owe their powers to the bromine, iodine, and sulphate of soda which they contain. Pliny and Dioscorides in their days extolled the qualities of various Sea Weeds; and practitioners of medicine on our sea coasts are now unanimous in pronouncing Sea Weed liniments, and poultices, as of undoubted value in reducing glandular swellings, and in curing obstinate sprains; whilst they administer the Bladderwrack, etc., internally for alterative purposes with no little success. Bits of Sea Weed, called Ladies' trees, are still to be seen as chimney ornaments in many a Cornish cottage, being fixed on small stands, and supposed to protect the dwelling from fire, or other mishaps.

Samphire, of the true sort, is a herb difficult to be gathered, because it grows only out of the crevices of lofty perpendicular rocks which cannot be easily scaled. This genuine Samphire (*Crithmum maritimum*) is a small plant, bearing yellow flowers in circular umbels on the tops of the stalks, which flowers are followed by seeds like those of the Fennel, but larger.

The leaves are juicy, with a warm aromatic taste, and may be put into sauce; or they make a good appetising condimentary pickle, which is wholesome for scrofulous subjects. Persons living by the coast cook this plant as a pot herb. Formerly, it was regularly cried in the London streets, and was then called Crest Marine.

Shakespeare alludes in well-known lines to the hazardous proceedings of the Samphire gatherer's "dreadful trade":—

> "How fearful
> And dizzy 'tis to cast one's eyes so low!
> The crows and choughs that wing the midway air
> Show scarce so gross as beetles: half-way down
> *Hangs one that gathers Samphire*: dreadful trade!
> Methinks he seems no bigger than his head."—*King Lear.*

And Evelyn has praised the plant for excellence of flavour, as well as for aromatic virtues against the spleen. Pliny says Samphire is the very herb that the good country wife Hecate prepared for Theseus when going against the Bull of Marathon.

Its botanic name is from the Greek *crithe*, "barley," because the seeds are thought to resemble that grain. The title Samphire is derived from the French *Herbe de St. Pierre*, because the roots strike deep in the crevices of rocks. St. Peter's Wort has become corrupted to Sampetre, Sampier, and Samphire.

A spurious Samphire, the *Inula crithmoides*, or Golden Samphire, is often supplied in lieu of the real plant, though it has a different flavour, and few of the proper virtues. This grows more abundantly on low rocks, and on ground washed by salt water. Also a Salicornia, or jointed Glasswort, or Saltwort, or Crabgrass, is sold as Samphire for a pickle, in the Italian oil shops.

Gerard says of Samphire: "It is the pleasantest sauce, most familiar, and best agreeing with man's body." "Preferable," adds Evelyn, "for cleansing the passages, and sharpening appetite, to most of our hotter herbs, and salad ingredients."

The Sea Holly (*Eryngium maritimum*), or Sea Hulver, is a well-known prickly sea-green plant, growing in the sand on many parts of our coasts, or on stony ground, with stiff leaves, and roots which run to a great length among the sand, whilst charged with a sweetish juice.

A manufactory for making candied roots of the Sea Holly was established at Colchester, by Robert Burton, an apothecary, in the seventeenth century, as they were considered both antiscorbutic, and excellent for health.

Gerard says: "The roots, if eaten, are good for those that be liver sick; and they ease cramps, convulsions, and the falling sickness. If condited, or preserved with sugar, they are exceeding good to be given to old and aged people that are consumed and withered with age, and which want natural moisture." He goes on to give an elaborate receipt how to condite the roots of Sea Holly, or Eringos (which title is, according to Liddell and Scott, the diminutive of *eerungos*, "the beard of a goat." Or, Eryngo has been derived from the Greek *eruggarein*, to eructate, because the plant is, according to herbalists, a specific against belching). With healthy provers, who have taken the Sea Holly experimentally in *toxical* doses of varying strength the sexual energies and instincts became always depressed. This accounts for the fact that during the Elizabethan era the roots of the plant used *in moderation* were highly valued for renovating masculine vigour, such as Falstaff invoked, and which classic writers have extolled:—

> "Non male tum graiis florens eryngus in hortis
> Quæritur; hunc gremio portet si nupta virentem
> Nunquam inconcessos conjux meditabitur ignes."
>
> —*Rapinus.*

These Eryngo roots, prepared with sugar, were then called "Kissing Comfits." Lord Bacon when recommending the yolks of eggs for giving strength if taken with Malmsey, or sweet wine, says: "You shall doe well to put in some few slices of Eringium roots, and a little Ambergrice: for by this means, besides the immediate facultie of nourishment, such drinke will strengthen the back."

Plutarch writes: "They report of the Sea Holly, if one goat taketh it into her mouth, it causeth her first to stand still, and afterwards the whole flock, until such time as the shepherd takes it from her. Boerhaave thought the root "a principal aperient."

Irish Moss, or *Carraigeen*, is abundant on our rocky coasts, and is collected on the north western shores of Ireland, while some of it comes to us from Hamburg. Its chief constituent is a kind of mucilage, which dissolves to a stiff paste in boiling water, this containing some iodine, and much sulphur. But before being boiled in water or milk, the Moss should be soaked for an hour or more in cold water. Officinally, a decoction is ordered to be made with an ounce of the Moss to a pint of water: of which from one to four fluid ounces may be taken for a dose.

This Lichen contains starchy, heat-giving nourishment, about six parts of the same to one of flesh-forming food; therefore its jelly is found to be specially sustaining to persons suffering from pulmonary consumption, with an excessive waste of the bodily heat. At one time the Irish Moss fetched as high a price as half-a-crown for the pound. It bears the botanical name of *Chondrus crispus*, and varies much in size and colour. When growing in small pools, it is shallow, pale, and stunted; whilst when found at the bottom of a deep pool, or in the shadow of a great rock, it occurs in dense masses of rich ruddy purple, with reddish green thick fronds.

Iceland Moss contains the form of starch called "lichenin." It is a British lichen found especially in Wales and Scotland. Most probably the Icelanders were the first to learn its helpful properties. In two kinds of pulmonary consumption this lichen best promotes a cure—that with active bleeding from the lungs, and that with profuse purulent expectoration. The Icelanders boil the Moss in broth, or dry it in cakes used as bread. They likewise make gruel of it mixed with milk: but the first decoction of it in water, being purgative, is always thrown away. An ounce of the Iceland Moss boiled for a quarter-of-an-hour in a pint of milk, or water, will yield seven ounces of thick mucilage. This has been found particularly useful in dysentery. Also contained in the Moss are cetrarin, uncrystallizable sugar, gum, and green wax; with potash, and phosphate of lime. It affords help in diabetes, and for general atrophy; being given also in powder, or syrup, or mixed with chocolate. Francatelli directs for making *Iceland Moss Jelly*. Boil four ounces of the Moss in one quart of water: then add the juice of two lemons, and a bit of the rind, with four ounces of sugar (and perhaps a gill of sherry ?). Boil up and remove the scum from the surface. Strain the jelly through a muslin bag into a basin, and set it aside to become cold. It may be eaten thus, but it is more efficacious when taken warm. A Sea-Moss, the *Lichen marinum*, is "a singular remedy to strengthen the weakness of the back." It is called "Oister-green."

In New England the generic term "Moss" is a cant word signifying money: perhaps as a contraction of Mopuses, or as a play on the proverb, "a rolling stone gathers no moss."

The Dulse is used in Scotland and Ireland both as food and medicine. Botanically it bears the name of *Iridea edulis*, or *Rhodymenia palmata* (the sugar *Fucus* of Iceland).

There is a saying in Scotland: "He who eats of the Dulse of Guerdie, and drinks of the wells of Kindingie, will escape all maladies except black death." This marine weed contains within its cellular structure much iodine, which makes it a specific remedy for scrofulous glandular enlargements, or morbid deposits.

In Ireland the Dulse is first well washed in fresh water, and exposed in the air to dry, when it gives out a white powdery substance, which is sweet and palatable, covering the whole plant. The weed is presently packed in cases, and protected from the air, so that being thus preserved, it may either be eaten as it is, or boiled in milk, and mixed with flour of rye. The powdery substance is "mannite," which is abundant likewise on many of our Sea Weeds.

Cattle and sheep are very fond of Dulse, for which reason in Norway it is known as Soudsell, or Sheep's Weed. This *Iridea edulis* is pinched with hot irons by the fishermen in the south west of England, so as to make it taste like an oyster. In Scotland it is roasted in the frying-pan.

The Maritime Sea Tang (*Laminaria digitata*) was belauded in the *Proverbial Philosophy* of Martin Tupper:—

> "Health is in the freshness of its savour; and it cumbereth the beach with wealth;
> Comforting the tossings of pain with its violet tinctured essence."

Tang signifies Anglo-Saxon "thatch," from Sea Weed having been formerly used instead of straw to cover the roofs of houses. When bruised and applied by way of a poultice to scrofulous swellings and glandular tumours, the Sea Tang has been found very valuable. The famous John Hunter was accustomed to employ a poultice of sea water and oatmeal.

This weed is of common marine growth, consisting of a wide smooth brown frond, with a thick round stem, and broad brown ribbons like a flag at the end of it. It is familiarly known as Seagirdles, Tangle, Sea Staff, Sea Wand, and Cows' Tails. Fisher boys cut up the stems as handles for knives, or hooks, because, after the haft of the blade is inserted within the stem, this dries, and contracts on the iron staple, becoming densely hard and firm.

The absorbent stem power of the *Laminaria* for taking up iodine is very large; and this element is afterwards brought out by fire in the kelp kilns of Ireland and Scotland. Sea Tang acts most beneficially against the various forms of scrofulous disease; and signally relieves some rheumatic affections. It is also used largely in the making of glass.

Likewise for scrofula, seawater, being rich in chlorides and iodides, has proved both curative and preventive. Dr. Sena, of Valencia, gave bread made with sea-water in the Misericordia Hospital for cases of scrofulous disease, and other states of defective nutrition, with singular success.

Another Laminaria (*Saccharina*), with a single olive yellow semi-transparent frond, yields an abundance of sweet "mannit" when boiled and evaporated.

The Bladderwrack (*Fucus vesiculosus*), Kelpware, or Our Lady's Wrack, is found on most of our sea coasts in heavy brown masses of coarse-looking Sea Weed, which cover, and shelter many small algæ. Kelp is an impure carbonate of soda containing sulphate, and chloride of sodium, with a little charcoal.

By its characteristic bladders, or vesicles studded about the blades of the branched narrowish fronds, this Sea Weed may be easily known.

These bladders are full of a glutinous substance, which makes the weed valuable both as a remedy for the glandular troubles of scrofula, and, when bottled in rum, as an embrocation, such as is specially useful for strengthening the limbs of rickety, or bandy-legged children. Against glandular swellings also the weed is taken internally as a medicine, when burnt to a black powder. An analysis of the Bladderwrack has shown it to contain an empyreumatic oil, sulphur, earthy salts, some iron, and iodine freely. Thus it is very rich in anti-scrofulous elements.

The fluid extract of this Sea Weed has the long standing reputation of safely diminishing an excess of personal fat. It is given for such a purpose three times a day, shortly after meals, in doses of from one to four teaspoonfuls. The remedy should be continued perseveringly, whilst cutting down the supplies of fat, starchy foods, sugar, and malt liquors. When thus taken (as likewise in the concentrated form of a pill, if preferred) the Bladderwrack will especially relieve rheumatic pains; and the sea pod liniment dispensed by many druggists at our chief marine health resorts, proves signally efficacious towards the same end. Furthermore, they prepare a sea-pod essence for applying on a wet compress beneath waterproof tissue to strumous tumours, goitre, and bronchocele; also for old strains and bruises.

This Sea Weed should not be obtained when too fully matured, as it quickly undergoes decomposition.

Wrack is Sea Weed thrown ashore, from *Vrage*, to reject. Wrack Grass (*Zostera Marina*), is a marine plant with long grass-like leaves.

There are four common *Fuci* on our coasts—the *Nodosus* (Knobbed Wrack), the *Vesiculosus* (Bladder Wrack), the *Serratus* (Saw-edged Sea Weed), and the *Caniculatus* (Channeled Sea Weed).

It is by reason of its contained bromine and iodine as safe medicinal elements, the *Fucus vesiculosus* acts in reducing fatness; these elements stimulating all the absorbent glands of the body to increased activity.

In common with the other *Fuci* it furnishes mannite, an odorous oil, a bitter principle, mucilage, and ash, this last constituent abounding in the bromine and iodine.

For internal use, a decoction may be made with from two to four drachms of the weed to a pint of water, boiled together for a few minutes; and for external application to enlarged or hardened glands, the bruised weed may be applied as a cold poultice.

This Bladder Wrack is reputed to be the *Anti-polyscarcique* nostrum of Count Mattæi.

Although diminishing fat it does no harm by inducing any atrophied wasting of the breast glands, or of the testicles.

The Bladderwrack yields a rich produce to the seaside agriculturist highly useful as manure for the potato field and for other crops: and it is gathered for this purpose all along the British coast. In Jersey and Guernsey it is called *vraic*. Among the Hebrides, cheeses, whilst drying, are covered with the ashes of this weed which abounds in salt. Patients who have previously suffered much from rheumatism about the body and limbs have found themselves entirely free from any such pains or trouble whilst taking the extract of *Fucus Vesiculosus* (Bladderwrack). This Sea Weed is in perfection only during early and middle summer. For fresh sprains and bruises a hot decoction of the Bladderwrack should be used at first as a fomentation; and, afterwards, a cold essence of the weed should be rubbed in, or applied on wet lint beneath light thin waterproof tissue, or oiled silk, as a compress: this to be changed as often as hot or dry.

Laver is the popular name given to some edible Sea Weeds—the *Porphyra lanciniata*, and the *Ulva latissima*. The same title was formerly bestowed by Pliny on an aquatic plant now unknown, and called also Sloke, or Sloken.

Porphyra, from a Greek word meaning "purple," is the true Laver, or Sloke. It is slimy, or semi-gelatinous of consistence when served at table, having been stewed for several hours until quite tender, and then being eaten with butter, vinegar, and pepper. At the London Reform Club Laver is provided every day in a silver saucepan at dinner, garnished with lemons, to flank the roast leg of mutton. Others prefer it cooked with leeks and onions, or pickled, and eaten with oil and lemon juice. The Englishman calls this Sea Weed, Laver; the Irishman, Sloke; the Scotchman, Slack; and the student, *Porphyra*. It varies in size and colour between tidemarks, being sometimes long and ribbon-like, of a violet or purple hue; sometimes long and broad, whilst changing to a reddish purple, or yellow.

It is very wholesome, and preventive of scurvy, being therefore valuable on sea voyages, as it will keep good for a long time in closed tin vessels.

The *Ulva latissima* is a deep-green Sea Weed, called by the fishermen Oyster Green, because employed to cover over oysters. This is likewise known as Laver, because sometimes substituted by epicures for the true Laver (*Porphyra*) when the latter cannot be got; but it is not by any means as good. The name *Ulva* is from *ul*, meaning "water."

Sea Spinach (*Salsolacea—Spirolobea*) is a Saltwort found growing on the shore in Hampshire and other parts of England, the best of all wild vegetables for the table, having succulent leaves shaped like worms, and being esteemed as an excellent antiscorbutic.

The Sea Beet—a Chenopod—which grows plentifully on our shores, gave origin to the cultivated Beetroot of our gardens. Its name was derived from a fancied resemblance borne by its seed vessels when swollen with seed to the Greek letter B (*beta*).

> "Nomine cum Graio cui litera proxima primœ
> Pangitur in cerâ docti mucrone magistri."
>
> "The Greeks gave its name to the Beet from their alphabet's second letter,
> As an Attic teacher wrote it on wax with a sharp stiletto."

By the Grecians the Beet was offered on silver to Apollo in his temple at Delphi. A pleasant wine may be made from its roots, and its juice when applied with a brush is an excellent cosmetic. The Mangel Wurzel, also a variety of Beet, means literally, "scarcity root."

Another Sea Weed, the Bladderlocks (*Alaria esculenta*), "henware," "honeyware," "murlins," is edible, the thick rib which runs through the frond being the part chosen. This abounds on the Northern coasts of England and Scotland, being of a clear olive yellow colour, with a stem as thick as a small goosequill, varying in length, with its fronds, from three to twenty feet. The fruit appears as if partially covered with a brown crust consisting of transparent spore cases set on a stalk in a cruciform manner.

Common Coraline (*Corallina Anglica*), a Sea Weed of a whitish colour, tinged with purple and green, and of a firm substance, is famous for curing worms.

The presence of gold in sea water, even as surrounding our own islands, has been sufficiently proved; though, as yet, its extraction is a costly and uncertain process. One analyst has estimated that the amount of gold contained in the oceans of the globe must be ten million tons, without counting the possible quantity locked up in floating icebergs about the Poles.

Professor Liveredge, of the Sydney University, examined sea water collected off the Australian coast, as also some from Northern shores, and obtained gold, from five-tenths to eight-tenths of a grain per ton of the sea water. It occurs as the chloride, and the bromide of gold; which salts, as recently shown by Dr. Compton Burnett, when administered in doses almost infinitesimally small, are of supreme value for the cure of epilepsy, secondary syphilis, sexual debility, and some disorders of the heart.

Dr. Russell wrote on the uses of sea water in diseases of the glands. He found the soapy mucus within the vesicles of the Bladderwrack an excellent resolvent, and most useful in dispersing scrofulous swellings. He advises rubbing the tumour with these vesicles bruised in the hand, and afterwards washing the part with sea water.

SELFHEAL.

SEVERAL Herbal Simples go by the name of Selfheal among our wild hedge plants, more especially the Sanicle, the common Prunella, and the Bugle.

The first of these is an umbelliferous herb, growing frequently in woods, having dull white flowers, in panicled heads, which are succeeded by roundish seeds covered with hooked prickles: the Wood Sanicle (*Europœa*).

It gets its name Sanicle, perhaps, from the Latin verb *sanare*, "to heal, or make sound;" or, possibly, as a corruption of St. Nicholas, called in German *St. Nickel*, who, in the *Tale of a Tub*, is said to have interceded with God in favour of two children whom an innkeeper had murdered and pickled in a pork tub; and he obtained their restoration to life.

Anyhow, the name Sanicle was supposed in the middle ages to mean "curative," whatever its origin:

thus, *Qui a la Bugle, et la Sanicle fait aux chirurgiens la nicle*—"He who uses Sanicle and Bugle need have no dealings with the doctor." Lyte and other herbalists say concerning the Sanicle: "It makes whole and sound all wounds and hurts, both inward and outward."

> "Celui qui Sanicle a
> De plaie affaire il n'a."
> "Who the Sanicle hath
> At the surgeon may laugh."

The name Prunella (which belongs more rightly to another herb) has been given to the Sanicle, perhaps, through its having been originally known as Brunella, Brownwort, both because of the brown colour of its spikes, and from its being supposed to cure the disease called in Germany *die braune*, a kind of quinsy; on the doctrine of signatures, because the corolla resembles a throat with swollen glands.

The Sanicle is popularly employed in Germany and France as a remedy for profuse bleeding from the lungs, bowels, womb, and urinary organs; also for the staying of dysenteric diarrhœa. The fresh juice of the herb may be given in tablespoonful doses.

As yet no analysis has been made of this plant; but evidence of tannin in its several parts is afforded by the effects produced when these are remedially applied.

The *Prunella vulgaris* is a distinct plant from the Self Heal, or Sanicle, and belongs to the labiate order of herbs. It grows commonly in waste places about England, and bears pink flowers, being sometimes called Slough heal. This is incorrect, as the surgical term "slough" was not used until long after the Prunella and the Sanicle became named Self-heal. Each of these was applied as a vulnerary, not to sloughing sores, but to fresh cut wounds.

The *Prunella vulgaris* has a flattened calyx, and whorls of purplish blue flowers, which are collected in a head. It is also known as Carpenter's Herb, perhaps, from its corolla, when seen in profile, being shaped like a bill hook ; and therefore, on the doctrine of signatures, it was supposed to heal wounds inflicted by edge tools ; whence it was likewise termed Hook-heal and Sicklewort, and in Yorkshire, Black man.

By virtue of its properties as a vulnerary it has also been called *Consolida ;* but the daisy is the true *Consolida minor.*

"The decoction of Prunell," says Gerard, "made with wine and water, doth join together and make whole and sound all wounds, both inward and outward, even as Bugle doth. To be short, it serveth for the same that the Bugle serveth ; and in the world there are not two better wound herbs, as hath been often proved."

The Bugle, or middle Comfrey, is also a Sanicle, because of its excellence for healing wounds, in common with the Prunella and the true Sanicle. It grows in almost every wood, and copse, and moist shadowy place, being constantly reckoned among the Consounds.

This herb (*Ajuga reptans*) is of the labiate order, bearing dark blue or purple flowers, whorled, and crowded into a spike. Its decoction, "when drunk, healeth and maketh sound all wounds of the body." "It is so singular good for all sorts of hurts that none who know its usefulness will be ever without it. If the virtues of it make you fall in love with it (as they will if you be wise), keep a syrup of it to take inwardly, and an ointment and plaister of it to use outwardly, always by you."

The chemical principles of the Prunella and the Bugle

resemble those of other Labiate herbs, comprising a volatile oil, some bitter principle, tannin, sugar, and cellulose. The Ladies' Mantle, Alchemilla—a common inconspicuous weed, found everywhere—is called Great Sanicle, also Parsley-breakstone, or Piercestone, because supposed to be of great use against stone in the bladder. It contains tannin abundantly, and is said to promote quiet sleep if placed under the pillow at night. "*Endymionis somnum dormire.*"

SHEPHERD'S PURSE.

THE small Shepherd's Purse (*Bursa Capsella Pastoris*) is one of the most common of wayside English weeds. The name *Capsella* signifies a little box, in allusion to the seed pods. It is a Cruciferous plant, made familiar by the diminutive pouches, or flattened pods at the end of its branching stems. This herb is of natural growth in most parts of the world, but varies in luxuriance according to soil and situation, whilst thickly strewn over the whole surface of the earth, facing alike the heat of the tropics, and the rigours of the arctic regions; even, if trodden underfoot, it rises again and again with ever enduring vitality, as if designed to fulfil some special purpose in the far-seeing economy of nature. It lacks the winged valves of the *Thlaspi*.

Our old herbalists called it St. James's Wort, as a gift from that Saint to the people for the cure of various diseases, St. Anthony's Fire, and several skin eruptions. In France, too, the plant goes by the title of *Fleur de Saint Jacques.* It flowers from early in Spring until Autumn, and has, particularly in Summer, an acrid bitter taste. Other names for the herb are, "Case weed," "Pick pocket," and "Mother's heart," as called so by children. If a pod is picked they raise the cry, "You've plucked out your mother's heart." Small birds are fond of the seeds.

Bombelon, a French chemist, has reported most favourably about this herb as of prompt use to arrest bleedings and floodings, when given in the form of a fluid extract, one or two teaspoonfuls for a dose. He explains that our hedge-row Simple contains a tannate, an alkaloid "bursine," (which resembles sulphocyansinapine), and bursinic acid, this last constituent being the active medicinal principle. English chemists now prepare and dispense the fluid extract of the herb. This is given for dropsy in the U. S. America as a diuretic; from half to one teaspoonful in water for a dose.

Dr. Von Ehrenwall relates a recent case of female flooding, which had defied all the ordinary remedies, and for which, at the suggestion of a neighbour, he tried an infusion of the Shepherd's Purse weed, with the result that the bleeding stopped after the first teacupful of the infusion had been taken a few minutes. Since then he has used the plant in various forms of hæmorrhage with such success that he considers it the most reliable of our medicines for staying fluxes of blood. "Shepherd's Purse stayeth bleeding in any part of the body, whether the juice thereof be drunk, or whether it be used poultice-like, or in bath, or any way else."

Besides the ordinary constituents of herbs, it is found to contain six per cent. of soft resin, together with a sulphuretted volatile oil, which is identical with that of Mustard, as obtained likewise from the bitter Candytuft, *Iberis amara*.

Its medicinal infusion should be made with an ounce of the plant to twelve ounces of water, reduced by boiling to half-a-pint; then a wineglassful may be given for a dose.

The herb and its seeds were employed in former times to promote the regular monthly flow in women.

It bears, further, the name of Poor Man's Permacetty (or Spermaceti), "the sovereignst remedy for bruises;"—"perhaps," says Dr. Prior, "as a joke on the Latin name *Bursa pastoris*, or 'Purse,' because to the poor man this is always his best remedy." And in some parts of England the Shepherd's Purse is known as Clapper Pouch, in allusion to the licensed begging of lepers at our crossways in olden times with a bell and a clapper. They would call the attention of passers-by with the bell, or with the clapper, and would receive their alms in a cup, or a basin, at the end of a long pole. The clapper was an instrument made of two or three boards, by rattling which the wretched lepers incited people to relieve them. Thus they obtained the name of Rattle Pouches, which appellation has been extended to this small plant, in allusion to the little purses which it hangs out by the wayside. Because of these miniature pockets the herb is also named Toy Wort; and Pick Purse, through being supposed to steal the goodness of the land from the farmer. In Queen Elizabeth's time leper hospitals were common throughout England; and many of the sufferers were banished to the Lizard, in Cornwall.

The Shepherd's Purse is now announced as the chief remedy of the seven "marvellous medicines" prepared by Count Mattæi, of Bologna, which are believed by his disciples to be curative of diseases otherwise intractable, such as cancer, internal aneurism, and destructive leprosy.

Count Mattæi professed to extract certain vegetable

electricities found stored up in this, and some other plants, and to utilize them for curative purposes with almost miraculous success. His other herbs, as revealed by a colleague, Count Manzetti, are the Knotgrass, the Water Betony, the Cabbage, the Stonecrop, the House-leek, the Feverfew, and the Watercress. Lady Paget, when interviewing Count Mattæi, gathered that Shepherd's Purse is the herb which furnishes the so-called "blue electricity," of extraordinary efficacy in controlling hæmorrhages.

Small birds are fond of the seeds: and the young radical leaves are sold in Philadelphia as greens in the Spring.

SILVERWEED.

Two *Potentillas* occur among our common native plants, and possess certain curative virtues (as popularly supposed), the Silverweed and the Cinquefoil. They belong to the Rose tribe, and grow abundantly on our roadsides, being useful as mild astringents.

The *Potentilla anserina* (Silverweed) is found, as its adjective suggests, where geese are put to feed.

Country folk often call it Cramp Weed: but it is more generally known as Goose Tansy, or Goose Gray, because it is a spurious Tansy, fit only for a goose; or, perhaps, because eaten by geese. Other names for the herb are Silvery Cinquefoil, and Moorgrass. It occurs especially on clay soils, being recognised by its pinnate white silvery leaves, and its conspicuous golden flowers.

In Yorkshire the roots are known as "moors," which boys dig up and eat in the winter; whilst swine will also devour them greedily. They have then a sweet taste like parsnips. In Scotland, also, they are eaten roasted, or boiled; and sometimes, in hard seasons, when other provisions were scanty, these roots have been known to support the inhabitants of certain islands for months together.

Both the roots and the leaves are mildly astringent; so that their infusion helps to stay diarrhœa, and the fluxes of women; making also with honey a useful gargle. The leaf is of an exquisitely beautiful shape, and may be seen carved on the head of many an old stall in Church, or Cathedral. By reason of its five leaflets, this gives to the plant the title "five leaf," or five fingered grass, *Pentedaktulon*. *Potentilla* comes from the Latin *potens*, as alluding to the medicinal virtues of the species.

In former days the Cinquefoil was much affected as a heraldic device through the number of the leaflets answering to the five senses of man; whilst the right to bear Cinquefoil was considered an honourable distinction to him who had worthily mastered his senses, and conquered his passions.

Silverweed tea is excellent to relieve cramps of the belly; and compresses, wrung out of a hot decoction of the herb, may at the same time be helpfully applied over the seat of the cramps. A potent Anglo-Saxon charm against crampy bellyache was to wear a gold ring with a Dolphin engraved on it, and bearing in Greek the mystic words:—"Theos keleuei mee keneoon ponois," "*God forbids the pains of colic.*" This acted doubtless by mental suggestion, as in the cure of warts. The knee-cap bone, or patella, of a sheep, known locally as the "cramp-bone," is worn in Northamptonshire for a like purpose; also the application of a gold wedding ring (first wetted with saliva, an ingredient in the holy salve of the Saxons), to a stye threatened in an eyelid is often found to disperse the swelling; but in this case it may be, that a sulphocyanide of gold is formed with the spittle, which promotes the cure by absorption.

A strong infusion, if used as a lotion, will check the bleeding of piles, the ordinary infusion being meantime taken as a medicine.

The good people of Leicestershire were accustomed in bygone days to prevent pitting by small-pox with the use of Silverweed fomentations. A distilled water of the herb takes away freckles, spots, pimples in the face, and sunburnings; whilst all parts of the plant are found to contain tannin.

The Creeping Cinquefoil (*Potentilla reptans*) grows also abundantly on meadow banks, having astringent roots, which have been used medicinally since the times of Hippocrates and Dioscorides.

They were found to cure intermittent fevers, such as used to prevail in marshy or ill-drained lands much more commonly than now in Great Britain; though country folk still use the infusion or decoction for the same purpose in some districts; also for jaundice.

Likewise, because of the tannin contained in the outer bark of the roots, their decoction is useful against diarrhœa; and their infusion as a gargle for relaxed sore throats. But, except in mild cases, other more positively astringent herbs are to be preferred. The roots afford a useful red dye.

SKULLCAP.

A useful medicinal tincture (H.) is made from the Skullcap (*Scutellaria*), which is a Labiate plant of frequent growth on the banks of our rivers and ponds, having bright blue flowers, with a tube longer than the calyx. This is the greater variety (*Galericulata*). There is a lesser variety (*Scutellaria minor*), which is infrequent, and grows in bogs about the West of England, with flowers of a dull purple colour. Each kind gets its name from the Latin *scutella,* "a little cap," which the calyx resembles, and is therefore called Hood Wort, or Helmet flower. The upper lip of the calyx bulges outward about its middle, and finally closes down like a lid over the fruit. When the seed is ripe it opens again.

Provers of the tincture (H.) in toxic doses experienced giddiness, stupor, and confusion of mind, twitchings of the limbs, intermission of the pulse, and other symptoms indicative of the epileptiform "petit mal"; for which morbid affection, and the disposition thereto, the said tincture, of a diluted strength, in small doses, has been successfully given.

The greater Skullcap contains, in common with most other plants of the same order, a volatile oil, tannin, fat, some bitter principle, sugar, and cellulose.

If a decoction of the plant is made with two ounces of the herb to eight ounces of water, and is taken for some weeks continuously in recent epilepsy, or when the disease has only functional causes, it will often prove very beneficial. Likewise, this decoction, in common with an extract of the herb, has been given curatively for intermittent fever and ague, as well as for some depressed, and disordered states of the nervous system.

A dried extract of the lesser Skullcap (*Lateriflora*) is made by chemists, and given in doses of from one to three grains as a pill to relieve severe hiccough, and as a nervine stimulant; also for the sleeplessness of an exhausted brain.

SLOE.

THE parent tree which produces the Sloe is the Blackthorn, our hardy, thorny hedgerow shrub (*Prunus spinosa*), Greek *Prounee*, common everywhere, and starting into blossom of a pinky white about the middle of March before a leaf appears, each branchlet ending in a long thorn projecting beyond the flowers at right angles to the stem. From the conspicuous blackness of its rind at the time of flowering, the tree is named Blackthorn, and the spell of harsh unkindly cold weather which prevails about then goes by the name of "blackthorn winter."

The term Sloe, or Sla, means not the fruit but the hard trunk, being connected with a verb signifying to slay, or strike, probably because the wood of this tree was used as a flail, and nowadays makes a bludgeon.

In the Autumn every branch becomes clustered with the oval blue-black fruit presently covered with a fine purple bloom: and until mellowed by the early frosts, this fruit is very harsh and sour.

The leaves, when they unfold late in the spring, are small and narrow. If dried, they make a very fair substitute for tea, and when high duties were placed on imported tea, it was usual to find the sloe trees stripped of their marketable foliage.

Furthermore, the dark ruby juice of Sloes enters largely into the manufacture of British port wine, to which it communicates a beautiful deep red colour, and a pleasant sub-acid roughness. Letters marked upon linen fabric with this juice, when used fresh, will not wash out.

If obtained by expression from the unripe fruit, it is very useful as an astringent medicine, and is a popular remedy for stopping a flow of blood from the nose. It may be gently boiled to a thick consistence, and will then keep throughout the year without losing its virtues. Winter-picks is a provincial name for the Sloe fruit, and winter-pick wine takes the place of port in the rustic cellar. The French call them Prunelles.

Sloe-blossoms make a safe, harmless, laxative medicine. To use these, "Boil them up, and drink a cup of the tea daily for three or four days; it will act gently, painlessly, but thoroughly." The syrup is especially useful for children.

Country people bury the Sloes in jars to preserve them for winter use; and the bush which bears this fruit is sometimes called, provincially, Scroggs.

Sloes may be gathered when ripe on a dry day, picked clean, and put into jars or bottles, without any boiling or other process, and then covered with loaf sugar; a tablespoonful of brandy should presently be added, and the jar sealed. By Christmas, the syrup formed from the juice, the sugar, and the spirit, will have covered and saturated the fruit, and then a couple of tablespoonfuls will not only make an agreeable dessert liqueur, but will act as an astringent cordial of a very pleasant sort.

In Somersetshire the Sloe is named Snag (as corrupted from "Slag," *i. e.*, Sloe). The juice is viscid, and when thickened to dryness, is the German Gum Acacia.

Those provers who have taken experimentally a tincture made from the wood and bark and leaves of the Blackthorn, all had to complain of sharp pains in the right eyeball; and accordingly the diluted tincture is found, when administered in small quantities, to give signal relief for ciliary neuralgia, arising from a functional disorder of the structures within the eyeball. Dr. Hughes says: "It not only relieves such pains, but also checks the inflammation, and clears the vision." The medicinal tincture is made (H.) with proof spirit of wine from the flower buds collected in early spring before they expand. The Sloe has been employed as a styptic ever since the time of Dioscorides. "From the effects," says Withering, "which I have repeatedly observed to follow a wound from the thorns, I find reason for believing that there is something poisonous in their nature, particularly in the autumn."

Next to the Sloe in order of development comes the Bullace (*Prunus insititia*), a shrub with fewer thorns, and bearing its flowers after the leaves have begun to unfold.

The fruit is five times as big as the Sloe, but likewise of a delicate bluish colour. It is named from the Latin plural *bullas*, meaning the round bosses which the Romans put on their bridles. Lydgate (1440) used the phrase, "As bright as Bullaces," in one of his poems. In Lincolnshire the blossom is known as "Bully bloom," and the fruit are "Bullies." After harvest the women and children go out gathering them for Bullace-wine. Boys in France call Sloes "*Sibarelles,*" because it is impossible to whistle immediately after eating them. Some writers say the signification of "Sloe" is "that which sets the teeth on edge."

Finally comes the true Wild Plum (*Prunus domestica*), which is far less common than the two preceding sorts. Its flowers are large, and in small clusters, whilst the leaves unfold with the blossom. The fruit is a small brownish plum, intensely sharp and acrid to the taste, and the tree is thorny. Only in this latter respect does it differ from an inferior kind of garden plum of which the cultivation has been neglected.

The cultivated Plum has been developed from the Wild Plum, and has been made to exhibit some fifty varieties of form and character. The fruit of Damascus was formerly much valued, being now known as Damascenes, (damsons), Damasin, or Damask prune.

All the Wild Plums develop thorns; but the cultivated kinds have entirely cast them off. The Plum, as a fruit, was known to the Romans in Cato's time, but not the tree.

"Little Jack Horner," says the familiar nursery rhyme, "sat in a corner, eating a Christmas pie; he put in his thumb, and he pulled out a plum, and said 'What a good boy am I.'"

> "Inquit, et unum extraheus prunum,
> Horner, quam fueris nobile pueris
> Exemplar imitabile"!

When ripe, cultivated Plums are cooling and slightly laxative, especially the French fruit, which is dried and bottled for dessert. They are useful for costive habits, and may be made into an electuary; but, when unripe, Plums provoke choleraic diarrhœa. The garden fruit contains less sugar than cherries, but a large amount of gelatinising pectose. Dr. Johnson was specially fond of veal pie with plums and sugar. He taunted Boswell about the need of gardeners to produce in Scotland what grows wild in England. "Pray, Sir," said he, "are you ever able to bring the Sloe to perfection there?" On Change a hundred thousand pounds are whimsically known as "a plum," and a million of money is "a marigold." Lately a Chicago physician whilst officiating at a Reformatory found that the boys behaved themselves much better when taking prunes in their diet than at any other time. These act, he supposes, on certain organs which are the seats, and centres of the passions.

From France comes the Greengage, named in that country (out of compliment to the Queen of Francis the First) *La Reine Claude*. It was brought to England from the Monastery of La Grande Chartreuse, about the middle of the eighteenth century, by the Rev. John Gage, brother to the owner of Hengrave Hall, near Coldham, Suffolk; and taking his name this fruit soon became diffused throughout England.

French Prunes are conveyed to England in their dried state from Marseilles. With their pulp, figs, tamarinds, and senna, the officinal "lenitive electuary" is made; and apothecaries prepare a medicinal tincture from the fresh flower-buds of the Blackthorn.

Culpeper says: "All Plumbs are under Venus, and are like women—some better, some worse."

In Sussex and some other counties, a superstitious fear attaches itself to the Blackthorn in bloom, because of the apparent union of life and death when the tree is clothed in early Spring with white flowers, but is destitute of leaves; so that to carry, or wear a piece of Blackthorn in blossom, is thought to signify bringing a death token.

SOAPWORT.

THE Soapwort (*Saponaria officinalis*) grows commonly in England near villages, on roadsides, and by the margins of woods, in moist situations. It belongs to the *Caryophyllaceæ*, or Clove and Pink tribe of plants; and a double flowered variety of it is met with in gardens. This is Miss Mitford's "Spicer" in *Our Village*. It is sometimes named "Bouncing Bet," and "Fuller's herb."

The root has a sweetish bitter taste, but no odour. It contains resin and mucilage, in addition to saponin, which is its leading principle, and by virtue of which decoctions of the root produce a soapy froth. Saponin is likewise found in the nuts of the Horse-chestnut tree, and in the Scarlet Pimpernel.

A similar soapy quality is also observed in the leaves, so much so that they have been used by mendicant monks as a substitute for soap in washing their clothes. This "saponin" has considerable medicinal efficacy, being especially useful for the cure of inveterate syphilis without giving mercury. Several writers of note aver that such cases have been cured by a decoction of the plant; though perhaps the conclusion has been arrived at through the resemblance between the roots of Soapwort and those of Sarsaparilla.

Gerard says: "Ludovicus Septalius, when treating of decoctions in use against the French poxes, mentions the singular effect of the Soapwort against that filthy disease"; but, he adds, "it is somewhat of an ungrateful taste, and therefore must be reserved for the poorer sort of patients." He employed it *sæpe et sæpius*.

The *Pharmacopœia Chirurgica* of 1794, teaches: "A decoction of this plant has been found useful for scrofulous, impetiginous, and syphilitic affections. Boil down half a pound of the bruised fresh herb in a gallon of distilled water to two quarts, and give from one to three pints in the twenty-four hours."

Formerly the herb was called Bruisewort, and was thought of service for contusions. It will remove stains, or grease almost as well as soap, but contains no starch.

Saponin, when smelt, excites long-continued sneezing; if injected or administered, it reduces the frequency and force of the heart's pulsations, paralyzing the cardiac nerves, and acting speedily on the vaso-motor centres, so as to arrest the movements of the heart; on which principle, when given in a diluted form, and in doses short of all toxic effects, it has proved of signal use in low typhoid inflammation of the lungs, where restorative stimulation of the heart is to be aimed at.

Also, likewise for passive suppression of the female monthly flow, it will act beneficially as a stimulant of the womb to incite its periodical function.

In a patient who took a poisonous quantity of Saponin at Saint Petersburg all the muscular contractile sensitiveness was completely abolished; whilst, nevertheless, all the bodily functions were normally performed. *Per contra*, this effect should be a curative guide in the use of Soapwort as a Simple.

Saponin is found again in the root and unripe seeds of the Corn Cockle, and in all parts of the Nottingham Catch-fly except the seeds; also in the wild Lychnis, and some others of the Pink tribe.

SOLOMON'S SEAL.

THE Solomon's Seal (*Convallaria polygonatum*) is a handsome woodland plant by no means uncommon throughout England, particularly in Berkshire, Bucks, Hants, Kent, and Suffolk.

It grows to the height of about two feet, bearing along its curved drooping branches handsome bells of pure white, which hang down all along the lower side of the gracefully weeping flower stalks.

The oval leaves are ribbed, and grow alternately from the stem, for which reason the plant is called Ladder-to-heaven; or, "more probably," says Dr. Prior, "from a confusion of *Seal de notre Dame* (our Lady's Seal), with *Echelle de notre Dame* (our Lady's Ladder). The round depressions resembling seal marks, which are found on the root, or the characters which appear when it is cut transversely, gave rise to the notion that Solomon, "who knew the diversities of plants, and the virtues of roots," had set his seal upon this in testimony of its value to man as a medicinal root. The rhizome and herb contain convallarin, asparagin, gum, sugar, starch, and pectin.

In Galen's time the distilled water was used by ladies as a cosmetic for removing pimples and freckles from the skin, "leaving the place fresh, fair, and lovely." During the reign of Elizabeth it had great medical celebrity, so that, as we learn from a contemporary writer, "The roots of Solomon's Seal, stamped whilst fresh and green, and applied, taketh away, in one night, or two at the most, any bruise, black or blue spots gotten by falls, or woman's wilfulness in stumbling upon their hasty husband's fists, or such like," and "that which might be trewly written of this herb as touching the knitting of bones, would seem to some well nigh incredible; yea, although they be but slenderly, and unhandsomely wrapped-up; but common experience teacheth that in the worlde there is not to be found another herbe comparable for the purpose aforesaid. It was given to the patients in ale to drink—as well unto themselves as to their cattle—and applied outwardly in the manner of a pultis."

The name Lady's Seal was conferred on this plant by old writers, as also St. Mary's Seal, *Sigillum sanctæ Mariæ.*

The Arabs understand by Solomon's Seal the figure of a six-pointed star, formed by two equilateral triangles intersecting each other, as frequently mentioned in Oriental tales. Gerard maintains that the name, *Sigillum Solomonis*, was given to the root "partly because it bears marks something like the stamp of a seal, but still more because of the virtue the root hath in sealing or healing up green wounds, broken bones, and such like, being stamp't and laid thereon."

The bottle of brass told of in the *Arabian Nights* as fished up was closed with a stopper of lead bearing the

"Seal of our Lord Suleyman." This was a wonderful talisman which was said to have come down from heaven with the great name of God engraved upon it, being composed of brass for the good genii, and iron for the evil jinn.

The names *Convallaria polygonatum* signify "growth in a valley," and "many jointed." Other titles of the plant are Many Knees, Jacob's Ladder, Lily of the Mountain, White wort, and Seal wort.

The Turks eat the young shoots of this plant just as we eat Asparagus.

SORREL.

(*See* "Dock," *page* 157.)

SOUTHERNWOOD.

SOUTHERNWOOD, or Southern Wormwood, though it does not flower in this country, is well known as grown in every cottage garden for its aromatic fragrance. It is the *Artemisia Abrotanum*, a Composite plant of the Wormwood tribe, commonly known as "Old Man." Pliny explains that this title is borne because of the plant being a sexual restorative to those in advanced years, as explained by Macer :—

> "Hœc etiam venerem pulvino subdita tantum
> Incitat."

Pliny says further that this herb is potent against syphilis, and *veneficia quibus coitus inhibeatur*. Its odour is lemon-like, and depends on a volatile essential oil which consists chiefly of absinthol, and is common to the other Wormwoods. "Abrotanum" is a Greek term. Another appellation of this plant is "Lad's love," and "Boy's love," from the making of an ointment with its ashes, to be used by youngsters for promoting the growth of the beard. "Cinis Abrotani barbam segnius tardiusque enascentem cum aliquo dictorum oleorum elicit." The plant is found in Spain and Italy as an indigenous herb. Its leaves and tops have a strong aromatic odour, and a penetrating warm, bitterish taste which is rather nauseous. An infusion, or tea, of the herb is agreeable: but a decoction is distasteful, having lost much of the aroma. The plant was formerly in great repute as a cordial against hysterics, and to strengthen the stomach of a weakly person. It will expel both round worms and thread worms, whilst its presence is hostile to moths; and hence has been got one of its French names, "Garde robe." Externally it will promote the growth of the hair. In Lincolnshire it is known as "Motherwood."

SOWBREAD, or CYCLAMEN.

(*See page* 450, "Primrose.")

SPEEDWELL.

THIS little plant, with its exquisite flowers of celestial blue, grows most familiarly in our hedgerows throughout the Spring, and early Summer. Its brilliant, gem-like blossoms show a border of pale purple, or delicate violet, marked with deeper veins or streaks. But the lovely circlet of petals is most fragile, and falls off at a touch; whence are derived the names Speedwell, Farewell, Good-bye, and Forget-me-not.

Speedwell is a Veronica (*fero*, "I bring," *nikee*, "victory"), which tribe was believed to belong especially to birds. So the plant bears the name "Birds' Eyes," as well as "Blue Eyes," "Strike Fires," and "Mammy Die" (because of the belief that if the herb were brought into a family the mother would die within the year). Turner calls the plant "Fluellin," or "Lluellin," a name "the shentleman of Wales have given it because it saved her nose, which a disease had almost gotten from her." Further, it is the Paul's Betony, called after Paulus Œgineta. The plant belongs to the Scrofula-curing order.

It is related that a shepherd observed how a stag, whose hind-quarters were covered with a scabby eruption brought about through the bite of a wolf, cured itself by rolling on plants of the Speedwell, and by eating its leaves. Thereupon he commended the plant to his king, and thus promoted his majesty's restoration to health.

In Germany it bears the title *Grundheele*, from having cured a king of France who suffered from a leprosy for eight years, which disease is named *grund* in German. At one time the herb was held in high esteem as a specific for gout in this country, but it became adulterated, and its fame suffered a downfall.

The only sensible quality of the Speedwell is the powerful astringency of its leaves, and this property serves to protect it from herbivorous foes.

It has been long held famous among countryfolk as an excellent plant for coughs, asthma, and pulmonary consumption. The leaves are bitter, with a rough taste; and a decoction of the whole plant stimulates the kidneys. The infusion promotes perspiration, and reduces feverishness. The juice may be boiled into a syrup with honey, for asthma and catarrhs.

When applied outwardly, it is said to cure the itch; and by some it has been asserted that a continued use of the infusion will overcome sterility, if taken daily as a tea. The French still distinguish the plant as the

Thé d'Europe; and a century ago it was used commonly in Germany in substitution for tea. As a medicine, by reason of its astringency, it became called *Polychresta herba veronica.*

"My freckles with the Speedwell's juices washed," says Alfred Austin, our Poet Laureate.

The Germans also name this plant *Ehren-preis*, or Prize of Honour, which fact favours the supposition of its being the true "Forget-me-not," or *souveigne vous de moy*, as legendary on knightly collars of yore to commemorate a famous joust fought in 1465 between the most accomplished champions of England and France.

The present Forget-me-not is a *Myosotis,* or Mouse Ear, or Scorpion Grass.

In Somersetshire, the pretty little Germander Speedwell is known as Cat's Eye: and because seeming to reflect by its azure colour the beautiful blue firmament above, this pure-tinted blossom has got its name of *veron eikon*, the "true image" (*Veronica*); just as the napkin with which a compassionate maiden wiped the face of Christ on the morning of His crucifixion, held imprinted for ever on its fabric a miraculous portrait, which led to her being afterwards canonised on this account as Saint Veronica.

The Emperor Charles the Fifth of Spain is said to have derived much relief to his gout from the use of this herb. It contains tannin, and a particular bitter principle.

SPINACH.

Spinach (*Lapathum hortense*) is a Persian plant which has been cultivated in our gardens for about two hundred years; and considerably longer on the Continent. Some say the Spinach was originally brought from Spain. It was produced by monks in France at the middle of the 14th century.

This is a light vegetable, easily digested, and rather laxative, besides having some wonderful properties ascribed to its use. Its sub-order, the Saltworts (*Salsolaceæ*), are found growing in marshes by the seashore, and as weeds by waste places, serving some of them to expel worms.

"Spinach," says John Evelyn, "if crude, the oft'ner kept out of sallets the better; but being boiled to a pulp, and without other water than its own moisture, is a most excellent condiment with butter, vinegar, or lemon, for almost all sorts of boiled flesh, and may accompany a sick man's diet. 'Tis laxative and emollient, and therefore profitable for the aged." Spinach is richer in iron than the yolk of the egg, which contains more than beef. Its juice produced in cooking the leaves without adding any water is a wholesome drink, and improves the complexion.

It was with a delicate offering of "gammon and spinach" in his hands, Mr. Anthony Roley, of nursery fame, went so sadly a wooing:—

> "Ranula furtivos statuebat quœrere amores:
> Me miserum! tristi Rolius ore gemit.
> Ranula furtivos statuebat quœrere amores,
> Mater sive daret, sive negaret iter."

A wild species of Spinach, the "Good King Henry," grows in England, and is popular as a pot herb in Lincolnshire.

SPINDLE TREE (Celastraceæ).

DURING the autumn, in our woody hedgerows a shrub becomes very conspicuous by bearing numerous rose-coloured floral capsules, strikingly brilliant, each with a scarlet and orange-coloured centre. This is the Spindle Tree (*Euonymus*), so called because it furnishes wood for spindles, or skewers, whence it is also named Prickwood, Skewerwood, and Gadrise, or Gad Rouge. The word "gad" is used in our western counties for a stick pointed at both ends to fasten down thatch. The Spindle Tree has a green bark, and glossy leaves, producing only small greenish flowers: whilst the pendulous ornaments so brilliantly borne in autumn are four-lobed capsules of a pale red hue, which open out and disclose ruddy orange-coloured seeds wrapped in a scarlet arillus. It is further known as the Louseberry Tree, from the fruit being applied to destroy lice in children's heads, whilst its powdered bark will kill nits, and serve to remove scurf. Other popular titles owned by this shrub are "gatter," "gatten," and "gatteridge." The ripe fruit, from which a medicinal tincture is prepared, furnishes euonymin, a golden resin, which is purgative and emetic. This acts specially on the liver, and promotes a free flow of bile. The plant also yields asparagin, and euonic acid. An ointment is made with the fruits: and the powdered resin is given in doses of from half-a-grain to two grains.

In the United States of America, this tree is the Wahoo, or Burning Bush. The green leaves of one species are eaten by the Arabs to induce watchfulness. In allusion to the actively irritating properties of the shrub, its name, *Euonymus*, is associated with that of Euonyme, the Mother of the Furies. The bark is mildly aperient and causes no nausea, whilst at the same time stimulating the liver somewhat freely. To make its decoction add an ounce to a pint of water, and boil together slowly. A small wineglassful may be given, when cool, for a dose two or three times in the day. Of the medicinal tincture made from the bark with spirit of wine, a dose of from five to ten drops may be taken with water in the same way. French doctors call the shrub Fusain, or *bonnet de prêtre* (birretta). They give the fruit, three or four for a dose, as a purgative in rural districts : and employ the decoction, whilst adding some vinegar, as a lotion against mange in horses and cattle. Also, they make from the wood when slightly charred a delicate crayon for artists.

SPURGE.

CONSPICUOUS in Summer by their golden green leaves, and their striking epergnes of bright emerald blossoms, the Wood Spurge, and the Petty Spurge, adorn our woodlands and gardens commonly and very remarkably. Together with many other allied plants, foreign and indigenous, they yield from their severed stems a milky juice of medicinal properties. The name *Euphorbiœ* has been given to this order from Euphorbus, the favourite physician of Juba, King of Mauritania. All the Spurges possess the same poisonous principle, which may, however, be readily dissipated by heat ; and then, in many instances, the root becomes a nourishing and palatable food. For example, the Manioc, a South American Spurge, furnishes a juice which has been known to kill in a few minutes. Nevertheless, its root baked, after first draining away the juice, makes a wholesome bread : and by washing the fresh pulp a starch is produced which we know as Tapioca for our table. This is so sustaining that half-a-pound a day is said to be sufficient of itself to support a healthy man. The Indian rubber and Castor oil plants belong also to this order of Euphorbiœ.

The Wood Spurge, seen so frequently during our country rambles, suggests by its spreading aspect a clever juggler balancing on his upturned chin a widely-branched series of delicate green saucers on fragile stems, which ramify below from a single rod. Each saucer is the bearer again of sub-divided pedicels which stretch out to support other brightly verdant little leafy dishes; so that the whole system of well poised flowering perianths forms a specially handsome candelabrum of emerald (cup-like) bloom. The botanical title Spurge is derived from *expurgare*, to act as a purgative, because of the acrid juice possessing this property. Gerard says "the juice of the Wood Spurge, if given as physic, must be ministered with discretion, and prepared with correctories by some honest apothecary." Furthermore, this juice, "if mixed with honey causeth hair to fall from that part which is anointed therewith, if it be done in the sun." Therefore, what better place may there be than a wooded English meadow on a sunny day for a clean and convenient natural shave by those of the fair sex who, unhappily, own hirsute facial appendages of which they would gladly be rid? *Euphorbia Peplus*, the Petty Spurge, is equally common, and often called "wart weed." It signifies, "Welcome to our house," and turns its flowers towards the sun. The Irish Spurge (*Hiberna*), is so powerful that a small bundle of its bruised plant will kill the fish for several miles down a river. Yet another Spurge (*Lathyris*), a twin brother, bears caper-like seeds which are sometimes dishonestly pickled and sold as a (dangerous) substitute for the toothsome flowerbuds taken in sauce with our boiled mutton. The whole tribe of Spurges contains two hundred genera, and forms, what we call now-a-days, "a large order." The roots of several common kinds are used in making quack medicines, which are unsafe, and violent in action. Because of its milk-white sap the Wood Spurge bears the name in Somersetshire of Virgin Mary's Nipple: and yet in other parts, for the like reason, this plant is known as Devil's Milk. Chemically, most of the Spurges contain caoutchouc, resin, gallic acid, and their particular acrid principle which has not been fully defined. In France the rustics sometimes purge themselves with a dose of from six to twelve grains of the dried Wood Spurge: and its juice is used in this country as an application to destroy warts; also, to be rubbed in behind the ear for ear-ache, or face-ache. The famous surgeon, Cheselden, employed a noted plaster made with the resin of Spurge for relieving disease of the hip joint by counterstimulation. But, to sum up, I would say with wise Gerard, "these herbes by mine advice should not be received into the body, considering there be so many other good and wholesome potions to be made with other herbes that may be taken without peril." Nevertheless, a tincture prepared (H.) from the Wood Spurge, with spirit of wine, may be given admirably in much diluted doses for curing the same severe symptoms which the plant produces when taken to a toxical degree. Offensive diarrhœa, with prolapse of the lowest bowel, will be certainly remedied by four or five drops of this tincture, first decimal strength, with water, every two or three hours: especially if, at the same time, there be a burning and stinging soreness of the throat. Said young Rosamond Berew (1460), in *Malvern Chase*, concerning "a tall gaunt figure," noted for her knowledge of herbs, sometimes called the Witch, but worshipped by the hinds and their children:—"There is Mary, of Eldersfield; I expect she has been on Berthill after Nettles to make a capon sit, or to gather Spurges for ointments."

STITCHWORT.

THE Stitchworts, greater and less (*Stellaria holostea*), grow very abundantly as herbal weeds in all our dry hedges and woods, having tough stems which run closely together, and small white star-like (*stellaria*) blossoms.

These plants are of the same order (Chickweed) as the Alsine and the small Chickweed. Their second name, *Holostea*, signifies "all bones," because the whole plant is very brittle from the flinty elements which its structures contain.

As its title declares, the great Stitchwort has a widespread reputation for curing the stitch, or sharp muscular pain, which often attacks one or other side of the body about the lower ribs.

In the days of the old Saxon leechdoms it was customary against a stitch to make the sign of the cross, and to sing three times over the part:—

> "Longinus miles lanceâ pinxit dominum:
> Restet sanguis, et recedat dolor!"
>
> "The spear of Longinus, the soldier, pierced our Saviour's side:
> May the blood, therefore, quicken: and the pain no longer abide!"

Or some similar form of charm.

Gerard said of folk, in his day: "They are wont to drink it in wine (with the powder of acorns) against the pain in the side, stitches, and such like." But according to Dr. Prior, the herb is named rather because curing the sting (in German *stich*) of venomous reptiles. In country places the Stitchwort is known as Adder's meat, and the Satin Flower: also Miller's Star, Shirtbutton, and Milk Maid, in Yorkshire: the early English name was Bird's Tongue.

About Plymouth, it is dedicated to the Pixies; whilst the lesser variety is called White Sunday, because of its delicate white blossoms, with golden-dusted stamens. These were associated with the new converts baptised in white garments on Low Sunday—the first Sunday after Easter—named, therefore, White Sunday.

But in some parts of Wales the Stitchwort bears the names of Devil's-eyes and Devil's-corn. Boys in Devonshire nickname the herb Snapjack, Snapcrackers, and Snappers.

Parkinson tells us that in former days it was much commended by some to clear the eyes of dimness by dropping the fresh juice into them. Again, Galen said: "The seed is sharp and biting to him that tastes it."

As a modern curative Simple, the Stitchworts, greater and less, stand related to silica, a powerfully remedial preparation of highly pulverised flint. This is because of the exquisitely subdivided flint found abundantly dispersed throughout the structures of Stitchwort plants; which curative principle is eminently useful in chronic diseases, such as cancer, rickets, and scrofula. It exercises a deep and slow action, such as is remedially brought to bear by the Bethesda waters of America, and the powdered oyster shells of Sir Spencer Wells.

The fresh infusion should be steadily taken, a teacupful three times daily, for weeks or months together. It may be made with a pint of boiling water to an ounce of the fresh herb. Likewise, the fresh plant should be boiled and eaten as "greens," so as to secure medicinally the insoluble parts of the silica. This further serves against albumen, and sugar in the urine.

STONE CROP (*See House Leek, page 273*).

STRAWBERRY.

PROPERLY, our familiar Strawberry plant is a native of cold climates, and so hardy that it bears fruit freely in Lapland. When mixed with reindeer cream, and dried in the form of a sausage, this constitutes Kappatialmas, the plum pudding of the Polar regions.

"Strawberry" is from the Anglo-Saxon *Strowberige*, of which the first syllable refers to anything *strewn*.

The wild woodland Strawberry (*Fragaria vesca*) is the progenitor of our highly cultivated and delicious fruit. This little hedgerow and sylvan plant has a root which is very astringent, so that when held in the mouth it will stay any flow of blood from the nostrils. Its berries are more acid than the garden Strawberry, and make an excellent cleanser of the teeth, the acid juice dissolving incrustations of tartar without injuring the enamel.

A medicinal tincture is ordered (H.) from the berries of this Woodland Strawberry, which is of excellent service for nettle rash, or allied erysipelas: also for a suffocative swelling of the swallowing throat. "*Ipsa tuis manibus sylvestri nata sub umbrâ: mollia fraga leges,*" says Ovid. An infusion of the leaves is of excellent service in dysentery.

It is incorrect to call the fruit a berry, because the edible, succulent pulp is really a juicy cushion over which numerous small seeds are plentifully dotted; whilst the name Strawberry is a corruption of Stray-berry, in allusion to the trailing runners, which stray in all directions from the parent stock.

Being of very ancient date, the Strawberry is found widely diffused throughout most parts of the world.

Among the Greeks its name *Komaros*, "a mouthful," indicated the compact size of the fruit. By the Latins it was termed *Fragaria*, because of its delicate perfume.

Virgil ranked it with sweet-smelling flowers; Ovid gave it a tender epithet; Pliny mentions the Strawberry as one of the native fruits of Italy; Linnæus declared he kept himself free from gout by eating plentifully of the fruit; and Hoffman says he has known consumption cured by the same means.

From Shakespeare we learn that in his day the fruit was grown in Holborn, now the centre of London. Gloster, when contemplating the death of Hastings, wishes to get the Bishop of Ely temporarily out of the way, and thus addresses him: –

"My Lord of Ely—when I was last in Holborn
I saw good Strawberries in your garden there;
I do beseech you send for some of them."

In Elizabeth's time doctors made a tea from the leaves to act on the kidneys, and used the roots as astringent.

All former Herbalists agreed in pronouncing Strawberries wholesome and beneficial beyond every other English fruit. Their smell is refreshing to the spirits; they abate fever, promote urine, and are gently laxative. The leaves may be used in gargles for quinsies and sore mouths, but, "if any one suffering from a wound in the head should partake of this fruit, it would certainly prove fatal," in accordance with a widespread superstition.

So wholesome are Strawberries, that if laid in a heap and left by themselves to decompose, they will decay without undergoing any acetous fermentation; nor can their kindly temperature be soured even by exposure to the acids of the stomach. They are constituted entirely of soluble matter, and leave no residuum to hinder digestion. It is probably for this reason, and because the fruit does not contain any actual nutriment as food, that a custom has arisen of combining rich clotted cream with it at table, whilst at the same time the sharp juices are thus agreeably modified.

"Mella que erunt epulis, et lacte fluentia fraga":—

"Then sit on a cushion, and sew up a seam;
And thou shalt have Strawberries, sugar, and cream."

Cardinal Wolsey regaled off this delicate confection with the Lords of the Star Chamber; and Charles Lamb is reported to have said, "Doubtless, God Almighty could have made a better berry, but He never did."

Parkinson advised that water distilled from Strawberries is good for perturbation of the spirits, and maketh the heart merry.

The fruit especially suits persons of a bilious temperament, being "a surprising remedy for the jaundice of children, and particularly helping the liver of pot companions, wetters, and drammers." "Some also do use thereof to make a water for hot inflammations in the eyes, and to take away any film that beginneth to grow over them. Into a closed glass vessel they put so many strawberries as they think meet for their purpose, and let this be set in a bed of hot horse manure for twelve or fourteen days, being afterwards distilled carefully, and the water kept for use."

The chemical constituents of the Strawberry are—a peculiar volatile aroma, sugar, mucilage, pectin, citric and malic acids in equal parts, woody fibre, and water.

The fruit is mucilaginous, somewhat tart and saccharine. It stimulates perspiration, and imparts a violet scent to the urine. When fermented for the purpose it yields an ardent spirit. If beaten into a pulp when ripe, and with water poured thereupon, it makes a capital cooling drink which is purifying, and somewhat laxative.

Strawberries are especially suitable in inflammatory and putrid fevers, and for catarrhal sore throats. French herbalists direct that when fresh, and recently crushed, the fruit shall be applied on the face at night for heat spots and freckles by the sun. From the juice, with lemon, sugar, and water, they concoct a most agreeable drink, *Bavaroise à la grecque;* also they employ the roots and leaves against passive hemorrhages, and in chronic diarrhœa.

In Germany, stewed strawberries, and strawberry jam are taken at dinner with roasted meats, or with chicken. This jam promotes a free flow of urine.

It is to be noticed that though most commonly wholesome and refreshing, yet with some persons, particularly those of a strumous bodily habit, Strawberries will often disagree. The late Dr. Armstrong held a very strong opinion that the seed grains which lie sprinkled all over the outer surface of each pulpy berry are prone to excite much intestinal irritation, and he advised his patients to suck their Strawberries through muslin, in order to prevent these diminutive seeds from being swallowed.

German legends dedicate Strawberries to the Virgin, with whom they are reputed to have been a favourite fruit. She went a berrying with the children on St. John's morning; and therefore no mother who has lost a young child, will taste the delicacy then. The Strawberries symbolise little children who have died when young, and the mothers suppose they ascend to heaven concealed in the fragrant pulp.

From the French, *fraise,* signifying the Strawberry

leaves borne on the family shield, is derived in Scotland the name of the Frazers. And eight of these (so called) leaves wrought in ornamental gold form a part of the coronet which our English dukes claim as one of their proud insignia, conferred by Henry the Fourth. Being desirous of adding fresh splendour to the Coronation of a Lancastrian Prince he introduced these leaves into the regal Crown. An earl's coronet has eight leaves: that of a marquis four.

SUCCORY.

THE Wild Succory (*Cichorium intybus*) is a common roadside English plant, white or blue, belonging to the Composite order, and called also Turnsole, because it always turns its flowers towards the sun.

It blows with a blue blossom somewhat paler than the Cornflower, but "bearing a golden heart."

Its fresh root is bitter, and a milky juice flows from the rind, which is somewhat aperient and slightly sedative, so that this specially suits persons troubled with bilious torpor, and jaundice combined with melancholy. An infusion of the herb is useful for skin eruptions connected with gout. If the root and leaves are taken freely, they will produce a gentle diarrhœa, their virtue lying chiefly in the milky juice; and on good authority the plant has been pronounced useful against pulmonary consumption. In Germany it is called Wegwort, or "waiting on the way." The Syrup of Succory is an excellent laxative for children.

The Succory or Cichorium was known to the Romans, and was eaten by them as a vegetable, or in salads. Horace writes (*Ode* 31):

> "Me pascunt olivæ,
> Me chicorea, levesque malvæ."

And Virgil, in his first *Georgic*, speaks of *Amaris intuba fibris.* When cultivated it becomes large, and constitutes Chicory, of which the taproot is used extensively in France for blending with coffee, being closely allied to the Endive and the Dandelion.

This is the *Chicorée frisée* when bleached, or the *Barbe de Capucin.* The cortical part of the root yields a milky saponaceous juice which is very bitter and slightly sedative. Some writers suppose the Succory to be the Horehound of the Bible. In the German story, *The Watcher of the Road*, a lovely princess, abandoned for a rival, pines away, and asking only to die where she can be constantly on the watch, becomes transformed into the wayside Succory.

This Succory plant bears also the name of *Rostrum porcinum.* Its leaves, when bruised, make a good poultice for inflamed eyes, being outwardly applied to the grieved place. Also the leaves when boiled in pottage or broths for sick and feeble persons that have hot, weak, and feeble stomachs, do strengthen the same.

It is said that the roots, if put into heaps and dried, are liable to spontaneous combustion. The taproot of the cultivated plant is roasted in France, and mixed with coffee, to which, when infused, it gives a bitterish taste and a dark colour.

The chemical constituents of Succory and Chicory are—in addition to those ordinarily appertaining to vegetables—inulin, and a special bitter principle not named.

Chicory, when taken too habitually or too freely, causes venous passive congestion in the digestive organs within the abdomen, and a fulness of blood in the head. Both it and Succory, if used in excess as a medicine, will bring about amaurosis, or loss of visual power in the retina of the eyes. Therefore, when given in a much diluted form they are remedial for these affections.

The only benefit of quality which Chicory gives to coffee is by increase of colour and body, with some bitterness, but not by possessing any aroma, or fragrant oil, or stimulating virtue. French writers say it is *contra-stimulante*, and serving to correct the excitation caused by the active principles of coffee, and therefore it suits sanguineo-bilious subjects who suffer from habitual tonic constipation. But it is ill adapted for persons whose vital energy soon flags; and for lymphatic, or bloodless people its use should be altogether forbidden.

The flowers of Succory used to rank among the four cordial flowers, and a water was distilled from them to allay inflammation of the eyes. The seeds contain abundantly a demulcent oil, whilst the petals furnish a glucoside which is colourless unless treated with alkalies, when it becomes of a golden yellow.

SUNDEW.

THE Sundew (*Ros solis*, or *Drosera rotundifolia*) is a little plant always eagerly recognised in marshy and heathy grounds by ardent young botanists. In the sun its leaves seem tipped with dew (*drosos*). It grows plentifully in Hampshire and the New Forest, bearing a cluster of hairy leaves in a stellate form, at the top of a slender stem. These leaves either from lack of other sustenance in so barren a soil, or more probably as an advance in plant evolution to a higher grade of development, excrete a sticky moisture or dew, which entangles unwary flies settling on the plant, and which serves to digest these victims therewith. Each of the long red hairs on the leaves is viscid, and possesses a small secreting gland at its top.

Some writers say the word Sundew means "sin" ever, moist (dew). The plant is also called Redrot, and Moor Grass, because the soil in which it grows is unwholesome for sheep.

It goes further by the additional names of Youthwort, and Lustwort—*quia acrimonia sua sopitum veneris desiderium excitat* (Dodœus). The fresh juice of the herb contains malic acid in a free state, various salts, and a red colouring matter; also glucose, and a peculiar crystallisable acid. Cattle of the female gender are said to have their copulative instincts excited by eating even a small quantity of the plant. Throughout Europe it has long been esteemed a remedy of repute for chronic bronchitis and asthma; and more recently, in the hands of homœopathic practitioners, it has acquired a fame for specifically curing whooping cough in its spasmodic stages, after the first feverishness of this malady has become subdued. It signally lessens the frequency and force of the spasmodic attacks, besides diminishing the sickness.

Provers who have pushed on themselves the administration of the Sundew in toxical quantities, developed hoarseness, with expectoration of yellow mucus from the throat and upper lungs, as well as a hacking cough, and loss of flesh, this combination of symptoms closely resembling the form of tubercular consumption which begins in the throat, and extends mischievously to the lungs. Regarded from such point the Sundew may be justly pronounced a homœopathic antidote to consumptive disease of the nature here indicated, when attacking spontaneously from constitutional causes.

Moreover, country folk notice that sheep who eat the Sundew in their pasturage have often a violent cough, and waste away. Dr. Curie, of Paris, fed cats with this plant, and they died subsequently with all the symptoms of lung consumption, their chest organs being afterwards found studded with tubercular deposit though cats are not ordinarily liable to tubercle.

So the Sundew may fairly be accepted as a medicinal Simple for laryngeal and pulmonary consumption in its early stages, as well as for whooping-cough, after the manner already explained. A tincture is made (H.) from the entire fresh plant, with spirit of wine, of which a couple of drops may be given in water several times a day, to a child of from four to eight years old, for confirmed whooping-cough; and if this dose seems to aggravate the paroxysms, or to provoke sickness, it must be reduced in strength, and dilution.

Also from four to ten drops of the tincture may be administered with a tablespoonful of cold water, two or three times a day, for several consecutive weeks, to a consumptive adult, in the early stages of this disease.

Dr. Hughes (Brighton) has employed a diluted tincture of the Sundew (one part of this tincture admixed with nine parts of spirit of wine) in doses of from three to five drops with water, to a child of from three to eight years of age, for spasmodic whooping-cough, several times in the day, with marked success; whilst a larger dose or the stronger tincture served only to increase the cough in violence and frequency. The same results may perhaps follow too strong or full a dose to a consumptive patient, so that it must be regulated by the effects produced. Externally, the juice of the fresh Sundew has been used for destroying warts.

SUNFLOWER.

THE Sunflower (*Helianthus annuus*), which is so popular and brilliant an ornament of cottage gardens throughout England in summer and autumn, is an importation of long standing, and has been called the Marigold of Peru.

Its general nature and appearance are so well known as scarcely to need any description. The plant is of the Composite order, indigenous to tropical America, but flourishing well in this country, whilst bearing the name of *Heli-anthus* (Sunflower), and smelling of turpentine when the disc of the flower is broken across.

The growing herb is highly useful for drying damp soils, because of its remarkable power of absorbing water; for which reason several acres of Sunflowers are now planted in the Thames Valley. Swampy districts in Holland have been made habitable by an extensive culture of the Sunflower, the malarial miasmata being absorbed and nullified, whilst pure oxygen is emitted abundantly.

An old rhyme declares, for some unknown reason:—

> "The full Sunflower blew
> And became a starre of Bartholomew."

The name Sunflower has been given as most persons think because the flowers follow the sun by day turning always towards its shining face. But Gerard says, about this alleged fact, he never could observe it to happen, though he spared no pains to observe the matter; he rather thought the flower to have got its title because resembling the radiant beams of the sun. Likewise, some have called it Corona Solis, and Sol Indianus, the Indian Sunne-floure : by others it is termed Chrysanthemum Peruvianum. In Peru this flower was much reverenced because of its resemblance to the radiant sun, which luminary was worshipped there. In their Temples of the Sun the priestesses were crowned with Sunflowers, and wore them in their bosoms, and carried them in their hands. The early Spanish invaders found in these temples numerous representations of the Sunflower wrought in pure virgin gold, the workmanship of which was so exquisite that it far out-valued the precious metal whereof they were made. Some country folk call it "Lady eleven o'clock."

If the buds of the Sunflower before expanding be boiled, and eaten with butter, vinegar and pepper, after the manner of serving the Jerusalem Artichoke, they are exceeding pleasant meat, surpassing the artichoke moreover in provoking the *desiderium veneris.*

The Chinese make their finest yellow dye from the Sunflower, which they worship because resembling the sun.

All parts of the plant contain much carbonate of potash ; and the fruit, or seed, furnishes a fixed oil in abundance. The kernels of the seeds contain helianthic acid, and the pith of the plant will yield nine per cent. of carbonate of potash. The oil of the Sunflower may be used as olive oil, and the cake after expressing away this oil makes a good food for cattle. A medicinal tincture (H.) is prepared from the seed with rectified spirit of wine ; also from the fresh juice with diluted spirit. Each of these serves admirably against intermittent fever and ague, instead of quinine. The Sunflower is adored by the Chinese as the most useful of all vegetables. From its seeds the best oil is extracted, and an excellent soap is made. This oil burns longer than any other vegetable oil, and Sunflower cake is more fattening to cattle than linseed cake.

The flowers furnish capital food for bees, and the leaves are of use for blending with tobacco. The stalk yields a fine fibre employed in weaving Chinese silk, and Evelyn tells of "The large Sunflower, ere it comes to expand and show its golden face, being dressed as an artichoke, and eaten as a dainty."

The plant is closely allied in its species to the Globe Artichoke, and the Jerusalem Artichoke (*girasole*), so named from turning *vers le soleil*, or *au soleil*, this being corrupted to "Jerusalem," and its soup by further perversion to "Palestine" soup. The original Moorish name was Archichocke, or Earththorn.

The Globe Artichoke (*Cinara maxima anglicana*) of our kitchen gardens, when boiled and brought to table, has a middle pulp which is eaten as well as the soft delicate pulp at the base of each prickly floret. "This middle pulp," says Gerard, "when boiled with the broth of fat flesh, and with pepper added, makes a dainty dish being pleasant to the taste, and accounted good to procure bodily desire. (It stayeth the involuntary course of the natural seed)." Evelyn tells us: "This noble thistle brought from Italy was at first so rare in England that they were commonly sold for crowns apiece." Pliny says: "Carthage spent three thousand pounds sterling a year in them." The plant is named Cinara, from *cinis*, "ashes," because land should be manured with these. It contains phosphoric acid, and is, therefore, stimulating.

The leaves of the Globe Artichoke afford somewhat freely on expression a juice which is bitter, and acts as a brisk diuretic in many dropsies. Such a constituent in the plant was known to the Arabians for curdling milk.

The Jerusalem Artichoke (*Helianthus tuberosus*) is of the Sunflower genus, having been brought at first from Brazil, and being now commonly cultivated in England for its edible tubers. These are red outside, and white within; they contain sugar, and albumen, with an aromatic volatile principle, and water. The tuber is the *Topinambour*, and *Pois de terre* of the French; having been brought to Europe in 1617. It furnishes more sugar and less starch than the Potato.

In 1620 the Jerusalem Artichoke was quite common as a vegetable in London: though, says Parkinson, when first introduced, it was "a dainty for a queen." Formerly, it was baked in pies with beef marrow, dates, ginger, raisins, and sack. The juice pressed out before the plant blossoms was used by the ancients for restoring the hair of the head, even when the person was quite bald.

The Sunflower has been from time immemorial a popular remedy for malarial fevers in Russia, Turkey, and Persia, being employed as a tincture made by steeping the stems and leaves in brandy. It is considered even preferable to quinine, sometimes succeeding when this has failed, and being free from any of the inconveniences which often arise from giving large doses of the drug: whilst the pleasant taste of the plant is of no small advantage in the case of children.

Cases in which both quinine and arsenic proved useless have been completely cured by the tincture of Sunflower in a week or ten days.

Golden Sunflowers are introduced at Rheims into the stained glass of an Apse window in the church of St. Remi, with the Virgin and St. John on either side of the Cross, the head of each being encircled with an aureole havng a Sunflower inserted in its outer circle. The flowers are turned towards the Saviour on the Cross as towards their true Sun.

TAMARIND.

THE Tamarind pod, though of foreign growth, has been much valued by our immediate ancestors as a household medicinal Simple; and a well stocked jar of its useful curative pulp was always found in the store cupboard of a prudent housewife. But of late years this serviceable fruit has fallen into the background of remedial resources, from which it may be now brought forward again with advantage. The natives of India have a prejudice against sleeping under the Tamarind; and the acid damp from the trees is known to affect the cloth of tents pitched under them for any length of time. So strong is this prejudice of the natives against the Tamarind tree that it is difficult to prevent them from destroying it, as they believe it hurtful to vegetation. The parent tree, Tamar Hindee, "Indian date," is of East, or West Indian growth; but the sweet pulpy jam containing shining stony seeds, and connected together by tough stringy fibres, may be readily obtained at the present time from the leading druggists, or the general provision merchant. It fulfils medicinal purposes which entitle it to high esteem as a Simple for use in the sick-room. Large quantities of this luscious date are brought to our shores from the Levant and Persia, but before importation the shell of the pod is removed; and the pulp ought not to exhibit any presence of copper, as shown on a clean steel knife-blade held within the same, though the fruit by nature possesses traces of gold in its composition. Chemically, this pulp contains citric, tartaric, and malic acids, as compounds of potassium ; with gum, pectin and starch. Boiled syrup has been poured over it as a preliminary. The fruit is sharply acid, and may be made into an excellent cooling drink by infusion with boiling water, being allowed to become cold, and then strained off as an agreeable tea, which proves highly grateful to a fevered patient.

The Arabians first taught the use of Tamarinds, which contain an unusual proportion of acids to the sweet constituents. They are anti-putrescent, and exert a laxative action corrective of bilious sluggishness. A capital whey may be made by boiling two ounces of the fruit with two pints of milk, and then straining. Gerard tells that " travellers carry with them the pulp mixed with sugar throughout the desert places of Africa."

Tamarinds are an efficient laxative if enough (from one to two ounces) can be taken at a time: but this quantity is inconvenient, and apt to clog by its excess of sweetness. Therefore a compressed form of the pulp is now in the market, known as Tamar Indien lozenges, coated with chocolate. These are combined, however, with a purgative of greatér activity, most probably jalap.

The fruit of the Tamarind is certainly antibilious, and by the virtue of its potash salts it tends to heal any sore places within the mouth. In India it is added as an ingredient to punch ; but the tree is superstitiously regarded as the messenger of the God of death.

When acids are indicated, to counteract septic fever, and to cool the blood, whilst in natural harmony with the digestive functions, the Tamarind will be found exceptionally helpful ; and towards obviating constipation a dessertspoonful, or more, of the pulp may be taken with benefit as a compôte at table, together with boiled rice, or sago. The name Tamarind is derived from *tamar*, the date palm ; and *indus*, of Indian origin. Formerly this fruit was known as Oxyphœnica (sour date). Officinally apothecaries mix the pulp with senna as an aperient confection. It is further used in flavouring curries on account of its acid.

TANSY.

THE Tansy (*Tanacetum vulgare*—" buttons,"—bed of Tansy), a Composite plant very familiar in our hedgerows and waste places, being conspicuous by its heads of brilliant yellow flowers, is often naturalized in our gardens for ornamental cultivation. Its leaves smell like camphor, and possess a bitter aromatic taste ; whilst young they were commonly used in times past, and are still employed, when shredded, for flavouring cakes, puddings, and omelets. The roots when preserved with honey, or sugar, are reputed to be of special service against the gout, if a reasonable quantity thereof be eaten fasting every day for a certain space. The fruit is destructive to round worms

The seed also of the Tansy is a singular and appropriate medicine against worms : for " in whatsoever sort taken it killeth and driveth them forth." In Sussex a peasant will put Tansy leaves in his shoes to cure ague ; and the plant has a rural celebrity for correcting female irregularities of the functional health. The name Tansy is probably derived from the Greek word *athanasia* which signifies immortality, either, as, says Dodœus, *quia non cito flos inflorescit*, " because it lasts so long in flower," or, *quia ejus succus, vel oleum extractum cadavera a putredine conservat* (as Ambrosius writes), " because it is so capital for preserving dead bodies from corruption." It was said to have been given to Ganymede to make him immortal. The whole herb contains resin, mucilage, sugar, a fixed oil, tannin, a colouring matter, malic or tanacetic acid, and water. When the camphoraceous bitter oil is taken in any excess it induces venous congestion of the abdominal organs, and increases the flow of urine.

If given in moderate doses the plant and its essential oil are stomachic and cordial, whether the leaves, flowers, or seeds be administered, serving to allay spasm, and helping to promote the monthly flow of women; the seeds being also of particular use against worms, and relieving the flatulent colic of hysteria. This herb will drive away bugs from a bed in which it is placed. Meat rubbed with the bitter Tansy will be protected from the visits of carrion flies.

Ten drops of the essential oil will produce much flushing of the head and face, with giddiness, and with heat of stomach; whilst half a drachm of the oil has been followed by a serious result. But from one to four drops may be safely given for a dose according to the symptoms it is desired to relieve. Cases of epilepsy (not inherited) have been successfully treated with the liquid extract of Tansy in doses of a drop with water four times in the day. The essential oil will toxically produce epileptic seizures.

The plant has been used externally with benefit for some eruptive diseases of the skin; and a hot infusion of it to sprained, or rheumatic parts will give relief from pain by way of a fomentation. In Scotland the dried flowers are given for gout, from half to one teaspoonful for a dose two or three times in the day; or an infusion is drank prepared from the flowers and seeds. This has kept inveterate gout at bay for years.

A medicinal tincture is made (H.) from the fresh plant with spirit of wine. From eight to ten drops of the same may be given with a tablespoonful of cold water to an adult twice or three times in the day.

Formerly this was one of the native plants dedicated to the Virgin Mary; and the "good wives" used to take a syrup of Tansy for preventing miscarriage. "The Laplanders," says Linnœus, "use Tansy in their baths to facilitate parturition."

At Easter also it was the custom, even by the Archbishops, the Bishops, and the clergy of some churches, to play at handball (so say the old chroniclers), with men of their congregations, whilst a Tansy cake was the reward of the victors, this being a confection with which the bitter herb Tansy was mixed. Some such a corrective was supposed to be of benefit after having eaten much fish during Lent.

The Tansy cake was made from the young leaves of the plant mixed with eggs, and was thought to purify the humours of the body. "This Balsamic plant" said Boerhaave, "will supply the place of nutmegs and cinnamon." In Lyte's time the Tansy was sold in the shops under the name of Athanasia.

TARRAGON.

THE kitchen herb Tarragon (*Artemisia dracunculus*) is cultivated in England, and more commonly in France, for uses in salads, and other condimentary purposes.

It is the "little Dragon Mugwort: in French, *Herbe au Dragon*"; to which, as to other Dragon herbs, was ascribed the faculty of curing the bites and stings of venomous beasts, and of mad dogs. The plant does not fructify in France.

It is of the Composite order, and closely related to

our common Wormwood, and Southern-wood, but its leaves are not divided. This herb is a native of Siberia, but has been long grown largely by French gardeners, and has since become widespread in this country as a popular fruit, also for making a vinegar, and for adding to salads. The word Tarragon is by corruption "a little dragon." French cooks commonly mix their table mustard with the vinegar of the herb.

Many strange tales have been told about the origin of the plant, one of which, scarce worth the noting, runs that the seed of flax put into a radish root, or a sea onion, and being thus set doth bring forth this herb Tarragon (so says Gerard).

In Continental cookery the use of Tarragon is advised to temper the coldness of other herbs in salads, like as a Rocket doth. "Neither," say the authorities, "do we know what other use this herb hath."

The volatile essential oil of Tarragon is chemically identical with that of Anise, and it is found to be sexually stimulating. Probably by virtue of its finely elaborated camphor it exercises its specific effects, the fact being established that too much camphor acts in the opposite direction.

John Evelyn says of the plant "'Tis highly cordial and friendly to the head, heart, and liver."

THISTLES.

THISTLES are comprised in a large mixed genus of our English weeds, and wild plants, several of them possessing attributed medicinal virtues. Some of these are Thistles proper, as the *Carduus*, the *Cnicus*, and the *Carlina*: others are Teasels, Eryngiums, and Globe Thistles, etc. Consideration should be given here to the *Carduus marianus*, or Lady's Thistle, the common

Carline Thistle, the *Carduus benedictus* (Blessed Thistle), the wild Teasel (*Dipsacus*), and the Fuller's Teasel, as Herbal Simples; whilst others of minor curative usefulness are to be incidentally mentioned.

As a class Thistles have been held sacred to Thor, because, say the old authors, receiving their bright colours from the lightning, and because protecting those who cultivate them from its destructive effects.

In Devon and Cornwall Thistles are commonly known as Dazzels, or Dashel flowers. As a rule they flourish best in hot dry climates.

The *Carduus marianus* (Lady's Thistle), Milk Thistle, or Holy Thistle, grows abundantly in waste places, and near gardens throughout the British Isles, but it is not a native plant. The term *Carduus*, or Cardinal, refers to its spring leaves, and the adjectives "Marianus," "Milk," and "Holy," have been assigned through a tradition that some drops of the Virgin Mary's milk fell on the herb, and became exhibited in the white veins of its leaves. By some persons this Thistle is taken as the emblem of Scotland.

Dioscorides told of the Milk Thistle, "the seeds being drunk are a remedy for infants that have their sinews drawn together." He further said: "The root if borne about one doth expel melancholy, and remove all diseases connected therewith." Modern writers do laugh at this: "Let them laugh that win! My opinion is that this is the best remedy that grows against all melancholy diseases."

The fruit of the *Carduus marianus* contains an oily bitter seed: the tender leaves in spring may be eaten as a salad; and the young peeled stalks, after being soaked, are excellent boiled, or baked in pies. The heads of this Thistle before the flowers open may be cooked like artichokes. The seeds were formerly thought to cure hydrophobia. They act as a demulcent in catarrh and pleurisy, being also a favourite food of Goldfinches. A decoction of the seeds when applied externally is said to have proved beneficial in cases of cancer.

Thistle down was at one time gathered by poor persons and sold for stuffing pillows. It is very prolific in germination, and an old saying runs on this score :—

> "Cut your Thistles before St. John,
> Or you'll have two instead of one."

This Milk Thistle (*Carduus marianus*) is said to be the empirical nostrum, *anti-glaireux*, of Count Mattæi.

"Disarmed of its prickles," writes John Evelyn, "and boiled, it is worth esteem, and thought to be a great breeder of milk, and proper diet for women who are nurses."

In Germany it is very popular for curing jaundice and kindred biliary derangements. When taken by healthy provers in varying quantities to test its toxic effects the plant has caused distension of the whole abdomen, especially on the right side, with tenderness on pressure over the liver, and with a deficiency of bile in hard knotty stools, the colouring matter of the fæces being found by chemical tests present in the urine: so that a preparation of this Thistle modified in strength, and considerably diluted in its doses proves truly homœopathic to simple obstructive jaundice through inaction of the liver, and readily cures the disorder. A tincture is prepared (H.) for medicinal use from equal parts of the root, and the seeds (with the hull on) together with spirit of wine.

The *Carduus benedictus* (Blessed Thistle) was first

cultivated by Gerard in 1597, and has since become a common medicinal Simple. It was at one time considered to be almost a panacea, and capable of curing even the plague by its antiseptic virtues.

This Thistle was a herb of Mars, and, as Gerard says: "It helpeth giddiness of the head: also it is an excellent remedy against the yellow jaundice. It strengthens the memory, cures deafness, and helps the bitings of mad dogs and venomous beasts." It contains a bitter principle "cnicin," resembling the similar tonic constituent of the Dandelion, this being likewise useful for stimulating a sluggish liver to more healthy action.

The infusion should be made with cold water: when kept it forms a salt on its surface like nitre. The herb does not yield its virtues to spirit of wine as a tincture. Its taste is intensely bitter.

The Carline Thistle (*Carlina vulgaris*) was formerly used in magical incantations. It possesses medicinal qualities very like those of Elecampane, being diaphoretic, and in larger doses purgative. The herb contains some resin, and a volatile essential oil of a camphoraceous nature, like that of Elecampane, and useful for similar purposes, as cordial and antiseptic. This Thistle grows on dry heaths especially near the sea, and is easily distinguished from other Thistles by the straw-coloured glossy radiate long inner scales of its outer floral cup. They rise up over the florets in wet weather. The whole plant is very durable, like that of the "everlasting flowers:" Cudweed (*Antennaria*).

The name Carlina was given because the Thistle was used by Charles the Great as a remedy against the plague. It was revealed to him when praying for some means to stay this pestilence which was destroying his army. In his sleep there appeared to him an angel who shot an arrow from a cross bow, telling him to mark the plant upon which it fell : for that with such plant he might cure his soldiers of the dire epidemic : which event really happened, the herb thus indicated being the said thistle. In Anglo-Saxon it was the ever-throat, or boar-throat.

On the Continent a large white blossom of this species is nailed upon cottage doors by way of a barometer to indicate the weather if remaining open or closing.

The wild Teasel (*Dipsacus sylvestris*) grows commonly in waste places, having tall stems or stalks, at the bottom of which are leaves (like bracts) united at their sides so as to form a cup, open upwards, around the base of the stalk, and hence the term "*Dipsacus*," thirsty. This cup serves to retain rain water, which is thought to acquire curative properties, being used, for one purpose, to remove warts. The cup is called Venus' basin, and its contents, says Ray, are of service *ad verrucas abigendas*; also it is named Barber's Brush, and Church Broom.

The Fuller's Teasel, or Thistle (*Dipsacus fullonum*) is so termed from its use in combing and dressing cloth, —*teasan*, to tease,—three Teaselheads being the arms of the Cloth Weavers' Company. This is found in the neighbourhood of the cloth districts, but is not considered to be a British plant. It is probably a cultivated variety of the wild Teasel, but differs by having the bristles of its receptacles hooked.

The Sow Thistle (*Sonchus oleraceus*), named *sonchus* because of its soft spikes instead of prickles, grows commonly as a weed in gardens, and having milky stalks which are reputed good for wheezy and short-winded folk, whilst the milk may be used as a wash for the face. It is named also "turn sole" because always facing the sun, and Hare's Thistle (the hare's panacea, says an old writer, is the Sow Thistle), or Hare's Lettuce because "when fainting with the heat she recruits her strength with the herb; or if a hare eat of this herb in the summer when he is mad he shall become whole." Another similar title of the herb is Hare's palace, since the creature was thought to get shelter and courage from it. Some suppose that the botanical term *Sonchus* signifies *apo tou soon ekein*, from its yielding a salubrious juice.

The Sow thistle has been named also Milkweed. According to tradition it sometimes conceals marvels, or treasures; and in Italian stories the words, "Open Sow Thistle" are used as of like significance with the magical invocation "Open sesame." Another name is "Du Tistel" or Sprout Thistle, because the plant may be used for its edible sprouts, which Evelyn says, were eaten by Galen as a lettuce. And Matthiolus told of the Tuscans in his day "*Soncho nostri utuntur hyeme in acetariis.*"

The Melancholy Thistle (*Carduus heterophyllus*) has been held curative of melancholy. It grows most frequently in Scotland and the North of England, and is a non-prickly plant.

THYME.

THE Wild English Thyme (*Thymus serpyllum*) belongs to the Labiate plants, and takes its second title from a Greek verb signifying "to creep," which has reference to the procumbent habit of the plant. It bears the appellation "Brotherwort."

Typically the *Thymus serpyllum* flourishes abundantly on hills, heaths, and grassy places, having woody stems, small fringed leaves, and heads of purple flowers which diffuse a sweet perfume into the surrounding air, especially in hot weather. Shakespeare's well known line alludes to this pleasant fact: "I know a bank where the wild Thyme grows."

The name Thyme is derived from the Greek *thumos*, as identical with the Latin *fumus*, smoke, having reference to the ancient use of Thyme in sacrifices, because of its fragrant odour: or, it may be, as signifying courage (*thumos*), which its cordial qualities inspire.

With the Greeks Thyme was an emblem of bravery, and activity; also the ladies of chivalrous days embroidered on the scarves which they presented to their knights the device of a bee hovering about a spray of Thyme, as teaching the union of the amiable and the active.

Horace has said concerning Wild Thyme:—

> "Impune tutum per nemus arbutos
> Quærunt latentes, et thyma deviæ
> Olentis uxores mariti."

Wild Thyme is subject to variations in the size and colour of its flowers, as well as in the habits of the varieties.

This wild Thyme bears also the appellation, "Mother of Thyme," which should be "Mother Thyme," in allusion to its medicinal influence on the womb, an organ which the older writers always termed the "Mother." Isidore tells that the wild Thyme was called in Latin, *Matris animula, quod menstrua movet.* Platearius says of it: *Serpyllum matricem comfortat et mundificat. Mulieres Saliternitanæ hoc fomento multum utuntur.*

Dr. Neovius writes enthusiastically in a Finnish Journal on the virtues of common Thyme in combating whooping cough. He has found that if given *fresh*, from an ounce and a half to six ounces a day, mixed with a little syrup, regularly for some weeks, it is practically a specific. If taken from the first, the symptoms vanish in two or three days, and in a fortnight the disease is expelled. The simplicity, harmlessness, and cheapness of this remedy are great supporters of its claims.

Other titles of the herb are Pulial mountain, and creeping Thyme. It is anti-spasmodic, and good for nervous or hysterical headaches, for flatulence, and the headache which follows inebriation. The infusion may be profitably applied for healing skin eruptions of various characters.

Virgil mentions (in *Eclogue* xi., lines 10, 11) the restorative value of Thyme against fatigue:—

> "Thestylis et rapido fessis messoribus œstu
> Allia, Serpyllumque herbas contundit olentes."

Or,

> "Thestlis for mowers tired with parching heat
> Garlic and Thyme, strong smelling herbs, doth beat."

Tournefort writes: "A conserve made from the flowers and leaves of wild Thyme (*Serpyllum*) relieves those troubled with the falling sickness, whilst the distilled oil promotes the monthly flow in women."

The delicious flavour of the noted honey of Hymettus was said to be derived from the wild Thyme there visited by the bees. Likewise the flesh of sheep fed on pasturage where the wild Thyme grows freely has been said to gain a delicate flavour and taste from this source: but herein a mistake is committed, because sheep are really averse to such pasturage, and refuse it if they can get other food.

An infusion of the leaves of Thyme, whether wild, or cultivated, makes an excellent aromatic tea, the odour of which is sweet and fragrant, whilst the taste of the plant is bitter and camphoraceous. There is in some districts an old superstition that to bring wild Thyme into the house conveys severe illness, or death to some member of the family.

In Grecian days the Attic elegance of style was said to show an odour of Thyme. Shenstone's schoolmistress had a garden :—

> " Where herbs for use and physic not a few
> Of grey renown within those borders grew,
> The tufted Basil, —*pun provoking* Thyme,
> The lordly Gill that never dares to climb."

Bacon in his *Essay on Gardens* recommends to set whole alleys of Thyme for the pleasure of its perfume when treading on the plant. And Dioscorides said Thyme used in food helps dimness of sight.

Gerard adds: "Wild Thyme boiled in wine and drunk is good against the wamblings and gripings of the belly": whilst Culpeper describes it as "a strengthener of the lungs, as notable a one as grows." "The Thyme of Candy, Musk Thyme, or Garden Thyme is good against the sciatica, and to be given to those that have the falling sickness, to smell to."

The volatile essential oil of Wild Thyme (as well as of Garden Thyme) consists of two hydrocarbons, with thymol as the fatty base, this thymol being readily soluble in fats and oils when heated, and taking high modern rank as an antiseptic. It will arrest gastric fermentation when given judiciously as a medicine, though an overdose will bring on somnolence, with a ringing in the ears. Officinally Thymol, the stearoptene obtained from the volatile oil of *Thymus vulgaris*, is directed to be given in a dose of from half to two grains.

Thymol is valued by some authorities more highly even than carbolic acid for destroying the germs of disease, or for disinfecting them. It is of equal service with tar for treating such skin affections as psoriasis, and eczema. When inhaled thymol is most useful against septic sore throat, especially during scarlet fever. At the hospital for throat diseases the following formula is ordered: Thymol twenty grains to rectified spirit of wine three drachms, and carbonate of magnesia ten grains, with water to three ounces; a teaspoonful to be used in a pint of water at 150° Fahrenheit for each inhalation.

Against ringworm an ointment made with one drachm of thymol to an ounce of soft paraffin is found to be a sure specific.

The spirit of thymol should consist of one part of thymol to ten parts of spirit of wine; and this is a convenient form for use to medicate the wool of antiseptic respirators. As a purifying and cleansing lotion for wounds and sores, thymol should be mixed in the proportion of five grains thereof to an ounce of spirit of wine, an ounce of glycerine, and six ounces of water.

The common Garden Thyme is an imported sort from the South of Europe. Its odour and taste depend on an essential oil known commercially as oil of origanum.

Another variety of the Wild Thyme is Lemon Thyme (*Thymus citriodorus*), distinguished by its parti-coloured leaves, and by its lilac flowers. Small beds of this Thyme, together with mint, are cultivated at Penzance, in which to rear millepedes, or hoglice, administered as pills for several forms of scrofulous disease. The woodlouse, sowpig, or hoglouse abounds with a nitrous salt which has long found favour for curing scrofulous disease, and inveterate struma, as also against some kinds of stone in the bladder.

The Hoglouse, or Millepede was the primitive medicinal pill. It is found in dry gardens under stones, etc., and rolls itself up into a ball when touched. These are also called Chiselbobs, and Cudworms. From three to twelve were formerly given in Rhenish wine for a hundred days together to cure all kinds of cancers; or they were sometimes worn round the neck in a small bag (which was absurd !). In the Eastern counties they are known as "Old Sows," or "St. Anthony's Hogs." Their Latin name is *Porcellus Scaber*. The Welsh call this small creature the "withered old woman of the wood," "the little pig of the wood," and "the little grey hog," also "Grammar Sows." Their word "gurach" like "grammar" means a dried up old dame.

Cat Thyme (*Teucrium marum verum*) was imported from Spain, and is cultivated in our gardens as a cordial aromatic herb, useful in nervous disorders. Its flowers are crimson, and its bark is astringent. The dried leaves may be given in powder or used in snuff. A tincture (H.) is made from the whole herb which is effectual against small thread worms. Provers of the herb in material toxic quantities have experienced troublesome itching and irritation of the fundament. For similar conditions, and to expel thread worms, two or three drops of the tincture diluted to its first decimal strength should be given with a spoonful of water three or four times in the day to a child of from four to six years.

TOADFLAX.

THE Toadflax, or Flaxweed (*Linaria vulgaris*) belongs to the scrofula-curing order of plants, getting its name from *linum*, flax, and being termed "toad" by a mistaken translation of its Latin title *Bubonio*, this having been wrongly read *bufonio*,—belonging to a toad,—or because having a flower (as the Snapdragon) like a toad's mouth: whereas "bubonio" means "useful for the groins."

It is an upright herbaceous plant most common in hedges, having leaves like grass of a dull sea green aspect, and bearing dense clusters of yellow flowers shaped like those of the garden Snapdragon, with spurs at their base. It continues in flower until the late autumn. The Russians cultivate the Snapdragon for the oil yielded by its seeds.

The Toadflax has a faint disagreeable smell, and a bitter saline taste. It acts medicinally as a powerful purge, and promoter of urine, and therefore it is employed for carrying off the water of dropsies, being in this respect a well known rural Simple. Waller says: "Country people boil the whole plant in ale, and drink the decoction; but the expressed juice of the fresh plant acts still more powerfully."

In many districts the herb is familiarly known as "butter and eggs;" and in Germany though dedicated to the Virgin it is called "devil's band."

Again in Devonshire it goes by the names of "Rambling," or "Wandering Sailor," "Pedler's Basket," "Mother of Millions" (the ivy-leaved sort), "Lion's Mouth" and "Flaxweed."

When used externally an infusion of the herb acts as an anodyne to subdue irritation of the skin, and it may be taken as a medicine to modify skin diseases. The fresh juice is attractive to flies, but at the same time it serves to poison them: so if it be mixed with milk, and placed where flies resort they will drink it and perish at the first sip.

As promoting a free flow of urine, the herb has been named "Urinalis," or sometimes "Ramsted." The flowers contain a yellow colouring matter, mucilage, and sugar. In Germany they are given with the rest of the plant for dropsy, jaundice, piles, and some diseases of the skin. Gerard says: "The decoction openeth the stoppings of the liver, and spleen: and is singular good against the jaundice which is of long continuance." He advises an ointment made from the plant stampt with lard for certain skin eruptions, and a decoction made with four drachms of the herb in eight ounces of boiling water. The bruised leaves are useful externally for curing blotches on the face, and for piles.

An old distich says of the Toadflax as compared with the Larkspur :—

"Esula lactescit: sine lacte Linaria crescit;"

or,

"Larkspur with milk doth flow:
Toadflax without milk doth grow,"

(alluding to the dry nature of the toadflax). To which the Hereditary Marshal of Hesse added the following line :—

"Escula nil nobis, sed dat linaria *taurum*,"

implying that the herb was of old valued for its good effects when applied externally to piles as an ointment, a fomentation, or a poultice, each being made from the leaves and the flowers. The originator of this ointment was a Dr. Wolph, physician to the Landgrave of Hesse, who only divulged its formula on the prince promising to give him *a fat ox* annually for the discovery.

TOMATO (or LOVE APPLE).

THOUGH only of recent introduction as a common vegetable in this country, and though grown chiefly under glass for the table in England, yet the Tomato is so abundantly imported, and so extensively used by all classes now-a-days throughout the British Isles that it may fairly take consideration for whatever claims it can advance as a curative Simple. Imported early in the present century from South America it remained for a while an exclusive luxury produced for the rich like pine apples and melons. But gradually since then the Tomato has steadily acquired an increasing popularity, and now large crops of the profitable fruit are brought from Bordeaux and the Channel Islands, to meet the demands of our English markets. Much of the favour which has become attached to this ruddy, polished, attractive-looking fruit is due to a widespread impression that it is good for the liver, and a preventive of biliousness. Nevertheless, rumours have also gone abroad that habitual Tomato-eaters are especially liable to cancerous disease in this, or that organ.

Belonging to the Solanums the Tomato (*Lycopersicum*) is a plant of Mexican origin. Its brilliant fruit was first known as *Mala æthiopica*, or the Apples of the Moors, and bearing the Italian designation *Pomi dei Mori*. This name was presently corrupted in the French to *Pommes d'amour*; and thence in English to the epithet Love Apples, a perversion which shows by what curious methods primary names may become incongruously changed. They are also called Gold Apples from their bright yellow colour before getting ripe. The term *Lycopersicum* signifies a "wolf's peach," because some parts of the plant are thought to excite animal passions.

The best fruit is supposed to grow within sight, or smell of the sea. It needs plenty of sunlight and heat. The quicker it is produced the fewer will be the seeds discoverable in its pulp.

Green when young, Tomatoes acquire a bright yellow hue before reaching maturity, and when ripe they are smooth, shining, furrowed, and of a handsome red.

Chemically this Love Apple contains citric and malic acids: and it further possesses oxalic acid, or oxalate of potash, in common with the Sorrel of our fields, and the Rhubarb of our kitchen gardens. On which account each of this vegetable triad is ill suited for gouty constitutions disposed to the formation of irritating oxalate of lime in the blood. With such persons a single indulgence in Tomatoes, particularly when eaten raw, may provoke a sharp attack of gout.

Otherwise there are special reasons for supposing the Tomato to be a wholesome fruit of remarkable purifying value.

Dr. King Chambers classifies it among remedies against scurvy, telling us that Tomatoes mixed with brown bread make a capital sauce for costive persons. And the fruit owns a singular property in connection with diseases of plants, suggesting its probable worth as protective against bacterial germs, and microbes of disease in our bodies when it is taken as food, or medicinally. If a Tomato shrub be uprooted at the end of the summer, and allowed to wither on the bough of a fruit tree, or if it be burnt beneath the fruit tree, it will not only kill any blight which may be present, but will also preserve the tree against any future invasion by blight. The hostility thus evinced by the plant to low organisms is due to the presence of sulphur, which the Tomato shrub largely contains, and which is rendered up in an active state by decay, or by burning. Now remembering that digestion likewise splits up the Tomato into its chemical constituents, and releases its sulphur within us, we may fairly assume that persons who eat Tomatoes habitually are likely to have a particular immunity from bacterial and putrefactive diseases.

Wherefore it is altogether improbable that Tomatoes will engender cancer, which is essentially a disease of vitiated blood, and of degenerate cell tissue. Possibly the old exploded doctrine of signatures may have suggested, or started this accusation against the maligned, though unguarded Tomato: for it cannot be denied the guileless fruit bears a nodulated tumour-like appearance, whilst showing, when cut, an aspect of red raw morbid fleshy structure strangely resembling cancerous disease.

Vegetarians who eat Tomatoes constantly and freely claim that cancer is a disease almost unknown among their ranks; but an Italian doctor writing from Rome gives it as the experience of himself and his medical brethren that cancer is as common in Italy and Sicily among vegetarians as with mixed eaters. Most of our American cousins, who are the enterprising fathers of this medicinal fruit, persuade themselves that they are never in perfect health except during the Tomato season. And with us the ruddy Solanum has obtained a wide popularity not simply at table as a tasty cooling sallet, or an appetising stew, but essentially as a supposed antibilious purifier of the blood. When uncooked it contains a notable quantity of Solanin, and it would be dangerous to let animals drink water in which the plant had been boiled. The Staff of the Cancer Hospital at Brompton have emphatically declared "they see no ground whatever for supposing that the eating of Tomatoes predisposes to cancer."

Nevertheless some country people in the remote American States attribute cancer to an excessively free use of the wild uncultivated tomato as food.

The first mention of this fruit by the London Horticultural Society occurred in 1818.

Chemically in addition to the acids already named the Tomato contains a volatile oil, a brown resinous extractive matter very fragrant, a vegeto-mineral matter, muco-saccharin, some salts, and in all probability an alkaloid. The whole plant smells unpleasantly, and its juices when subjected to heat by the action of fire emit a vapour so powerful as to provoke vertigo and vomiting.

The specific principles furnished by the Tomato will, when concentrated, produce, if taken medicinally, effects very similar to those brought about by taking mercurial salts, viz., an ulcerative state of the mouth, with a profuse flow of saliva, and with excessive stimulation of the liver: peevishness also on the following day, with a depressing backache in men, suggesting paralysis, and with a profuse fluor albus in women. When given in moderation as food, or as physic, the fruit will remedy this chain of symptoms.

By reason of its efficacy in promoting an increased flow of bile if judiciously taken, the Tomato bears the name in America of Vegetable Mercury, and it has almost superseded calomel there as a biliary medicinal provocative. Dr. Bennett declares the Tomato to be the most useful and the least harmful of all known medicines for correcting derangements of the liver. He prepares a chemical extract of the fruit and plant which will, he feels assured, depose calomel for the future.

Across the Atlantic an officinal tincture is made from the Tomato for curative purposes by treating the apples, and the bruised fresh plant with alcohol, and letting this stand for eight days before it is filtered and strained. A teaspoonful of the tincture is a sufficient dose with one or two tablespoonfuls of cold water, three times in the day.

The fluid extract made from the plant is curative of any ulcerative soreness within the mouth, such as nurses' sore mouth, or canker. It should be given internally, and applied locally to the sore parts.

Spaniards and Italians eat Tomatoes with pepper and oil. We take them as a salad, or stewed with butter, after slicing and stuffing them with bread crumb, and a spice of garlic.

The green Tomato makes a good pickle, and in its unripe state is esteemed an excellent sauce with rich roast pork, or goose. The fruit when cooked no longer exercises active medicinal effects, as its volatile principles have now become dispelled through heat.

By the late Mr. Shirley Hibberd, who was a good naturalist, it was asserted with seeming veracity that the cannibal inhabitants of the Fiji Islands hold in high repute a native Tomato which is named by them the *Solanum anthropophagorum*, and which they eat, *par excellence*, with "Cold Missionary." Nearer home a worthy dame has been known with pious aspirations to enquire at the stationer's for "Foxe's book of To-Martyrs."

"Chops and Tomato sauce" were ordered from Mrs. Bardell, in Pickwick's famous letter. "Gentlemen!" says Serjeant Buzfuz, in his address to the jury, "What does this mean?" But he missed a point in not going on to add—"I need not tell you, gentlemen, the popular name for the Tomato is *love apple!* "Is it not manifest, therefore, what the base deceiver intended?"

"A cucumber in early spring
Might please a sated Cæsar,
Rapture asparagus can bring,
And dearer still green peas are:
Oh! far and wide, where mushrooms hide,
I'll search, as wide and far too
For watercress; but all their pride
Must stoop to thee,—Tomato!"

TORMENTIL.

THE Tormentil *(Potentilla Tormentilla)* belongs to the tribe of wild Roses, and is a common plant on our heaths, banks, and dry pastures. It is closely allied to the *Potentilla*, but bears only four petals on its flowers, which are of bright yellow. The woody roots are medicinally useful because of their astringent properties. Sometimes the stem is trailing, making this the *Tormentilla Reptans*, but more commonly it ascends. The name comes from *tormina*, which signifies such griping of the intestines as the herb will serve to relieve, as likewise the twinges of toothache. The root is employed both for tanning leather, and for dyeing it by the thickened red juice. Furthermore through its astringency this root is admirable for arresting bleedings. Vesalius considered it to be as useful against syphilis as Guiacum, and Sarsaparilla. A decoction of Tormentil makes a capital gargle, and will heal ulcers of the mouth if used as a wash. If a piece of lint soaked therein be kept applied to warts, they will wither and disappear. Chemically the herb contains "*Tormentilla Red,*" identical with that of the Horse Chestnut, also tannic, and kinoric acids. The decoction should be made with four drams to half-a-pint of water boiled together for ten minutes, adding half a dram of Cinnamon stick at the end of boiling; one or two tablespoonfuls will be the dose, or of the powdered root (dried) the dose will be from five to thirty grains.

"*In fluxu sanguinis, fluore albo, et mictu involuntario Tormentilla valet.*" Dr. Thornton (1810) tells of a labouring botanist who learnt the powers of this root, and by its decoction, sweetened with honey, cured intractable agues, severe diarrhœas, and scorbutic ulcers (which had been turned out of hospitals as inveterate), also many fluxes. Lord William Russell heard about this, and allowed the poor man a piece of his park in which to cultivate the herb. "*Non est vegetabile quod in fluxionibus alvi efficacius est.*" The root is so rich in tannin that it may be used instead of oak bark.

TURNIP.

THE Turnip (*Brassica Rapa*) belongs to the Cruciferous Cabbage tribe, being often found growing in waste places, though not truly wild. In this state it is worth nothing to man or beast; but, by cultivation, it becomes a most valuable food for cattle in the winter, and a good vegetable for our domestic uses. It exercises some aperient action, and the liquid in which turnips are boiled will increase the flow of urine. It is called also "bagie," and was the "gongyle" of the Greeks, so named from the roundness of the root.

When mashed, and mixed with bread and milk, the Turnip makes an excellent cleansing and stimulating poultice for indolent abscesses or sores.

The Scotch eat small, yellow-rooted Turnips as we do radishes. "Tastes and Turnips proverbially differ."

At Plymouth, and some other places, when a girl rejects a suitor, she is said to "give him turnips," probably with reference to his sickly pallor of disappointment.

The seventeenth of June—as the day of St. Botolph, the old turnip man,—is distinguished by various uses of a Turnip, because in the Saga, which figuratively represents the seasons, the seeds were sown on that day.

It is told that the King of Bithynia in some expedition against the Scythians during the winter, and when at a great distance from the sea, had a violent longing for a small fish known as *aphy*—a pilchard, or anchovy. His cook cut a Turnip to a perfect imitation of its shape, which, when fried in oil, well salted, and powdered with the seeds of a dozen black poppies, so deceived the king that he praised the root at table as an excellent fish.

Being likely to provoke flatulent distension of the bowels, Turnips are not a proper vegetable for hysterical persons, or for pregnant women. The rind is acrimonious, but the tops, when young and tender, may be boiled for the table as a succulent source of potash, and other mineral salts in the Spring.

The fermented juice of Turnips will yield an ardent spirit. When properly cooked they serve to sweeten the blood. An essential volatile oil contained in the root, chiefly in the rind, disagrees, by provoking flatulent distension. This root is sometimes cut up and partly substituted for the peel and pulp of oranges in marmalade.

If Turnips are properly grown in dry, lean, sandy earth, a wholesome, agreeable sort of bread can be made from them, "of which we have eaten at the greatest persons' tables, and which is hardly to be distinguished from the best of wheat." Some persons roast Turnips in paper under the embers, and serve them with butter and sugar. The juice made into syrup is an old domestic remedy for coughs and hoarseness.

A nice wholesome dish of Piedmontese Turnips is thus prepared: Half boil your Turnip, and cut it in slices like half-crowns; butter a pie dish, and put in the slices, moisten them with a little milk and weak broth, sprinkle over lightly with bread crumbs, adding pepper and salt; then bake in the oven until the Turnips become of a light golden colour.

The Turnip, a navew, or variety of Rape (*navus*), should never be sown in a rich soil, wherein it would become degenerate and lose its shape as well as its dry agreeable relish. Horace advised field-grown Turnips as preferable at a banquet to those of garden culture. They may be safely eaten when raw, having been at one time much consumed in Russia by the upper classes.

Turnips have been introduced into armorial bearings to represent a person of liberal disposition who relieves the poor.

Dr. Johnson's famous illustration of false logic ran thus :—

> "If a man fresh Turnips cries :
> But cries not when his father dies,
> Is this a proof the man would rather
> Possess fresh Turnips than a father?"

TURPENTINE.

FROM our English Pines, if their stems be wounded, the oleo-resin known as Turpentine, can be procured. This is so truly a vegetable product, and so readily available for medical uses in every household, being withal so valuable for its remedial and curative virtues that no apology is needed for giving it notice as a Herbal Simple. The said oleo-resin which exudes on incising the bark furnishes our oil, or so-called spirit of Turpentine. But larger quantities, and of a richer resin, can be had from abroad than it is practicable for England to provide, so that our Turpentine of commerce is mainly got from American and French sources.

The oleo-resin consists of a resinous base and a volatile essential oil, which is usually termed the spirit.

The *Pinus Picra*, or Silver Fir-tree, yields common

Turpentine; and to sleep on a pillow made from its yellow shavings is a capital American device for relieving asthma. Fir cones are called "buntins," and "oysters."

"Tears," or resin drops, which trickle out on the stems of the Pine, if taken, five or six of these tears in a day, will benefit chronic bronchitis, and will prove useful to lessen the cough of consumption.

When swallowed in a full dose, Turpentine gives a sensation of warmth, and excites the secretion of urine, to which it imparts a violet hue. It also promotes perspiration, and stimulates the bronchial mucous membrane. From eight to twenty drops may be given as a dose to produce these effects; but an immoderate dose will purge, or intoxicate, and stupefy, causing strangury, and congestion of the kidneys.

For bleeding from the lungs, five drops may be given, and repeated at intervals of not less than half-an-hour, whilst needed. The dose may be taken in milk, or on sugar, or bread.

With the object of meeting for a curative purpose such symptoms occurring as disease which large doses of this particular drug will produce, as if by poisoning, in a healthy person, quite small doses of Turpentine oil will promptly relieve simple congestion of the kidneys, when occurring as illness, it may be from exposure to cold, and accompanied by some feverishness, with frequent urination, as well as a dragging of the loins. On which principle three or four drops of a diluted tincture of Turpentine (made with one part of Turpentine to nine parts of spirit of wine), given in a spoonful of milk every four hours, will speedily dispel the congestion, thus acting as an infallible specific, and a similar dose of the same tincture will quickly subdue rheumatic inflammation of the eyes.

A pleasant form in which to administer Turpentine, whether for chronic bronchitis or for kidney congestion from cold, is a confection. This may be made by rubbing up one part of oil of turpentine, with one part of liquorice powder, and with two parts of clarified honey. Combine the first two together, then add the honey. If the Turpentine separates, pour it off, and add it again with plenty of rubbing until it unites. From half to one teaspoonful of this confection, when mixed with two tablespoonfuls of peppermint-water, will be found palatable, and may be repeated two or three times in the day.

What is called Terebene, a most useful medicine for winter cough, is produced by the action of sulphuric acid on Turpentine. From five to ten drops may be taken on sugar three or four times in the day, and its vapour acts by inhalation as a very useful antiseptic sedative in consumptive disease of the lungs.

Externally, Turpentine is stimulating and counter-irritating, and derivative. When applied to the skin, unless properly diluted, Turpentine will cause redness and smarting to a painful degree, with an outbreak of small blisters. As an embrocation, the oil of turpentine mixed with spirit of wine and camphor, together with soap liniment, proves very efficacious for the relief of sciatica, and for the chronic rheumatism of joints. Also, when compounded with wax and resin, it makes an excellent healing ointment for indolent, and unhealthy sores.

In Dublin, Turpentine is commingled with peppermint water, and used as an external stimulant for chronic bronchitis.

The famous liniment of St. John Long consisted of oil of turpentine one part, acetic acid one part, and liniment of camphor one part. This was of admirable service for rubbing along the spine to relieve the irritability of the spinal nerves, and it has proved effectual to modify or prevent epileptic attacks, by being thus applied. In cases of colic attending obstinate constipation, with strengthless distension of the bowels, Turpentine mixed with starch or thin gruel, an ounce to the pint, and administered as a clyster, makes one of the most reliable and safe evacuants. Also as a remedy for round worms, six or eight drops (more or less according to age) may be safely and effectively given to a child on one or more nights in milk.

Pills made from Chian Turpentine, which is got from Cyprus, were extolled by Dr. Clay of Manchester, in 1880, as a cure for cancer of the womb, and for some other forms of cancerous disease. From five to ten grains were to be given in a pill, or mixed with mucilage as an emulsion, so that in all daily, after food, and in divided doses, one hundred and eighty grains of this Turpentine were swallowed; and the quantity was gradually increased until five hundred grains a day were taken. In many cases this method of treatment proved undoubtedly useful.

A small quantity of powdered sulphur was also incorporated by Dr. Clay in his Chian pills. About the fourth day the pain was relieved, and the cancerous growth would melt away in a period of from four to thirteen weeks. The arrest of bleeding and the continued freedom from glandular infection after a prolonged use of this Chian Turpentine were highly important points in the improvement produced.

From the *Pinus Sylvestris* an oil is distilled by steam, and of this from ten drops to a teaspoonful may be given for a dose, in milk, for chronic rheumatism or chronic bronchitis

It is most useful in the treatment of diphtheria to burn in the room, near the patient, a mixture of turpentine and tar in a pan or deep dish. The fumes serve to dissolve the false membrane, and have helped to effect a cure in desperate cases.

This tree had the Anglo-Saxon name Pimm, from pen, or pin, a sharp rock,—"*ab acumine foliorum*," or perhaps as a contraction of *picinus*—pitchy. It furnishes from its leaves an extract, and the volatile oil. Wool is saturated with the latter, and dried, being then made into blankets, jackets, spencers, and stockings, for the use of rheumatic sufferers. There are establishments in Germany where the Pine Cure is pursued by the above means, together with medicated baths. Pine cones were regarded of old by the Assyrians as sacred symbols, and were employed as such in the decoration of their temples. From the tops of the Norway Spruce fir a favourite invigorating drink is brewed which is known in the north as spruce beer. This has an excellent reputation for curing scurvy, chronic rheumatism, and cutaneous maladies. Laplanders make a bread from the inner bark of the Pine.

Tar (*pix liquida*) is furnished abundantly by the *Pinus Sylvestris*, or Scotch Fir, and is extracted by heat. The tree is cut into pieces, which are enclosed in a large oven constructed for the purpose: fire is applied, and the liquid tar runs out through an opening at the bottom. It is properly an empyreumatic oil of turpentine, and has been much used in medicine both externally and internally. Tar water was extolled in 1744, by Bishop Berkley, almost as a panacea. He gave it for scurvy, skin eruptions, ulcers, asthma, and rheumatism. It evidently promotes the secretions, especially the urine.

Tar yields pyroligneous acid, oil of tar, and pitch: as well as guiacol and creasote.

Syrup of tar is an officinal medicine in the United States of America for chronic bronchitis, and winter cough. By this the expectoration is made easier, and the sleep at night improved. From one to two tea-spoonfuls are given as a dose, with or without water. Also tar pills are prepared of pitch and liquorice powder in equal parts, five grains in the whole pill. Two or three of these may be taken twice or three times in the day.

Tar ointment is highly efficacious against some forms of skin disease; but in eczema and allied maladies of the skin, no preparation of tar should be employed as long as the skin is actively inflamed, or any exudation of moisture is secreted by it.

Dr. Cullen met with a singular practice respecting Tar. A leg of mutton was put to roast, being basted during the whole process with tar instead of butter. Whilst roasting, a sharp skewer was frequently thrust into the substance of the meat to let the juices escape, and with the mixture of tar and gravy found in the dripping pan, the body of the patient was anointed all over for three or four nights consecutively, throughout all this time the same body linen being worn. The plan proved quite successful in curing obstinate lepra.

A famous liquor called "mum" was concocted by the House of Brunswick, some of which was sent to General Monk. It was chiefly brewed from the rind and tops of firs, and was esteemed very powerful against the formation of stone, and to cure all scorbutick distempers. Various herbs, as best approved by the maker, were infused with the mum in concocting it, such as betony, birch, burnet, brooklime, elder-flowers, horse-radish, marjoram, thyme, water-cress, pennyroyal, etc., together with several eggs, "the shells not cracked or broken"! The Germans, especially in Saxony, have so great a veneration for mum that they fancy their bodies can never decay as long as they are lined, and embalmed with so powerful a preserver. The Swedes call the fir "the scorbutick tree" to this day.

Tar is soluble in its own bulk of spirit of wine, rectified, but separates when water is added. Inhaled, its vapour is very useful in chronic bronchitis.

Tar water should be made by stirring a pint of tar with half a gallon of water for fifteen minutes, and then decanting it. From half-a-pint to a pint may be taken daily, and it may be used as a wash. Or from twenty to sixty drops of tar are to be swallowed for a dose several times in the day, whether for chronic catarrhal affections, or for irritable urinary passages. Tar ointment is prepared with five parts of tar to two pounds of yellow wax. It is an excellent application for scald head in a child.

Juniper tar oil is known as "oil of Cade," and Birch tar is got from the Butcher's Broom. A recognised plaster and an ointment are made with Burgundy pitch (from the *Picus Picea*) and yellow wax.

Probably the modern employment of carbolic acid, and its various combinations—all derived from tar—for neutralising the septic elements of disease, and for acting as germicides, was unknowingly forestalled by the sagacious Right Reverend Lord Bishop of Cloyne, in his *Philosophical Reflections and Inquiries concerning the virtues of Tar Water*, two centuries ago, when the cup which "cheers but not inebriates" was first told of by him, long before Cowper. Bishop Berkley said, "I do, verily, think there is not any other medicine whatsoever so effectual to restore a crazy constitution and to cheer a dreary mind: or so likely to subvert that gloomy empire of the spleen which tyranniseth over the better sort."

In *Great Expectations*, by Charles Dickens, the wife of Joe Gargery is described as possessed of great faith in the curative virtues of Tar water.

VALERIAN.

THE great Wild Valerian, or Heal-all (from *valere*, to be well), grows abundantly throughout this country in moist woods, and on the banks of streams. It is a Benedicta, or blessed herb, being dedicated to the Virgin Mary, as preservative against poisons; and it bears the name of Capon's tail, from its spreading flowers.

When found among bushes, in high pastures, and on dry heaths, it is smaller, with the leaves narrower, but the roots more aromatic, and less nauseous.

The Valerian family of plants is remarkable for producing aromatic and scented genera, which are known as "Nards" (the Spikenard of Scripture), and which are much favoured in Asiatic harems under several varieties, according to the situation of growth. Judas valued the box of ointment made from the Spikenard (*Valeriana Jatamansi*), with which Mary anointed the feet of our Saviour at two hundred denarii (£6: 9s : 2d.).

We have also the small Marsh Valerian, which is wild, and the cultivated Red Valerian, of our cottage gardens.

The roots of our Wild Valerian exercise a strange fascination over cats, causing an ecstasy of delight in these animals, who become almost intoxicated when brought into contact with the Simple. And rats strangely exhibit the same fondness for these roots which they grub up. It has been suggested that the Pied Piper of Hamelin may have carried one of such roots in his wallet.

They have been given from an early period with much success for hysterical affections, and for epileptic attacks induced by strong emotional excitement, as anger or fear: likewise, they serve as a safe and effectual remedy against habitual constipation when active purgatives have failed to overcome this difficulty.

The plant is largely cultivated for the apothecary's uses about the villages near Chesterfield, in Derbyshire. It is named Setwall in the North of England; and, says Gerard, "No broths, pottage, or physicall meats be worth anything if Setwall (a corruption from Zedoar), be not there":—

"They that will have their heale,
Must put *Setwall* in their keale."

The Greeks employed one kind of Valerian named *Phu* for hanging on doors and windows as a protective charm. But some suppose this to have been a title of aversion, like our English "faugh" against any thing which stinks. Dr. Uvedale introduced the Valerian into his garden, at Eltham Palace, before 1722; and Uvedale House still exists in Church Street, at Chelsea. The herb is sometimes called Cut-heal, not because, as Gerard thought, it is "useful for slight cuts and wounds," but from its attributed efficacy in disorders of the womb (kutte cowth). Joined with Manna, Valerian has proved most useful in epilepsy; and when combined with Guiacum it has resolved scrofulous tumours. In Germany imps are thought to be afraid of it.

At Plymouth, the broad-leaved Red Valerian goes by the name of Drunken Sailor, and Bovisand Soldier, the larger sort being distinguished as Bouncing Bess, whilst the smaller, paler kind is known as Delicate Bess throughout the West of Devon.

An officinal tincture is made from the rhizome of Valerian with spirit of wine, of which from one to two teaspoonfuls may be given for a dose, with a little water. Also a tincture (ammoniated) is prepared with aromatic spirit of ammonia on the rhizome, and this is considerably stronger; from twenty to forty drops is a sufficient dose with a spoonful or two of water.

The essential oil of Valerian lessens the sensibility of the spinal cord after primary stimulation of its nervous substance. A drop of this oil in a spoonful of milk will be a proper dose: especially in some forms of constipation.

Used externally, by friction, the volatile oil of Valerian has proved beneficial as a liniment for paralyzed limbs. The powdered root mixed in snuff is of efficacy for weak eyes.

The cultivated plant is less rich in the volatile oil than the wild herb. On exposure to the air Valerian oil becomes oxidised, and forms valerianic acid, which together with an alcohol, "borneol," constitutes the active medicinal part of the plant.

The root also contains malic, acetic, and formic acids, with a resin, tannin, starch, and mucilage. It is by first arousing and then blunting the reflex nervous activities of the spinal cord, that the oil of Valerian overcomes chronic constipation.

Preparations of Valerian act admirably for the relief of nervous headache associated with flatulence, and in a person of sensitive temperament. They likewise do good for infantine colic, and they diminish the urea when the urine contains it in excess.

The Greek Valerian is another British species, found growing occasionally in the North of England and in Scotland, being known as the blue Jacob's Ladder. It is also named "Make bate," because said to set a married couple quarrelling if put in their bed. This must be a play on its botanical name *Polemonium*, from the Greek *polemos*, war. It is called Jacob's Ladder from its successive pairs of leaflets.

VERBENA.

THE Verbena, or Common Vervain, is a very familiar herb on waste ground throughout England, limited to no soil, and growing at the entrance into towns and villages, always within a quarter of a mile of a house, and hence called formerly the Simpler's joy. Of old, much credit for curative virtues attached itself to this plant, though it is without odour, and has no taste other than that of slight astringency. But a reputation clings to the Vervain because it used to be held sacred, as "Holy Herb," and was employed in sacrificial rites, being worn also around the neck as an amulet. It was called "Tears of Isis," "Tears of Juno," "Persephonion," and "Demetria." The juice was given as a remedy for the plague. Vervain grew on Calvary: and Gerard says "the devil did reveal it as a secret, and divine medicine."

It is a slender plant with but few leaves, and spikes of small lilac flowers, when wild; but its cultivated varieties, developed by the gardener, are showy plants, remarkable for their brilliant colours.

The name Frogfoot has been applied to the Vervain because its leaf somewhat resembles in outline the foot of that creature. Old writers called the plant *Verbinaca* and *Peristerium* :—

> "Frossis fot men call it,
> For his levys are like the frossy's fet."

The practice of wearing it round the neck became changed from a religious observance to a medicinal proceeding, for which reason it was ordered that the plant should be *bruised* before being appended to the person; and thus it gained a name for curing inveterate headaches. Presently also it was applied to other parts as a cataplasm.

Nevertheless, the Vervain has fallen of late years into disfavour as a British Herbal Simple, though a pamphlet has recently appeared, written by a Mr. Morley, who strongly advises the revived use of the herb for benefiting scrofulous disease. Therein it is ordered that the root of Vervain shall be tied with a yard of white satin ribband round the neck of the patient until he recovers. Also an infusion and an ointment are to be prepared from the leaves of the plant.

The expressed juice of Verbena will act as a febrifuge; and the infusion by its astringency makes a good lotion for weak and inflamed eyes, also for indolent ulcers, and as a gargle for a relaxed sore throat. The Druids gathered it with as much reverence as they paid to the Mistletoe. It was dedicated to Isis, the goddess of birth, and formed a famous ingredient in love philtres.

Pliny saith: "They report that if the dining chamber be sprinkled with water in which the herb Verbena has been steeped, the guests will be the merrier."

Geoffrey St. Hilaire and Pasteur praise the Vervain highly as beneficial against ailments of the hair, the fresh juice being especially used.

Other names of the plant are Juno's tears, Mercury's moist blood, Pigeons' grass, and Columbine—the two latter being assigned because pigeons show a partiality for the herb.

Verbena plants were named *Sagmina*, of old, because

cut up by the Prætor in the Capitol. When borne by an Ambassador Verbena rendered his person inviolable. All herbs used in sacred rites were probably known as Verbena. They were reported as of singular force against the tertian and quartan agues; "but one must observe Mother Bombie's rules—to take just so many knots, or sprigs, and no more, lest it fall out that it do you no good, if you catch no harm by it."

VINE.

THE fruit of the Vine (*Vitis vinifera*) has already been treated of here under the heading "Grapes," as employed medicinally whether for the purgation of the bilious—being then taken crude, and scarcely ripe,—or for imparting fat and bodily warmth in wasting disease by eating the luscious and richly-saccharine berries.

It should be added that the fumes exhaled from the wine-presses whilst the juice is fermenting, prove highly beneficial as a restorative for weakly and delicate young persons (an example which might be followed perhaps at our home breweries).

Consumptive patients are sent with this view to the Gironde, where the vapour from the wine vats is more stimulating and curative than in Burgundy. Young girls who suffer from atrophy are first made to stand for some hours daily in the sheds when the wine pressing is going forward. After a while, as they become less weak, they are directed to jump into the wine press, where, with the vintagers and labourers they skip about and inhale the fumes of the fermenting juice, until they sometimes become intoxicated, and even senseless. This effect passes off after one or two trials, and the girls return to their labour with renewed strength and heightened colour, hopeful, joyous, and robust. The vats of the famous *Chateau d'yquem* are the most celebrated of all for the wondrous cures they have effected even in cases considered past human aid.

VIOLET.

THE Wild Violet or Pansy (*Viola tricolor*) is found commonly throughout Great Britain on banks and in hilly pastures, from whence it has come to be cultivated in our gardens.

Viola, a corruption of "Ion," is a name extended by old writers to several other different plants. But the true indigenous representative of the Violet tribe is our Wild Pansy, or Paunce, or Pance, or Heart's ease; called also "John of my Pink," "Gentleman John," "Meet her i' th' entry; kiss her i' th' buttery" (the longest plant name in the English language), and "Love in idleness."

> "A little Western flower,
> Before milk-white, now purple with love's wound,
> And maidens call it—'Love in idleness.'"

From its coquettishly half hiding its face, as well as from some fancied picture in the throat of the corolla it has received various other amatory designations, such as "cuddle me to you," "tittle my fancy," "jump up and kiss me," and "garden gate": also it is called "Flamy," because its colours are seen in the flame of burning wood, and Flame Flower.

The term "heart's ease" has signified a cordial which is comforting to the heart. But the fact is that Pansies, "pretty little Puritans," produce anything but heart's ease if eaten, and their roots provoke sickness so speedily that these are sometimes employed as an emetic.

Dr. Johnson derived the word Pansy from Panacea,

as curing all diseases; but this was a mistake. The true derivation is from the French *pensée*, "thoughts," as Shakespeare knew, when making Ophelia say: "There is pansies—that's for thoughts."

From its three colours it has been called the herb Trinity. A medicinal tincture is made (H.) from the *Viola tricolor* with spirit of wine, using the entire plant. Hahnemann found that the Pansy violet, when taken by provers, served to induce cutaneous eruptions, or to aggravate them, and he reasoned out the curative action of the plant in small diluted doses for the cure of these symptoms, when occurring as disease.

"For milk crust and scald head," says Dr. Hughes (Brighton)—the plague of children, "I have rarely needed any other medicine than this *Viola tricolor*; and I have more than once given it in recent impetigo (pustular eczema) for adults, with very satisfactory effects." For the first of these maladies the tincture should be given in doses of from three to six drops, to a child of from two to six or eight years, three times a day in water.

Again, "for curing scalled (from *scall*, a shell) head in children, a small handful of the fresh plant, or half a drachm of the dried herb, boiled for two hours in milk, is to be taken each night and morning; also a bread poultice made with this decoction should be applied to the affected part.

"During the first eight days the eruption increases, and the urine, when the medicine succeeds, has a nauseous odour like that of the cat, which presently passes off; then, as the use of the plant is continued, the scabs disappear, and the skin recovers its natural clean condition."

The root of the *Viola tricolor* has similar properties

to that of Ipecacuanha, and is often used beneficially as a substitute by country doctors. An infusion thereof is admirable for the dysentery of young children. It loves a mixture of chalk in the soil where it grows.

The Pansy contains an active chemical principle, "violin," resin, mucilage, sugar, and the other ordinary constituents of plants. When bruised the plant, and especially its root, smells like peach kernels, or prussic acid. It acts as a slight laxative: and "the distilled water of the flowers" says Gerard—"cureth the French disease."

The Germans style the Pansy *Stief-mutter*, because figuratively the mother-in-law appears in the flower predominant in purple velvet, and her own two daughters gay in purple and yellow, whilst the two poor little Cinderellas, more soberly and scantily attired, are squeezed in between. Again, another fable says, with respect to the five petals and the five sepals of the Pansy, two of which petals are plain in colour, whilst each has a single sepal, the three other petals being gay of hue, one of these (the largest of all) having two sepals; that the Pansy represents a family of husband, wife, and four daughters, two of the latter being step-children of the wife.

The plain petals are the step-children, with only one chair; the two small gay petals are the daughters, with a chair each; and the large gay petal is the wife, with two chairs. To find the father, one must strip away the petals until the stamens and pistils are bare. These then bear a fanciful resemblance to an old man with a flannel wrapper about his neck, having his shoulders upraised, and his feet in a bath tub. The French also call the Pansy "The Step-mother"

The chemical principle, "violin," contained in the

flowering Wild Pansy resembles emetin in action. If the dried plant is given medicinally, from ten to sixty grains may be taken as a dose, in infusion.

The Sweet Violet (*Viola odorata*) is well known for its delicious fragrance of perfume when growing in our woods, pastures, and hedge banks. The odour of its petals is lost in drying, but a pleasant syrup is made from the flowers which is a suitable laxative for children.

A conserve, called "violet sugar," prepared from the flowers, has proved of excellent use in consumption. This conserve was made in the time of Charles the Second, being named "Violet plate." Also, the Sweet Violet is thought to possess admirable virtues as a cosmetic. Lightfoot gives a translation from a Highland recipe in Gaelic, for its use in this capacity, rendered thus: "Anoint thy face with goat's milk in which violets have been infused, and there is not a young prince upon earth who will not be charmed with thy beauty."

There is a legend that Mahomet once compared the excellence of Violet perfume above all other sweet odours to himself above all the rest of creation: it refreshes in summer by its coolness, and revives in winter by its warmth.

The Syrup of Sweet Violets should be made as follows: To one pound of sweet violet flowers freshly picked, add two-and-a-half pints of boiling water: infuse these for twenty-four hours in a glazed china vessel, then pour off the liquid, and strain it gently through muslin; afterwards add double its weight of the finest loaf sugar, and make it into a syrup, but without letting it boil.

Violets are cultivated largely at Stratford-on-Avon for the purpose of making the syrup, which when mixed with almond oil, is a capital laxative for children, and will help to soothe irritative coughs, or to relieve a sore throat.

The flowers have been commended for the cure of epilepsy and nervous disorders; they are laxative when eaten in a salad. The seeds are diuretic, and will correct gravel. The Sweet Violet contains the chemical principle "violin" in all its parts. A medicinal tincture (H.) is made from the entire fresh plant with proof spirit. It acts usefully for a spasmodic cough, with hard breathing; also for rheumatism of the wrists especially the right one.

This Violet is highly esteemed likewise in Syria, chiefly because of its being chosen for making the violet sugar used in sherbet. That which is drunk by the Grand Signior himself is compounded of sweet violets, and sugar.

From the flower may be pleasantly contrived a pretty miniature bird, by carefully removing the calyx and corolla, leaving only the stamens and pistil attached to the receptacle; then the stigma forms the head and neck, whilst the anthers make a golden breast, and their tongues appear like a pair of green wings.

Mademoiselle Clarion, a noted French actress, had a nosegay of violets sent her every morning of the season for thirty years; and to enhance the value of the gift, she stripped off the petals every evening, being passionately devoted to the flower, and took them in an infusion as tea.

Pliny recommended a garland of sweet violets as a cure for headache. The Romans made wine of the flowers; and Napoleon the Great claimed the Violet as *par excellence* his own, for which reason he was often styled, *Le pere la violette*. This floral association took date from the time of his exile to Elba. The Emperor's return was alluded to among his adherents by a pass word, "*Aimez vous la Violette? Eh, bien! reparaitra au printemps.*"

The scentless Dog Violet (*Viola canina*) is likewise mildly laxative, and possesses the virtues of the *Viola odorata* in a lesser degree.

The Water Violet is "feather foil" (*Hottonia palustris*).

VIPER'S BUGLOSS.

THE Simpler's passing consideration should be given to this tall handsome English herb which grows frequently in gravel pits, and on walls. It belongs to the Borage tribe (see page 60), and, in common with the Lungwort (*Pulmonaria*), the Comfrey, and the ordinary Bugloss, abounds in a soft mucilaginous saline juice. This is demulcent to the chest, or to the urinary passages, being also slightly laxative. Bees favour the said plants, which are rich in honey. Each herb goes by the rustic name of "Abraham, Isaac, and Jacob," because bearing spires of tricoloured flowers, blue, purple, and red. The Viper's Bugloss is called botanically *Echium*, having been formerly considered antidotal to the bite of (*Echis*) a viper: and its seed was thought to resemble the reptile's head: wherefore such a curative virtue became attributed to it after the doctrine of signatures. "*In Echio, herba contra viperarum morsus celeberrima, natura semen viperinis capitibus simile procreavit.*" Similarly the Lungwort (or Jerusalem Cowslip), because of its spotted leaves, was held to be a remedy for diseased lungs. This rarely grows wild, but it is of frequent cultivation in cottage gardens, bearing also the rustic name, "Soldiers and Sailors," "To-day and to-morrow," and "Virgin Mary." From either of these herbs a fomentation of the flowers, or a decoction of the whole bruised plant, may be employed with benefit locally to sore or raw surfaces:

whilst an infusion made with three dramsof the dried herb to a pint of boiling water will be good in feverish pulmonary catarrh. By our ancestors viper broth was thought to be highly invigorating : and vipers cooked like eels were given to patients suffering from ulcers. The Sardinians still take them in soup. Marvellous powers were supposed to be acquired by the Druids through their possession of a viper's egg, laid in the air, and caught before reaching the earth. All herbs of the Borage order are indifferently "of force and virtue to drive away sorrow and pensiveness of the mind : also to comfort and strengthen the heart." With respect to the Comfrey (see page 120), quite recently the President of the Irish College of Surgeons has reported the gradual disappearance of a growth ("malignant, sarcomatous, twice recurrent, and of a bad type"), since steadily applying poultices of this root to the tumour. "I know nothing," says Professor Thomson, "of the effects of Comfrey root : but the fact that this growth has simply disappeared is one of the greatest surprises and puzzles I have met with."

WALLFLOWER.

THE Wallflower, or Handflower (*Cheiranthus cheiri*), or Wall-gilliflower, has been cultivated in this country almost from time immemorial, for its fragrance and bright colouring. It is found wild in France, Switzerland, and Spain, as the Keiri or Wallstock. Formerly this flower was carried in the hand at classic festivals Herrick, in 1647, gave a more romantic origin to the name Wallflower :—

> "Why this flower is now called so
> List, sweet maids, and you shall know :
> Understand this wilding was
> Once a bright and bonny la

Who a sprightly springal loved,
And to have it fully proved
Up she got upon a wall
Tempting to slide down withal:
But the silken twist untied,
So she fell: and, bruised, she died.
Love, in pity of the deed,
And such luckless eager speed,
Turned her to this plant we call
Now the 'Floweret of the Wall.'"

It is the only British species belonging to the Cruciferous order of plants, and flourishes best on the walls of old buildings, flowering nearly all the summer, though scantily supplied with moisture. We may presume it was one of the earliest cultivated flowers in English gardens, as it is discovered on the most ancient houses.

Turner, an early writer on Plants, calls it Wall-gelouer, or "Hartisease;" and by Spencer it was termed Cherisaunce, as meaning a cordial to the heart, this being really the herb to which the name Heart's-ease was originally given. By rustics it is known also as the "Beeflower."

But the common Stock likewise bore the appellation, "Gilliflower": and the probability is, there was in old days, as Cotgrave suggests, a popular medicine or food "for the passions of the heart," called "gariofile," from the cloves which it contained, the Latin for a clove being *caryophyllum*. Hence it came about that the Wall-flower, the Pansy, and the Stock, by virtue of their cordial qualities, were alike called Gilliflowers, or Heart's-ease.

There are two varieties of the cultivated Wallflower, the Yellow and the Red; those of a deep colour growing on old rockeries and similar places, are often termed

Bloody Warriors, and Bleeding Heart. The double Wallflower has been produced for more than two centuries. If the flowers are steeped in oil for some weeks, they contribute thereto a stimulating warming property useful for friction to limbs which are rheumatic, or neuralgic. Gerard suggests that the "oyle of Wallflowers is good for use to annoint a paralyticke." An infusion of the flowers, made with boiling water, will relieve the headache of debility, and is cordial in nervous disorders, by taking a small wineglassful immediately, and repeating it every half-hour whilst required. The aromatic volatile principles of the flowers are *caryophyllin* and *eugenol*. "This Wallflower," adds Gerard, "and the Stock Gilliflower are used by certain empiricks and quack salvers about love and lust, —matters which for modesty I omit."

WALNUT.

THE Walnut tree is known of aspect to most persons throughout Great Britain as of stately handsome culture, having many spreading branches covered with a silvery grey bark, which is smooth when young, though thick and cracked when old.

The flowers occur in long, hanging, inconspicuous spikes or catkins, of a brownish green colour.

This tree is a native of Asia Minor, but is largely grown in England. The Greeks called it "Karuon," and the Latins "Nux." Its botanical title is *Juglans regia*, a corruption of *glans*, the acorn, *jovis*, of Jupiter, or the "royal nut of Jupiter," food fit for the Gods! Its fruit is also named Ban nut, or Ball nut, and Welsh nut, or Walnut—the word Wal, or Welsh, being Teutonic for "stranger." "As for the timber," said Fuller, "it may be termed the English Shittim Wood."

The London Society of Apothecaries has directed that the unripe fruit of the Walnut should be used pharmaceutically on account of its worm-destroying virtues. It is remarkable that no insects will prey on the leaves of this tree. In good seasons the produce of nuts is weighty enough to pay the rent of the land occupied by the trees.

The vinegar of the pickled fruit makes a very useful gargle for sore throats, even when slightly ulcerated: and the green husks, or early buds of the blossom, being dried to powder, serve in some places for pepper.

The kernel of the nut (or the part of the inside taken at dessert) affords an oil which does not congeal by cold, and which painters find very useful on such account. This oil has proved useful when applied externally for troublesome skin diseases of the leprous type. Indeed, the Walnut has been justly termed vegetable arsenic, because of its curative virtues in eczema, and other obstinately diseased conditions of the skin.

The tincture when made (H.) from the rind of the green fruit and the fresh leaves, with spirit of wine, and given in material doses, will determine in a sound person a burning itching eruption of the skin, of an eczematous character, lasting a long time, and leaving the parts which have been affected afterwards blue and swollen. Reasoning from which it has been found that the tincture, in a reduced form, and of a diminished strength, proves admirably curative of eczema, impetigo, and ecthyma.

The unripe fruit is laxative, and of beneficial use in thrush, and in ulcerative sore throat. The leaves are said to be anti-syphilitic: likewise the green husk, and unripe shell. Obstinate ulcers may be cured with sugar well moistened in a strong decoction of the leaves.

Well kept, kiln-dried Walnuts, of some age, are better digested than newer fruit; in contrast to old gherkins, about which it has been humorously said, "avoid stale Q-cumbers: they will W-up." In many parts of Germany the peasants literally subsist on Walnuts for several months together; and a young farmer before he marries has to own a certain number of flourishing Walnut trees.

The bark or yellow skin which clothes the inner nut is a notable remedy for colic, being given when dried and powdered, in a dose of thirty or forty grains mixed with some carminative water; and the same powder will help to expel worms.

According to the Salernitan maxim, if the fruit of the Walnut be eaten after fish, the digestion of the latter is promoted:—

> Post pisces nux sit: post carnes caseus esto.

Or,

> "Take Welsh nuts after fish: take cheese after flesh meat."

But with some persons coughing is excited by eating Walnuts.

The roots, leaves, and rind yield a brown dye which is supposed to contain iodine, and which gipsies employ for staining their skins. It also serves to turn the hair black. "A custom prevails (says a Latin sentence) among certain country folk to thrash the nuts out of their husks while still on the trees, so that they may grow more abundantly the following year. In allusion to which practice the lines run thus:—

> "Nux, asinus, mulier, simili sunt lege ligata;
> Hæc tria nil fructûs faciunt si verbera cessant."

> "A woman, a donkey, a walnut tree—
> The more you beat them, the better they be."

It is a fact, that by acting in this way, the barren ends of the branches are knocked off, and fresh fruit-bearing twigs spring out at each side in their stead.

Walnut cake, after expressing out the oil from the kernels, is a good food for cattle, these kernels being the crumpled cotyledons or seed leaves. They contain oil, mucilage, albumen, mineral matter, cellulose, and water.

The rook has a most abiding affection for Walnuts. As soon as there is any fruit on the trees worth eating, this bird finds it out, and brings it to the ground, choosing only those nuts which are soft enough for him to penetrate.

Ovid has left a charming little poem, *Nucis Elegia*—the plaint of the Walnut tree—because beaten with sticks and pelted with stones, in return for the generosity with which it bestows on mankind its fair produce.

A valuable medicinal spirit is distilled by druggists from the fruit of the Walnut. It is an admirable remedy for spasmodic indigestion, and to relieve the morning sickness of pregnancy. A teaspoonful of the spirit (*Spiritus nucis juglandis*) may be given with half a wine-glassful of water every hour or two, for most forms of sickness, and the dose may be increased if necessary.

"Nucin," or "juglon," is the active chemical principle of the several parts of the tree and its fruit.

The leaves, when slightly rubbed, emit a rich aromatic odour, which renders them proof against the attacks of insects. Qualities of this odoriferous sort commended the tree to King Solomon, whose "garden of nuts" was clearly one of Walnuts, according to the Hebrew word *eghōz*. The longevity of the tree is very great. There is at Balaclava, in the Crimea, a Walnut tree believed to be a thousand years old.

The shade of the Walnut tree was held by the Romans to be baneful, but the nuts were thought propitious, and favourable to marriage as a symbol of fecundity. The ceremony of throwing nuts, for which boys scrambled at a wedding, was of Athenian origin :—

> "Let the air with Hymen ring
> Hymen ! Io ! Hymen sing !
> Soon the nuts will now be flung :
> Soon the wanton verses sung."
>
> —*Catullus.*

In Italy this is known as the "Witches tree." It is hostile to the oak.

The leaves of the American Black Walnut tree, which grows naturally in Virginia, are of the highest curative value for scrofulous diseases and for strumous eruptions. Chronic, indolent sores have been healed by these after every other remedy has failed. The parts should be washed several times a day with a strong decoction of the leaves, and an infusion of the same should be taken internally; also of the extract made from the leaves, four grains in a pill each night and morning. For such purposes the leaves of our English Walnut are almost equally efficacious. To make an infusion one ounce should be used to twelve ounces of boiling water. For a syrup mix eight grains of the extract with an ounce of simple syrup : and give one teaspoonful of this twice a day with water. Also apply to any sore some of the powdered leaves on lint soaked in the decoction. For scrofulous joints, or glands, this treatment is invaluable. A green English Walnut, boiled in syrup and preserved in the same, is an excellent homely remedy for constipation. It will be noticed that the fruit becomes black by boiling. The Chinese put the raw kernels into their tea to give it a flavour.

By the Romans Walnuts were scattered among the people when a marriage was celebrated, as an intimation that the wedded couple henceforth abandoned the frivolities of youth.

The "titmouse" walnut produces very delicate fruit, rich in oil, and with thin shells, so that the little creatures can pierce the husks and shells while the fruit is still on the bough.

Nuts of various kinds, being charged with carbon and oil, are highly nutritious, but on account of this oil abounding, they are not readily digested by some persons. In Southern Europe, the Chestnut is a staple article of food. The title "nut" signifies a hard round lump, from *nodus*, a knot.

Leigh Hunt wrote meaningly of the "inexorably hard cocoa nut—*milky at heart.*" In Devonshire a plentiful crop of hazel nuts is believed to portend an unhealthy year:—

"Many nits (nuts)
Many pits (graves)."

When eating almonds and raisins at dessert we get the nitrogenous food of the nuts with the saccharine nourishment of the grapes.

WART-WORT, OR WART-WEED.

THIS name has been commonly applied to the Petty Spurge, or to the Sun Spurge, a familiar little weed growing abundantly in English gardens, with umbels of a golden green colour which "turn towards the sun." Its stem and leaves yield, when wounded, an acrid milky juice which is popularly applied for destroying warts, and corns. But our Greater Celandine (see page 92) or Swallow-wort is better known abroad as the Wart-wort: and its sap is widely given in Russia for the cure, not only of warts, but likewise of cancerous outgrowths, whether occurring on the skin surface, or assailing membranes inside the body. Conclusive evidence has been adduced of cancerous disease within the gullet and the stomach —as well as on the external skin—being healed by this herb. Its sap, or juice, contains chemically, "chelidonine," and "sanguinarine," which latter principle (obtained heretofore from the Canadian "blood root"), is of long established repute for repressing fungoid granulations of indolent ulcers, when powdered over them, and of quickly advancing their cure. Each principle exercises a narcotic influence on the nervous system, and will, thereby, relieve spasmodic coughs. Healthy provers have taken the fresh juice of the Greater Celandine in doses of from twenty to two hundred drops, at repeated intervals; the results of the larger portions being drastic purgation, with persistent nervous torpor, and with an outbreak on the skin of irritating, sore, itching eruptions. In some of the provers active inflammatory congestion of the right lung ensued, with turgidity of the liver. The root beaten into a conserve with sugar will operate by stool, and by urine. For cancerous excrescences from five to ten drops of the fresh juice, or of the mother tincture (H.) should be given steadily three times a day, this quantity being reduced if it should move the bowels too freely. Some of the sap, or tincture, should be also used outwardly as a lotion, either by itself, or diluted with an equal quantity of cold water.

WATER PLANTS (Other).

(Water Dropwort, Water Lily, Water Pepper.)

THE Water Dropwort—Hemlock (*Œnanthe crocata*) is an umbelliferous plant, frequent in our marshes and ditches.

It is named from *oinos*, wine, and *anthos*, a flower, because its blossoms have a vinous smell. A medicinal tincture is made (H.) from the ripe fruit.

The leaves look like Celery, and the roots like parsnips. A country name of this plant is Dead-tongue, from its paralyzing effects on the organs of the voice. Of eight lads who were poisoned by eating the root, says Mr. Vaughan, five died before morning, not one of them having spoken a word. Other names are Horsebane, from its being thought in Sweden to cause in horses a kind of palsy; (due, as Linnæus thought, to an insect, *curculio paraplecticus*, which breeds in the stem); and Five-fingered-root, from its five leaflets. The roots contain a poisonous, milky juice, which becomes yellow on exposure to the air, and which exudes from all parts of the plant when wounded. It will be readily seen that because of so virulent a nature the plant is too dangerous for use as a Herbal Simple, though the juice has been known to cure obstinate and severe skin disease. It yields an acrid emetic principle. The root is sometimes applied by country folk to whitlows, but this has proved an unsafe proceeding. The plant has a pleasant odour. Its leaves have been mistaken for Parsley, and its root for the Skirret.

The *Œnanthe Phellandrium* (Water Fennel) is a variety of the same species, but with finer leaves. Pliny gave the seeds, twenty grains for a dose, against stone, and disorders of the bladder. Also they have been commended for cancer.

In this country Water Lilies, or Pond Lilies, comprise the White Water Lily—a large native flower inhabiting clear pools and slow rivers—and the Yellow Water Lily, frequent in rivers and ditches, with a yellow, globose flower smelling like brandy, so that it is called "Brandy bottle" in Norfolk and other parts. Its root and stalks contain much tannin.

This latter Yellow Lily (*Nuphar lutea*) possesses medicinal virtues against diarrhœa, such as is aggravated in the morning, and against sexual weakness. A tincture is made (H.) from the whole plant with spirit of wine. The second title, *lutea*, signifies growing in the mud; whilst the large white Water Lily is called *Nymphæa*, from occurring in the supposed haunts of the nymphs: and Flatter-dock.

The root stocks of the Yellow Water Lily, when bruised, and infused in milk, will destroy beetles and cockroaches. The smoke of the same when burnt will get rid of crickets.

The small Yellow Pond Lily bears the name of Candock, from the shape of its seed vessel, like that of a silver can or flagon, and this perhaps has likewise to do with the appellations, "Brandy bottle" and "Water can:" which latter may be given because of the half unfolded leaves floating on the water like cans.

The root of the larger white Water Lily is acrid, and will redden the skin if the juice is applied thereto.

An Ointment may be made with this juice to stimulate the scalp so as to prevent falling out of the hair. The root contains tannin and mucilage, it is therefore astringent and demulcent. Also the expressed juice from the fresh leaves of this white Water Lily, the "one sinless flower," if used as a head wash, will preserve the hair.

> "Oh, destinée des choses d'ici bas! descendre des austerités du cloitre dans l'officine Cancanière du perruquier!"

Dutch boys are said to be extremely careful about plucking or handling the Water Lily, for, if a boy fall with the flowers in his possession, he is thought to immediately become subject to fits.

The Water Pepper (*Polygonum Hydropiper*) or Arsmart, grows abundantly by the sides of lakes and ditches in Great Britain. It bears a vulgar English name signifying the irritation which it causes when applied to the fundament; and its French sobriquet, *Culrage*, conveys the same meaning :—

> "An erbe is the cause of all this rage,
> In our tongue called *Culrage.*"

The plant is further known to rustics as Cyderach, or Ciderage, and as Red-knees, from its red angular points. It possesses an acrid, biting taste, somewhat like that of the Peppermint, which resides in the glandular dots sprinkled about its surface, and which is lost in drying. Fleas will not come into rooms where this herb is kept. It is called also "lake weed." A tradition says that the plant when placed under the saddle will enable a horse to travel for some long time without becoming hungry or thirsty. The Scythians knew this herb (*Hippice*) to be useful for such a purpose.

The Water Pepper had its virtues first taught by a beggar of Savoy. It is admirable against syphilis, and to arrest sexual losses : being long adored because "healing the original sin."

Farriers use it for curing proud flesh in the sores of animals, and when applied to the human skin, the leaves will serve the purpose of a mustard poultice. Also, a piece of the plant may be chewed to relieve toothache, as well as to cure small ulcers of thrush in the mouth, and pimples on the tongue.

The expressed juice of the freshly-gathered plant has been found very useful in jaundice. From one to three tablespoonfuls may be taken for a dose. A hot decoction made from the whole herb (Water Persicaria) has a sheet soaked in it as an American remedy for cholera, the patient being wrapped therein immediately when seized. This herb, together with the *Thuja Occidentalis* (*Arbor vitæ*) makes the *Anti-venereo* of Count Mattæi.

Another *Polygonum*, the great Bistort, or Snakeweed, and Adderswort, is a common wild plant in the northern parts of Great Britain, having bent or crooked roots, which are difficult to be extirpated, and are strongly astringent.

This Bistort, "twice twisted," on account of its snake-like root, was at one time called *Serpentaria, Columbrina,* and *Dracunculus.*

It has been thought to be the *Oxylapathum Britannicum* and *Limonium* of the ancients.

The dose of the root in substance is from twenty to sixty grains. In the North of England the plant is known as Easter Giant, and its young shoots are eaten in herb pudding. About Manchester they are substituted for greens, under the name of Passion's dock. The root may be employed both externally as a poultice, and inwardly as a decoction, when an astringent is needed. It is most useful for a spongy state of the gums, attended with looseness of the teeth.

This plant grows in moist meadows, but is not common. Its roots are reddish of colour inside.

The Bistort contains starch, and much tannin; likewise its rhizome (crooked root) furnishes gallic acid. The decoction is to be made with an ounce of the bruised root boiled in a pint of water; one tablespoonful of this may be given every two hours in passive bleedings, and for simple diarrhœa. Other names for the plant are Osterick, and Twice writhen (*bis tort*), Red legs, and Man giant, from the French *mangeant*, eatable.

WHITETHORN.

(*See* "Hawthorn," *page 245.*)

WHORTLEBERRY.

(*See* "Bilberry," *page 52.*)

WOODRUFF.

CONCERNING the Sweet Woodruff (*Asperula odorata*), it is a favourite little plant growing commonly in our woods and gardens, with a pleasant smell which, like the good deeds of the worthiest persons, delights by its fragrance most after death. This herb is of the Rubiaceous order, and gets its botanical name from the Latin *asper*, rough, in allusion to the rough leaves possessed by its species.

It may be readily recognised by its small white flowers set on a slender stalk, with narrow leaves growing round it in successive whorls, just as in the Cleaver (Goosegrass), which belongs to the same order.

The name Woodruffe has been whimsically spelt Woodderowffe, thus:—

> Double U, double O, double D, E
> R, O, double U, double F, E.

Its terminal syllable, "ruff," is derived from *rofe*, a wheel,—with the diminutive *rouelle*, a little wheel or rowel, like that of an ancient spur,—which the verticillate leaves of this herb closely resemble. They serve to remind us also of good Queen Bess, and of the high, starched, old-fashioned ruff which she is shown to wear in her portraits. Therefore, the plant is known as Woodrowel.

When freshly gathered, it has but little odour, but when dried it exhales a delightful and lasting aroma, like the scent of meadow grass, or of peach blossoms.

A fragrant and exhilarating tea may be made from the leaves and blossoms of the sweet Woodruffe, and this is found to be of service in correcting sluggishness of the liver. "When it is desired," says Mr. Johns, "to preserve the leaves merely for their scent, the stem should be cut through just below and above a joint, and the leaves pressed in such a way as not to destroy their star-like arrangement."

Gerard tells us: "The flowers are of a very sweet smell, as is the rest of the herb, which, being made up into garlands or bundles, and hanged up in houses, in the heat of summer, doth very well attemper the air, cool and make fresh the place, to the delight and comfort of such as are therein."

The agreeable odour of this sweet Woodruffe is due to a chemical principle named "coumarin," which powerfully affects the brain; and the plant further contains citric, malic, and rubichloric acids, together with some tannic acid.

Another species of the same genus is the Squinancy Woodruff (*Asperula cynanchica*), so called from the Greek *cynanche*, which means quinsy, because an excellent gargle may be made from this herb for the troublesome throat affection here specified, and for any severe sore throat. Quinsy is called cynanche, from the Greek words, *kuon*, a dog, and *ancho*, to strangle, because the distressed patient is compelled by the swollen state of his highly inflamed throat, to gasp with his mouth open like a choking dog.

This plant is found growing in dry pastures, especially on a chalky or limestone soil, but it is not common; it has very narrow leaves, and tufts of lilac flowers.

Reverting to the Sweet Woodruff, the dried herb may be kept amongst linen, like lavender, to preserve it from insects.

> She—"Fresh Woodruff soaks
> To brew cool drink, and keep away the moth."
> —*A. Austin, Poet Laureate.*

It was formerly employed for strewing churches, littering chambers, and stuffing beds. Withering declares that its strongly aromatic flowers make an infusion which far exceeds even the choice teas of China. The powdered leaves are mixed with fancy snuffs, because of their enduring fragrance.

WOODSORRELL (*See also "Docks."*)

THIS elegant little herb, called also French Sorrel, Rabbits' food, Shamrock, and Wood Sour (*Oxalis acetosella*), is abundant throughout our woods, and in other moist, shady places. It belongs to the natural order of Geraniums, and bears the provincial names of Sour trefoil, Cuckoo's bread, or Gowk's-meat, and Stubwort (from growing about the stubs of hewn trees). Its botanical title is got from the Greek word *oxus*, sharp, or acid, because of its penetrating sour taste. This is due to the acid oxalate of potash which it contains abundantly, in common with the Dock Sorrel, and the Garden Rhubarb.

By reason of this chemical salt being present in combination with less leafy matter than in the other plants which are akin to it, the Wood Sorrel makes a lighter and more palatable salad.

In olden days the Monks named this pretty little

woodland plant *Alleluia*, because it blossoms between Easter and Whitsuntide, when the Psalms—from the 113th to the 117th, inclusive—which end with the aspiration, "Hallelujah!" were sung.

St. Patrick is said to have shown on the ternate leaf of the Wood Sorrel to his rude audience the possibility of a Trinity in Unity.

The herb has been long popular as a Simple for making a fever drink, which is thought to be somewhat sedative to the heart, and for helping to cure scurvy. Also, it has proved useful against intermittent fever.

Towards assisting to digest, by their free acid, the immature fibre of young flesh meats, the Wood Sorrel leaves are commonly eaten as a dressing with veal, and lamb. But too habitual use of such a salad or sauce has led to the formation of gouty crystals (oxalate of lime) in the urine, with considerable irritation of the kidneys. Externally, the bruised leaves are of excellent service for cleansing and stimulating foul sores and ulcers, being first macerated in a Cabbage leaf with warmth.

This familiar harbinger of Spring, with its three delicate leaflets on a long stalk, and its tiny white flowers, having purple veins like those of the Wood Anemone, bears the fanciful name of Fairy-bells in Welsh districts.

Fra Angelico placed the claret-stained flowers in the foreground of his pictures representing the Crucifixion. After the doctrine of signatures, because of its shape like a heart, the leaf of the Wood Sorrel was formerly esteemed as a cordial medicine. It was called in Latin *Panis Cuculi*, meaning the "Cuckoo's bread and cheese." The leaves, when bruised, make with sugar a capital conserve which is refreshing to a fevered stomach, or, if boiled in milk, they form an agreeable sub-acid whey.

Twenty pounds of the fresh plant will yield four ounces of the oxalate of potash, commonly known as salt of lemons or salt of sorrel, which is often used for taking ink stains out of linen. Francus, an old classical author, concluded by experiment that the herb is of value (*cordis vires reparare*) to recruit the energies of the heart, and (*anginum abigere*) to dispel the quinsy. Its infusion makes an excellent anti-putrescent gargle. There is also a yellow variety of the Wood Sorrel.

WORMWOOD.

THE common Wormwood (*Artemisia absinthium*) has been partly considered here together with Mugwort, to which it is closely allied. It is a Composite herb of frequent growth on waste ground, being a bushy plant with silky stems, and collections of numerous small heads of dull yellow flowers. The name Wormwood is from *wehren*, to keep off—*mought*, a maggot or moth; and *absinthium*, from-*a*-negative—*psinthos*, delight, in allusion to the very bitter taste.

The whole plant is of an aromatic smell and bitter flavour. The flowers, when dried and powdered, destroy worms more effectually than worm seed, whilst the leaves resist putrefaction and help to make capital antiseptic fomentations.

Wormwood tea, or the powdered herb in small doses, mixed in a little soup, will serve to relieve bilious melancholia, and will help to disperse the yellow hue of jaundice from the skin.

This herb was formerly thought to possess the power of dispelling demons, and was thus associated with the ceremonials of St. John's Eve, owning the name, on the Continent, of St. John's Herb, or St. John's Girdle. Both it, and the Mugwort were dedicated to Diana:

and Venus gave thereof (Ambrose) to Œneas. It bears the provincial name "old woman." The smell of common Wormwood is very refreshing, and its reviving qualities in heated Courts are almost equal to a change of air.

Dioscorides declared it a preventive of intoxication, and a remedy for the ill-effects of any such excess; for which reason the *poculum absinthiacum* was a favourite beverage.

Gerard says: "The plant voideth away the worms, not only taken inwardly, but applied outwardly; it withstandeth all putrefactions, and is good against the stinking breath." It keepeth garments also from the moths—*A tineis tutam reddit quá conditur arcam* (Macer); and Dr. W. Bulleyne says "it keepeth clothes from moths and wormes." This is the great preventive used by cloth manufacturers. "Furthermore," adds Gerard, "taken in wine it is good against the biting of the shrew mouse, and of the sea dragon. It may be applied against the Squincie, or inflammation of the throat, with honey and water: likewise, after the same manner, to dim eyes, and mattery ears."

The characteristic odour of the plant is due to a volatile oil which consists mainly of absinthol; and the intensely bitter taste resides in "absinthin."

The plant also contains tannin, resin, starch, succinic, malic, and acetic acids, with nitrate of potash, and other salts. In some districts it is popularly called "green ginger."

Wormwood is of benefit for strengthless flatulent indigestion. An infusion may be made of an ounce of the dried plant to a pint of boiling water, and given in doses of from one to two tablespoonfuls three times during the day.

This infusion with a few drops of the essential oil will prevent the hair from falling off.

Absinthe, a liqueur concocted from Wormwood, is used largely in France, and the medical verdict pronounced there about its effects shows that it exercises through the pneumogastric nerve a painful sensation, which has been taken for that of extreme hunger. This feeling goes off quickly if a little alcohol is given, though it is aggravated by coffee, whilst an excessive use of absinthe from day to day is not slow in producing serious symptoms: the stomach ceases to perform its duty, there is an irritative reaction in the brain, and the effects of blind drunkenness come on after each debauch. The French Military call absinthe *un perroquet.* The daily taking even for a short while only of a watery infusion of Wormwood shows its bad effects by a general languor, with obscurities of the sight, giddiness, want of appetite, and painful indigestion.

When indulged-in as an appetiser by connoisseurs, absinthe, the "fairy with the green eyes," is modified by admixture with anisette, noted as an "agreeable and bronchitis-palliating" liqueur.

As a result of his experiments on animals, Dr. Maignan has come to the conclusion that absinthe (Wormwood) determines tremblings, dulness of thought, and epileptiform convulsions,—symptoms which alcohol alone will not produce. Hence it may be inferred that absinthe contains really a narcotic poison which should prevent its being employed as a liqueur, or as a homely medicament, to any excess.

Dogs are given to eat the Wormwood as a remedy for their ailments. Its medicinal and curative uses have been already partly discussed, together with those of *Mugwort.*

WOUNDWORT.

The Hedge Woundwort (*Stachys sylvatica*) is a common Labiate plant in our hedges and woods, branched and hairy, with whorls of small dull purple flowers on a spike two feet high or more. There are other varieties of the herb, such as the Marsh (March) Woundwort, the Corn Woundwort, and the Downy Woundwort.

The Hedge Woundwort was named by Gerard, Clown's all heal, or the Husbandman's Woundwort, because a countryman who had cut his hand to the bone with a scythe, healed the wound in seven days with this plant.

It is called by some the Hedge Dead Nettle, from its nettle-like leaves, and the place of its growth.

"The leaves," says Gerard, "stampt (pounded) with hog's grease, and applied unto green wounds in the manner of a poultice, heal them in such short time and such absolute manner, that it is hard for any one that hath not had the experience thereof to believe. For instance, a deep and grievous wound in the breast with a dagger, and two others in the abdomen (or nether belly), so that the fat commonly named the caul, issued forth, the which mortal wounds, by God's permission, and the virtues of this herb, I perfectly cured within twenty days—for the which the name of God be praised."

The name *Stachys* given to this herb, is from the Greek *stakos*, a bunch, because of the arrangement of the flowers. It contains a volatile oil, and a bitter principle undetermined.

The *Stachys Germanica* (Downy Woundwort) is so called from its soft, downy leaves having been employed instead of lint as a surgical dressing to wounds. The plant grows on a chalky soil in Bedfordshire, Berkshire, and Oxfordshire: being named also "Lamb's Ear."

This *Stachys lanata* (Woolly Woundwort) is known as Saviour's blanket, in Sussex; also in Devonshire and Somersetshire, as Mouse's ear, Donkey's ear, and Lamb's tongue.

The Knights' Water Woundwort (*Statiotes aloides*) was supposed from its blade-like leaves, acting on the doctrine of signatures, to heal sword wounds.

YARROW.

THE Yarrow, from *hiera*, holy herb (*Achillea millefolium*), or Milfoil, is so called from the very numerous fine segments of its leaves. It is a Composite plant very common on waysides and in pastures throughout Britain.

The name *Achillea* has been bestowed thereupon because the Greek warrior, Achilles, is said to have disclosed its virtues which he had been taught by Chiron, the Centaur. This herb is the *Stratiotes chiliophullos* of the Greek botanists, by whom it was valued as an excellent astringent and vulnerary. But Gerard supposes it may have been the *Achillea millefolium nobile*, which grows with a thick root and longer leaves, on a fat and fruitful soil, a stranger in England, "and the very same with which Achilles cured the wounds of his soldiers." But, he adds, "the virtues of each sort of Milfoil are set to be both alike."

The flowers of the Common Yarrow or Nosebleed are white or pink; those of the *Nobile* are yellow.

The popular name of Nosebleed has been given to the Yarrow because the hairy filaments of the leaves, when put up the nose, provoke an exudation of blood, and will thus afford relief to headache, caused by a passive fulness of the vessels. Parkinson says "if it be put into the nose, assuredly it will stay the bleeding of it," which must be the effect of action according to similars. Or if using Yarrow in the same way as a love charm, the following lines were repeated :—

> "Green 'arrow! green 'arrow!
> You bear a white blow;
> If my love love me
> My nose will bleed now."

The leaves have a somewhat fragrant smell, and a bitterish taste. The odour of the flowers, when rubbed between the fingers, is aromatic. In consequence of this pungent, volatile principle, the herb has proved useful in hysteria, flatulence, heartburn, colic, and epilepsy; also, it is employed in Norway for the cure of rheumatism, and sometimes chewed for toothache.

Yarrow is one of the few aboriginal English plants, having held the primitive title, *Gearwe.* Greek botanists seem to have known the identical species which we now possess, and to have used it against hæmorrhagic losses. It yields, chemically, a dark-green volatile oil, and achilleic acid, which is said to be identical with aconitic acid; also resin, tannin, gum; and earthy ash consisting of nitrates, phosphates, and chlorides of potash and lime.

For preparing an infusion of the plant, half an ounce should be boiled down in half a pint of water to six ounces; one tablespoonful for a dose.

Sir John Hill says the best way of giving Yarrow is in a strong decoction of the whole plant. A hot infusion of the herb taken freely on going to bed at night seldom fails to make short work of a cold.

A medicinal tincture (H.) is prepared from the whole plant with spirit of wine. This, when employed in a diluted form of the first or third decimal strength, and in small doses of from five to ten drops in a table-spoonful of cold water, will act admirably in arresting nocturnal losses in the male; likewise bleeding from the lungs, the kidneys, or the nose, especially in florid, hectic subjects. It has been found by healthy provers that stronger, and larger doses of any preparation of the herb will induce or aggravate one or another of these bleedings.

The fresh juice of the plant may be had, a dessert-spoonful three times in the day; or of the volatile essential oil, from three to five drops for a dose. These medicines greatly stimulate and promote the appetite. "For ague," says Parkinson, "drink a decoction of the herb warm before the fit, and so for two or three fits together."

Externally, a strong decoction of the leaves has been used as an injection into the nostrils to stay bleeding from the nose. It is similarly of service tor piles, and for female floodings, because exerting a special local action on the organs within the middle trunk. The bruised herb, or an ointment made from it, is applied by rustics to heal fresh cuts and contusions.

Even in ancient times it was famous as a topical remedy for piles. It is further of benefit for sore nipples as a lotion, and for a relaxed sore throat as a gargle: also as a hair wash.

The leaves were applied in former days as a poultice to wounds; and because of its healing and astringent virtues when so used, the plant gained the names Sanguinary, Thousand leaf, Old Man's pepper, Soldiers' Woundwort. Other local names for it are Staunch grass, Carpenters' weed, and Bloodwort: also, "Old Man's Mustard," "Bad Man's Plaything," and "Devil's Plaything." In Gloucestershire and some other parts, the double-flowered Yarrow is brought to a wedding by bridesmaids as "seven years' love." In Cheshire, children draw the herb across the face to produce a tingling sensation, and they call it "Devil's nettle."

Culpeper spoke of the same as a profitable herb in cramps, and therefore called *Militaris*.

Yarrow, worn in a little bag over the stomach, was the secret (confided to Boyle) of a great lord against ague. A famous physician had used it with strange efficacy.

Similarly a charmed packet containing dried Yarrow has been credited with bringing success to its bearer, if at the same time he were admitted to the knowledge of a traditional secret (only whispered to the initiated) that this was the first herb our Saviour had put into His hand when a child.

Again, Elspeth Reoch, in 1616, when tried for witchcraft, acknowledged to having employed the Yarrow in her incantations. She "plucked one herbe called Meleflower, sitting on her right knee, and pulling it betwixt the mid-finger and thumbe, and saying: *In nomine Patris, Filii, et Spiritus Sancti.*" The Meleflower is the *Achillœa Ptarmica* or Sneezewort.

By the plant so gathered, she was enabled to cure distempers, and to impart the faculty of prediction.

YEW.

ALTHOUGH the Yew—a Conifer—which is so thoroughly English a tree, is known to be highly poisonous as regards its leaves to the human subject, and as concerning its loppings or half-dead branches, to oxen, horses, and asses, yet a medicinal tincture (H.) is made from the young shoots, which has distinct and curative uses. Both the Yew and the Ivy were called *abiga*, because causing abortion. From which word when corrupted was formed *iua*; and under this latter name, says Dr. Prior, the Ivy and the Yew became inextricably mixed up.

Moreover, the red berries, or their coloured fleshy cups, are not poisonous when taken in moderation, but rejecting the seeds.

Gerard says: "When I was yong, and went to schoole, divers of my school-fellows and likewise myself, did eat our fils of the berries of this tree, and have not only slept under the shadow thereof, but among the branches also, without any hurt at all, and that not one time, but many times."

Yet Leo Grindon says, much more recently: "Though the juice and pulp of the sweet and viscid berries are not harmful, still the *seeds* of the Yew, and the *leaves* are deadly poison."

In the *Herbal* of 1578, Lyte tells us the Yew is altogether venomous, and against man's nature. Such as do but only sleep under the shadow thereof become sick, and sometimes they die;" and, "the extract of yew is used by ignorant apothecaries to the great peril and danger of the poor diseased people."

The Yew tree (*Taxus baccata*) occurs in mountainous woods and rocky glens about Britain, but is rare as of native growth. Its name, *Taxus*, is a corruption of *toxos*, an arrow, since arrows in the old time were poisoned with the juice of yew.

The tree was planted frequently by our forefathers in churchyards, because of its value in the manufacture of bows. It is exceedingly long lived, and often attains great magnitude of girth.

A ghastly superstition was attached to the Yew when thus growing in a churchyard, that it would prey upon the dead bodies lying beneath its sombre shade. So Tennyson writes (*In Memoriam*) :—

> " Old Yew ! which graspest at the stones
> That name the underlying dead,
> Thy fibres net the dreamless head,
> Thy roots are wrapped about the bones."

The juice of the tree and of its leaves is a rapidly fatal poison, the symptoms corresponding in a very remarkable way with those which follow the bites of venomous snakes.

No known poison but the Yew produces the lazar-like ulcerations upon the body, on which Marlowe lays such stress—(Jew of Malta) :—

> " In few, the blood of Hydra—Herne's bane,
> The juice of *Hebron*, and Cocytus' breath,
> And all the poisons of the Stygian pool."

The witches in *Macbeth* include it in their accursed brew :—

> " Liver of blaspheming Jew,
> Gall of goat, and *Slips of Yew*."

The Yew tree is called " Hebon " by Spencer, and " Jew of Malta " by other writers of Shakespeare's time. The leaves are bitter, nauseous, and acrid. The succulent covering of the fruit is soft and slimy, mawkishly sweet, and mucilaginous. The leaves have a dangerous effect on the circulation of the heart, and when taken with any freedom are as fatal as the Foxglove.

Before the new Shakespeare Society, 1882, it was contended and proved to the satisfaction of the Society, that "the cursed Hebena," the "leperous distilment poured into the chambers of mine ears," told of, so pathetically, by the sad ghost of Hamlet's father, was the poison of the Yew, and identical with Marlow's juice of Hebron.

Ray mentions that a gardener employed in clipping a Yew tree at Pisa, could not proceed with his work for more than half-an-hour at a time without being seized with a violent pain in the head. Nevertheless, deer, sheep, and goats can eat the foliage with impunity.

The fresh leaves were administered to three children near Manchester for worms. Yawning and listlessness came on, and the eldest vomited a little, but neither of them complained of any pain. They all died within a few hours of each other.

Because being then green, on the Sunday next before Easter, the branches of the Yew tree have been used as a substitute for the Palms which symbolise the entry of Jesus into Jerusalem.

The symptoms induced by provings of the leaves and juice in toxic quantities, have been sick headache, with giddiness, feeble, faltering pulse, coldness of the extremities, diarrhœa, and general prostration. So that for this combination of symptoms, as in severe biliousness, or as in the auditory vertigo of Menière's disease, small doses of the diluted tincture are found to give prompt and effectual relief. The leaves contain a volatile oil, tannin, and a bitter principle "taxina," which is also furnished by the seeds. An extract of Yew has been pronounced a useful narcotic by more than one physician of repute: and in some parts of Germany a decoction of the wood is a well-known remedy against hydrophobia.

A jelly prepared from the berries has been given for chronic bronchitis, and the leaves have been used for epilepsy; likewise they have been taken by ignorant persons to induce abortion, but with serious injury to the experimenter. In some rural districts the berries are known as "Snots"; whilst the wood and roots are "Wire thorn."

By an old statute of Edward the First, trees were required to be placed in churchyards to defend the church from high winds, the clergy being allowed to cut them down for repairing the chancel when necessary. Perhaps, partly for this reason, the Yew was commonly planted by the side of a newly-built church. That its wood was certainly employed for making bows, we learn from Shakespeare :—

> "Thy very beadsmen learn to bend their bows
> Of double-fatal Yew against thy state."

It was "double-fatal," because the leaves and fruit seeds are poisonous, and the bows made from its branches, as well as arrows armed with its deadly juice, were instruments of death.

Against the maladies which have been specified as indicating the tincture of Yew for their cure, from five to ten drops of the third decimal tincture should be given, with a spoonful of water, every two, three, or four hours, whilst required.

In Switzerland the Yew is known as William's tree, in memory of Tell. Formerly the name was spelt "Eugh," "Yeugh," and "Ewgh."

Spenser says :—

> "The Eugh—obedient to the bender's will."

In olden times the Olitory, or Herb-garden, formed an important annex to all demesnes having any pretensions to completeness, and was under "My Lady's" special charge. In fact, the culture and preparing of Simples formed a part of every lady's education.

"My Lord's" retainers and tenants, when out of sorts, were treated with these wholesome remedies, and were directed to find in Simples the cure for all ordinary ailments.

Good George Herbert, of *Country Parson* celebrity, taught, 1620:—"In the knowledge of *Simples*, wherein the manifold wisdom of God is wonderfully to be seen, one thing should be carefully observed, which is, to know what herbs may be used instead of drugs of the same nature, and to make the garden the shop; for, home-bred medicines are both more easy for the Parson's purse, and more familiar for all men's bodies. So where the Apothecary useth either for loosing, Rhubarb, or for binding, Bole Armena; the Parson useth Damask, or White Roses for the one, and Plantain, Shepherd's Purse, or Knotgrass for the other: and that with better success. As for Spices, he doth not only prefer home-bred things before them, but condemns them for vanities, and so shuts them out of his family, esteeming that there is no spice comparable of herbs to Rosemary, Thyme, Savory, Mints: and of seeds to Fennel and Carraway. Accordingly for salves his wife seeks not the city, but prefers her garden and fields, before all outlandish gums. And, surely, Hyssop, Valerian, Mercury, Adder's tongue, Yarrow, Melilot, and St. John's Wort, made into a salve, and Elder, Camomile, Mallows, Comphrey, and Smallage, made into a poultice, have done great, and rare cures!"

INDEX.